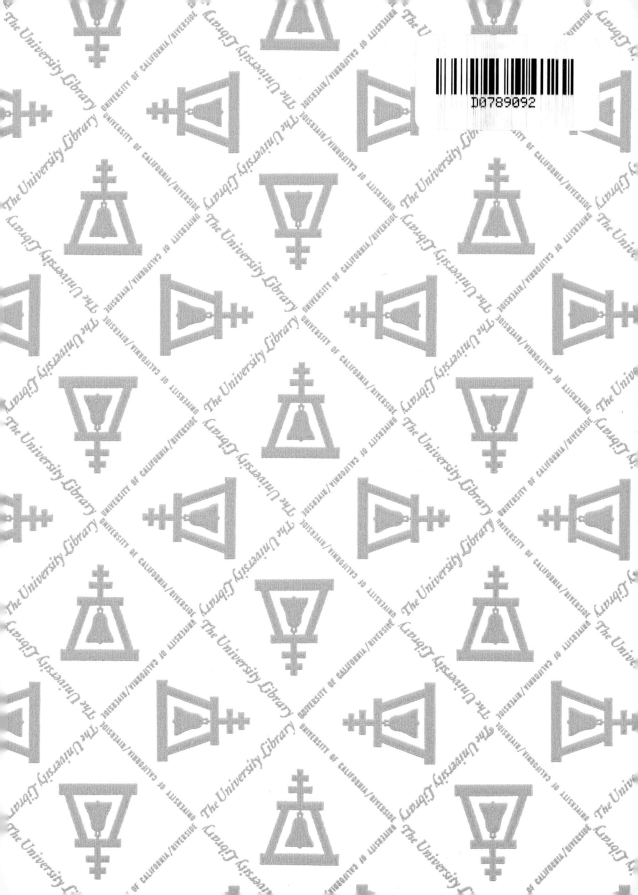

Parasitic Disease in Man

Parasitic Disease in Man

Richard Knight

B.A., M.B., Ph.D., F.R.C.P., D.T.M. & H.

Senior Lecturer, Department of Tropical Medicine,
Liverpool School of Tropical Medicine

Honorary Consultant Physician (Tropical Medicine),
Liverpool Area Health Authority, Liverpool, England

CHURCHILL LIVINGSTONE

EDINBURGH LONDON MELBOURNE AND NEW YORK 1982

CHURCHILL LIVINGSTONE
Medical Division of Longman Group Limited

Distributed in the United States of America by Churchill
Livingstone Inc., 19 West 44th Street, New York, N.Y.
10036, and by associated companies, branches and
representatives throughout the world.

© Longman Group Limited 1982

First published 1982

ISBN 0 443 01952 5

British Library Cataloguing in Publication Data
Knight, Richard
  Parasitic disease in man.
  1. Parastic diseases
  I. Title
  616.9'6   RC119

Library of Congress Catalog Card Number 80–42184

Printed in Singapore by Selector Printing Co Pte Ltd

Preface

A proper understanding of parasitic disease requires familiarity with the disciplines of applied zoology, immunopathology, epidemiology and clinical practice. This book departs from the more formal and conventional approach of dealing with parasitic diseases in a zoological sequence organism by organism. The new approach adopted in this work allows the viewpoints of these different disciplines to be presented in a more realistic manner.

After introducing the biological principles of parasitism the organisms themselves, the *dramatis personae*, are briefly presented in their ecological contexts. The text then covers the general characteristics of parasite epidemiology and the circumstances under which disease is produced; there follows an account of the complexities of the host – parasite relationship and the mechanisms of disease pathogenesis. A major part of the book, a series of six chapters, describes the local and systemic manifestations of parasitic diseases seen as clinical problems affecting various body systems. Details are given regarding differential diagnosis, pathology and practical management.

Further chapters deal with the currently used diagnostic methods, and the chemotherapy of these infections including drug schedules and toxicity. An account is given of the methods used to study these organisms at the community level and the ways in which such data are analysed. Finally the practical measures available for the control of these infections within human populations are described.

Throughout this work emphasis is given to those aspects of the subject that have practical importance or are of particular biological interest. Although this is an introductory text assuming no previous knowledge of the subject, the coverage is comprehensive and self-sufficient. It aims to provide medical, public health and other personnel with enough theoretical and practical information to deal effectively with the many problems posed by these fascinating and important infections.

1982   R.K.

Contents

1

Parasitism and related phenomena

Clinical parasitology is concerned with the diseases produced by the many species of parasitic animals that can use man as their host. Zoologically these parasites are very complex for they show great diversity in their size, structure, life cycles and taxonomic affinities. However, to the clinician or public health worker, who sees the outcome of the host-parasite relationship in man, it is soon evident that the diseases caused by these organisms share many clinical and epidemiological characteristics, and pose many similar problems in diagnosis and therapy.

PARASITES AND PARASITISM

Parasitism will be defined as the ecological relationship between two species in which one species, the parasite, is physically and physiologically dependent upon the other, the host, for at least part of its life cycle. Other essential features of the relationship are that the parasite is smaller than the host and has a shorter life span; in addition the greater reproductive potential of the parasite means that its population size will normally be much larger than that of the host. These latter features distinguish parasitism from predation. This definition mentions nothing about damage to the host or the production of disease for such an outcome is dependent upon several factors relating to the parasite, a particular host and the circumstances of infection. The parasitic relationship defined ecologically is not, of course, unique to animal parasites for it applies equally to bacteria, viruses and all other agents of infectious disease. Later in this chapter we will review the reasons why the discipline of parasitology, and hence the

clinical speciality relating to it, has become limited to those organisms that are members of the animal kingdom. For convenience we shall adopt this limitation in the scope of the word 'parasite' at this stage and use the term accordingly.

Three ways of classifying parasites

1. Zoological classification

An outline of the zoological classification of human parasites is given in the Appendix; they belong to five of the major groupings or **phyla** that make up the animal kingdom. Even the simplest, the unicellular PROTOZOA, are structurally advanced when compared with bacteria for they have a nucleus and a number of cell organelles that enable them to perform many of the functions of separate tissues and organs in higher organisms. Functionally protozoa can be regarded as non-cellular since they are complete animals which have not adopted the strategy of dividing their body into separate units or cells. The main limitation of a noncellular body structure is a small maximum size. The important protozoan diseases are malaria, amoebiasis, the various types of leishmaniasis, African and American trypanosomiasis, toxoplasmosis, giardiasis and trichomoniasis; but there are other less common ones, some of which can cause death.

The adult stages of members of the phylum PLATYHELMINTHES are more or less flattened, hence their common appellation 'flatworms'; the parasitic members of the group are the flukes (**trematodes**) and the tapeworms (**cestodes**). Most adult trematodes are hermaphroditic organisms living in the biliary tract, gut or lung to produce, in man, such diseases as fascioliasis, clonorchiasis, fasciolopsiasis and paragonimiasis; however one very important group, the schistosomes that live in the venous circulation of the gut and urinary tract, are unisexual. Cestode parasites infect man either as relatively benign adult tapeworms that live in the gut as in taeniasis, or as cystic larval forms that develop in the tissues to produce such serious conditions as hydatid cyst (echinococcosis) and cysticercosis. The cylindrical 'round worms' belong to the phylum NEMATODA and these cause a number of important infections including hookworm infection, ascariasis, the filarial infections, strongyloidiasis, guinea worm infection and trichinosis. The parasitic platyhelminthes and nematodes are often referred to as **helminths** or simply as the parasitic worms. There is another group of helminths, the ACANTHOCEPHALA or thorny-headed worms, but these are such rare accidental parasites of man that they will not be included in this book.

The only human parasites within the phylum ANNELIDA are the blood-sucking leeches. The phylum ARTHROPODA includes numerous members of importance to man. Many of these are biting insects, ticks and mites, whose relationships with man show varying degrees of intimacy. In addition there are the parasitic mites, the larval flies (order Diptera) that cause myiasis, and some very peculiar parasites known as pentastomes.

2. Ecological classifications

One of the simplest classifications of parasites is their division into internal or **endoparasites** that live within the host's body, and the external or **ectoparasites** that live on the body surface. All the protozoan and helminthic parasites of man are endoparasites, but this is not true of some other host species. Leeches are usually ectoparasitic but they may sometimes become internal parasites. The arthropods include both ectoparasites and endoparasites; it will be noted that all blood-feeding, or **haematophagous**, arthropods fall within the definition of parasitism.

Nearly all human parasites are **obligate** parasites, for they must practice the parasitic way of life during at least part of their life cycle. However there are a few examples of free-living organisms that can adopt parasitism in special circumstances; they are known as **facultative** parasites, the best examples being some of the myiasis-producing flies and free-living amoebae of the genus *Naegleria* that occasionally invade the human nervous system. One nematode parasite *Strongyloides stercoralis* can live, at least for several generations, as a free-living organism in the soil.

The apparently simple distinction between harmless or non-pathogenic parasites and disease-producing, **pathogenic** ones, cannot always be applied. However there are some protozoan species that infect the mouth and lumen of the gut, that never produce disease; these are **commensal** parasites and they occupy the same ecological niche as the many kinds of commensal bacteria with which they live. Sometimes a parasite can live either as a commensal or as a pathogen; for example the amoeba *Entamoeba histolytica* may live for many years as a commensal in the lumen of the colon and then suddenly become an invasive pathogen to produce amoebic dysentery. Multicellular parasites always have some direct contact with tissues; they are never true commensals since they inevitably cause some host damage, however minimal this may be in some light infections.

Some parasites which normally have a relatively low pathogenicity can become dangerous and sometimes life threatening pathogens when host immune mechanisms are impaired; these are **opportunistic** parasites and important examples are *Toxoplasma* and *Pneumocystis*.

3. The distinction between Protozoan and Metazoan parasites

There are a number of useful and important biological and conceptual differences between infections caused by unicellular protozoa, and those caused by the multicellular parasites, collectively known as the **metazoa**, a term that includes all non-protozoan animals.

a. Modes of multiplication Protozoa are predominently asexual animals that multiply by binary or multiple fission. The exceptions among the human parasitic species are a rather brief obligatory sexual phase in the coccidian parasites, and the optional and rather sporadic sexual conjugation indulged in by the ciliate *Balantidium*. The asexual multiplication of protozoa normally proceeds in an exponential manner, until it is slowed down or arrested by host defence mechanisms or other environmental factors. This implies that a single asexual infecting organism of a pathogenic protozoan species has the potential to kill its host. In this context protozoa behave in a manner similar to that seen in microbial infections, such as those caused by bacteria.

In contrast all metazoan parasites have sexually reproducing adult stages, which may be unisexual or hermaphroditic; and a developmental sequence passing from the egg and embryo, through various larval or nymphal stages to the sexually mature adult. A particular host may be infected by the larval stages of some parasite species and by the adult stages of others; commonly a host will be infected by both the larval and the adult stages of a parasite species. However it is very rare for all the life cycle stages of a metazoan parasite to be completed in one host, without at least one stage of the cycle occurring outside the host; hence in the absence of new infection, the number of parasites does not increase. The principal exception to this statement, among vertebrate hosts, are the larval cestodes which often multiply asexually; thus a hydatid cyst derived from a single ingested egg of the tapeworm *Echinococcus granulosus* may contain, when it is mature, many thousands of infective forms called protoscoleces each one of which could form a daughter cyst should the primary cyst rupture within the host. In addition there are a very small number of worm species, *Strongyloides stercoralis* being the most important, that can by internal self-infection of the host increase their numbers without the parasite entering the external environment.

The usual absence of multiplication within the host by metazoan parasites means that infections are built up by continued re-exposure and the entry into the host of further infective forms. The number of metazoan parasites, of a particular species, within a host is called the **intensity** of infection.

This fundamental distinction between protozoan and metazoan parasites can be summarised by the statement that protozoa multiply within their hosts, while the metazoa accumulate within theirs.

b. Rates of multiplication Most parasitic protozoa have generation times of between six and 24 hours which implies that large populations can build up in a week or so. Normally the host, by one method or another, soon controls population growth; nevertheless for various reasons the control mechanisms often do not eliminate the infection. Hence despite their relatively rapid multiplication many protozoan infections are of long duration.

The life cycles of metazoan parasites are much longer and the adult forms themselves often show considerable longevity. Thus at one end of the spectrum the pre-adult stages of a mosquito may last a week and those of the threadworm *Enterobius* three weeks, at the other extreme the filarial worm *Onchocerca volvulus* takes 18 months to mature, and some larval tapeworms even longer. Similarly adult longevity ranges from a few days in the case of a head louse *Pediculus h. capitis*, about one year for the 'roundworm' *Ascaris lumbricoides*, and up to 20 years for *O. volvulus* or even 40 years in the case of the liver fluke *Clonorchis sinensis*. The longevity of many helminths explains the length of many worm infections even in the absence of re-exposure.

The length of the generation time has important genetic consequences. Thus drug resistance by the selection of resistant mutants will take a very long time to appear when the generation time is long. So far, acquired drug resistance has not been reported among helminths while it is quite common among parasitic protozoa, and very common among ectoparasitic arthropods which also have relatively short life cycles. Protozoa are genetically more plastic than helminths and they can sometimes adapt to changing circumstances.

THE HOST-PARASITE RELATIONSHIP

A. The host as an environment for the parasite

For a host to be a suitable ecological niche for a parasite it must provide certain basic requirements.

1. Developmental stimuli

Most parasites have a fairly complex life cycle during which the organism undergoes a series of transformations in body form and function. These changes are necessary if the parasite is to survive in the external environment, gain entry into its host, maintain itself within that host, reproduce and discharge its infective forms. Protozoan parasites must achieve these specialisations within the context of a single cell, while metazoa can employ different stages of the development cycle. Parasites achieve these transformations by the reciprocal expression and suppression of different parts of their genome, or genetic constitution, in response to specific environmental triggers. Studies of parasites *in vitro* have identified some of these stimuli; they include changes in temperature, pH, redox potential, carbon dioxide tension, the concentration of certain ions, and the presence of bile. Knowledge of these factors not only assists in the maintenance of parasites in the laboratory but will also perhaps eventually explain the various tissue tropisms that parasites display. Many parasitic protozoa can be maintained in the laboratory indefinitely as replicating organisms at one stage of the life cycle. Transformation can then be elicited by changing the cultural conditions; and with some species it is possible to reverse the process. Helminthic parasites are much more stereotyped in their development for this must follow the normal sequence; nevertheless, specific triggers operate at each of the critical points in the life cycle and the transformations appear to be mediated by neuro-endocrine mechanisms. The uniqueness of the physiology of different host species explains the relative **host specificity** of many parasites. Sometimes, as in the head louse *P.h. capitis*, only one host species is infected; but at the other end of the spectrum *Toxoplasma gondii* can infect nearly all vertebrates.

2. *A source of nutrients*

The degree to which a parasite is nutritionally and metabolically dependent upon its host varies. Thus the blood fluke *Schistosoma mansoni* living in the mesenteric veins of the gut obtains all its nutrients, electrolytes and oxygen from its host who also disposes of its excretory products, while the head louse obtains its blood meals from its host, but breathes atmospheric oxygen and discharges its faeces onto the host's body surface.

The different organs of a host vary not only in physico-chemical ways but also in their potential supply of nutrients; the latter may determine their suitability for different stages of the parasite. Adult tapeworms have no gut but need to maintain very high rates of metabolism because of their enormous production of eggs; the small bowel of the host provides a perfect environment since abundant predigested nutrients, derived from the host's food, are available for rapid uptake across the worm's tegument. In contrast some larval tapeworms grow very slowly and are metabolically very inactive; they can therefore survive in nutritionally poor locations such as connective tissues, body cavities and subcutaneous tissue.

3. *A means of exit for infective forms from the body*

A parasite must be located in its host's body at a site that allows transmission of infective forms to other hosts. The usual routes of exit from a vertebrate host are the faeces, urine, sputum or the skin surface. Alternatively they may be picked up from the blood and upper dermis by a haematophagous arthropod. Lastly they may be transmitted by **carnivory** when one host, the prey, is eaten by another, the predator; clearly when transmission is by this means the location of the parasite within the body of the prey species is usually of less consequence.

When a host is potentially infectious to other hosts the infection is said to be **patent**; the interval between initial infection and the onset of patency is the **prepatent period**, and ranges in length from a few days in the case of amoebic infection of the bowel to 18 months or more in onchocerciasis and larval cestode infections. Some infections never become patent either because of host immunity, or because the parasite is in the wrong host and cannot complete its maturation. Sometimes after a period of patency the host becomes noninfectious, although viable parasites persist in the host's body, this is known as **latency**; periods of latency may alternate with patency, and frequently changes in the host's immune status are responsible for this. Opportunistic infections are sometimes due to a reactivation of a previously latent infection.

B. Modes of transmission

A successful parasite must have efficient mechanisms for transferring itself, or its progeny, to a new host. This presents little difficulty to the ectoparasite as many of these are partly free-living, and those that are exclusively parasitic like the scabies mite (*Sarcoptes scabiei*) or louse (*P. humanus*), can easily transfer when hosts are in bodily contact. For internal parasites, the problem is more difficult; although these organisms have evolved to occupy nearly every tissue of the host's body, the number of ways of achieving dispersal is limited. The tremendously varied life cycles used by different parasites fall naturally into two groups.

Direct life cycles

These involve no intermediate host; they are simple but usually not very efficient solutions to the problem of transmission. Besides the ectoparasites, the direct life cycles are limited to two groups (*see also Isospora belli* p. 17, 18); the lumen-dwelling protozoa, and the so called 'soil-transmitted helminths'. Most lumen-dwelling protozoa live in the gut, they are transmitted by the faeco-oral route, usually by means of resistant cysts; less common means of dispersal being genital contact, kissing and respiratory aerosols. The soil-transmitted helminths are all parasites of the gut in their adult stages; and with one exception, the dwarf tapeworm *Hymenolepis nana*, they are all nematodes. All the nematode species must undergo a period of development in the external environment, this may take only a few hours or it may require several weeks. Local soil conditions, such as temperature, moisture content, particle size and texture, are important determinants of the transmission efficiency of these parasites.

Two other forms of direct transmission should be mentioned. Firstly the protozoa found in the blood may be accidentally transmitted by blood transfusion. Secondly some parasites can be transmitted transplacentally from the mother to her foetus; this is known as **vertical transmission** because it passes from one generation to the next, it is to be contrasted with **horizontal transmission** which includes all the more usual modes of transmission.

Indirect life cycles

A greater number of parasites have cycles that involve one or more **intermediate hosts**; the latter being various species of vertebrate or invertebrate. Some indirect cycles are very complicated and it is not always apparent which hosts are intermediate ones and which are not. For this reason it is necessary to introduce the term **definitive host** and to stipulate that this is the host in which the adult parasite, or the sexual part of the life cycle, occurs. Protozoa with indirect life cycles always multiply within their intermediate hosts and they transform into stages which are quite different in structure and behaviour to those in the definitive host. Similarly metazoa undergo development and various transformations within their intermediate hosts; in the case of the trematodes and some of the cestodes, the transformations include asexual multiplication. Thus in both protozoan and helminthic infections the intermediate host is not infective to the next host until the necessary biological changes have occurred.

When one of a pair of host species in an indirect cycle is much smaller and more mobile than the other it is referred to as the **vector** of the infection it transmits. In practice, this term is only applied to blood-feeding arthropods; it is not used for relatively sedentary animals such as the aquatic snails that act as intermediate hosts for schistosome flukes. Indirect life cycles of the protozoa infecting man are either transmitted by blood-feeding arthropods, and are thus vector-borne; or they are transmitted faeco-orally by means of cysts from the definitive host to the intermediate host, and then by carnivory from the intermediate host to the definitive one. Many different types of indirect life cycle occur among the metazoa; transfer between hosts may not only be by vector, carnivory or the ingestion of eggs and cystic stages, but it may also involve motile larval stages that live in the external environment.

Transfer between hosts by vector or carnivory usually involves little or no direct exposure to the external environment; this increases its efficiency. Intermediate hosts in which parasites undergo multiplication are known as **amplifier hosts**; this is another way of increasing the efficiency of a life cycle.

Life cycles sometimes involve animal species in which the parasite does not undergo transformations, grow or multiply; these should not be referred to as intermediate hosts or true vectors. When an arthropod is involved it is termed a **mechanical vector** and the passive carriage of amoebic cysts from human faeces to food by the house fly (*Musca domestica*) is a good example; another is the direct transfer between hosts of certain trypanosomes on the contaminated mouthparts of biting flies. True vectors are sometimes known as **biological vectors** to distinguish them from mechanical ones (p. 82). When the species is not an arthropod it is termed a transport or **paratenic host**. This phenomenon occurs especially in prey-to-predator food chains; larval worms being transferred from one host to the next. Although the worm becomes an internal parasite in the paratenic host, it undergoes no growth or development. Examples among human parasites are to be found among the pseudophyllidean tapeworms (p. 72) and the nematode infection gnathostomiasis (p. 76); in both these examples, man himself becomes an accidental paratenic host.

As will be seen when individual parasite life cycles are described, man acts as a definitive host for some infections, and as a potential intermediate host in others.

ZOONOSES AND RESERVOIR HOSTS

Those parasitic infections that are normally maintained in nature by non-human vertebrates are known as **zoonoses**. In most cases man only becomes infected by zoonotic parasites when he is inadvertently exposed to the infective forms of a parasite that would normally infect other vertebrates. Man thus becomes an **accidental host** while the normal vertebrate species that keep the cycle going in nature are known as the **reservoir hosts**. In these circumstances, man may be acting either as a definitive or as an intermediate host. Quite often the parasite is unable to complete its development in man and this may produce unusual clinical manifestations, and also diagnostic difficulties because the infective forms of the parasite may never appear. In only two zoonotic infections, the beef and pork tapeworms, does man form an

essential link in the life cycle. In these infections, man is the only known definitive host and the cycle can only persist if man continues to become infected, and continues to disperse the infective eggs. Parasite species that are normally maintained by man alone are termed **anthroponoses**; while the beef and pork tapeworms, which occupy a unique intermediate position, are sometimes referred to as **zooanthroponoses**.

Many species of vertebrate can act as sources of zoonotic infection to man but they fall ecologically into two more or less distinct groups. Firstly, there are the so-called **feral** or **sylvatic** zoonoses that primarily involve wild animals with no close relationship to man. Humans become infected only when populations move into infected areas or individuals become exposed in the course of hunting, and other occupational or recreational pursuits. The second group comprise the **domestic zoonoses** and involve man's own domesticated animals, his dogs and cats, and the rats and mice that so frequently take up residence in man-made structures. The frequency of human infections of this type will depend upon methods of animal husbandry, house structure, hygiene, and the intimacy of association with pets and other animals.

We can now look at the modes of transmission of one parasite, *Trypanosoma cruzi*, the cause of Chagas' disease or American trypanosomiasis, and see how different cycles may be inter-related (Fig. 1.1).

In the rain forest this infection is maintained by numerous species of mammalian reservoir hosts. They are fed upon by large, nocturnal, blood-feeding reduviid bugs of the subfamily Triatominae, which act as intermediate hosts and biological vectors. The mammal hosts are apparently unharmed by the infection and trypanosomes can be found circulating in their blood for long periods. Burrowing mammals, such as the armadillo, are particularly important as both host and vector live together in the same burrow. This stable ecosystem constitutes the sylvatic zoonosis (1) and very rarely affects man directly. However, infected bugs can enter the domestic ecosystem and set up infection in dogs and cats, among whom it is maintained as a domestic zoonosis (2) by different species of triatomine vector. In Peru

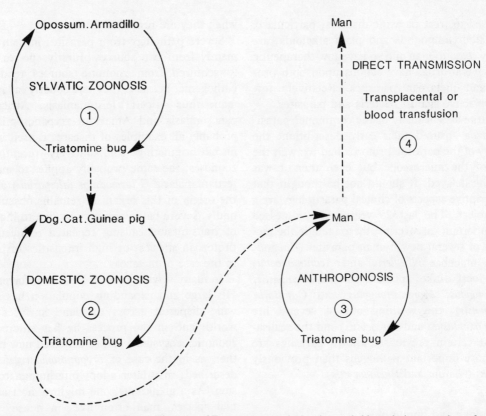

Fig. 1.1 Relationship between the different life cycles of *Trypanosoma cruzi*, showing probable evolutionary pathway from sylvatic zoonosis to direct man–to–man transmission (stages 1 to 4 as described in text).

and Bolivia, guinea pigs are raised for food and these also become an important reservoir. Man is infected by bugs from the domestic zoonosis and this in turn sets up infection in the bugs that live within the wall fabric of his own bedrooms. At this stage the cycle may become independent of animal reservoirs and then continues as an anthroponosis (3). In semi-urban communities this type of transmission is the most important, but it is amplified by direct transmission (4) that occurs transplacentally or by blood transfusion. This sequence illustrates the pathway along which an infective process can evolve, for it is virtually certain that the sylvatic zoonosis existed before man appeared in the Americas. The human species has entered an ecosystem and amplified the infectious process by creating a new domestic environment that is ideal for bug multiplication and well-stocked with mammals that provide blood meals for the bugs and hosts for the trypanosomes.

The normal **host range** of each parasite is deter-mined not only by the specific physiological fac-tors that underlie host specificity, but also by the access that different host species have to infection within the various ecosystems they occupy.

GENERAL CHARACTERISTICS OF PROTOZOAN AND METAZOAN INFECTIONS

1. Zoology

Protozoa like metazoa are eukaryotes, that is they have a well differentiated nucleus that usually con-tains all their genetic material; furthermore pro-tozoa are holozoic and derive their energy, like all animals, from other living organisms. Hence it is not surprising that the fine structure and biochemistry of protozoa are similar in many respects to the cells of metazoa throughout the animal kingdom, including man. Because of the biochemical similarity of all animal cells, many drugs used to treat parasitic diseases, particularly the metallic compounds and plant alkaloids, are relatively toxic to man and so have low therapeutic ratios. Several drugs have actions upon both protozoan and metazoan parasites. Relatively few drugs are active against bacteria and parasites.

The large size of many of the commoner parasitic metazoa ensured their early description; the discovery of the parasitic protozoa had to await the advent of the microscope but even then it was often long delayed. It should not be thought that the descriptive aspects of clinical parasitology are a dead subject. The last 25 years have witnessed many important discoveries; these include the recognition of several new human parasites (*Babesia*, the soil amoebae *Naegleria* and *Acanthamoeba*, several local fluke species, *Dirofilaria immitis*, *Angiostrongylus*, *Morerastrongylus* and *Capillaria philippinensis*), the working out of several life cycles (*Toxoplasma* and *Sarcocystis*) and the realisation that certain previously known parasites are much more important pathogens than previously suspected (*Giardia* and *Pneumocystis*).

2. Pathology and immunology

No internal parasites produce toxins and in their normal hosts many species are relatively non-pathogenic, having become well adapted by a long process of natural selection. Many pathogenic bacteria and fungi normally live as surface commensals or are free-living opportunistic organisms. However only a few pathogenic parasites, an example being *Entamoeba histolytica*, live mainly as commensals; the majority live continuously in intimate contact with their host's tissues. They can only do this because they have evolved a number of mechanisms for evading the host's immune responses. As a consequence many parasitic infections are of long duration, either because the parasites themselves are long-lived, or because low levels of host immunity allow the parasites to continue their multiplication. There is often little protection against reinfection. No effective vaccines have yet been produced against human parasites; two of the reasons for this are the low immunogenicity of many parasite antigens, and the low lethal effects of antibodies and cellular immune systems against most parasites

when they are produced.

Severe pathology from parasites in man derives mainly from two sources. Firstly species recently acquired from zoonotic sources tend to be pathogenic because they are poorly adapted to man; thus visceral leishmaniasis, African trypanosomiasis and American trypanosomiasis are probably all examples of diseases caused by organisms originating comparatively recently from zoonoses; the same probably applies to malignant tertian malaria (*Plasmodium falciparum*) although the origin of this organism remains obscure. Secondly, severe pathology may be due to high levels of transmission causing repeated reinfections by protozoan species, or high intensities of infection in the case of metazoa.

In many ways man is an ideal host for parasites. His large and expanding population has ensured wide dispersal across the land surfaces of the world; and in the process he has entered many zoonotic ecosystems and so acquired new parasites that, as in the case of *Trypanosoma cruzi* already described, may later adopt interhuman transmission. As a gregarious, one might almost say colonial species, man often lives in dense crowded conditions, which favour the transmission of parasites with direct life cycles, and also create poor living conditions and malnutrition which increase the morbidity due to parasites. The domestication by man of many animal species for food, companionship, as means of transport or as beasts of burden, has created many new zoonotic cycles, some of them with high levels of transmission. Man-made environments sometimes favour the breeding of insect vectors and intermediate hosts; thus peridomestic breeding by mosquitoes can create intense transmission of malaria and filariasis, and the breeding of aquatic snails in irrigation systems supports the transmission of schistosomiasis. Lastly man's very omnivorous dietary behaviour exposes him, through carnivory to many parasites acquired from animal tissues, and also to the numerous infections acquired by eating contaminated vegetable foods.

3. Parasite ecology

Compared with bacterial and other microbial infections, a higher proportion of parasites have indirect life cycles involving intermediate hosts or vectors; in addition many parasitic infections are zoonoses. Field studies of endemic parasites often involve what has become known as landscape ecology; this is a detailed study of the topographical, hydrological, demographic, edaphic and faunal characteristics of an ecosystem that enable predictions to be made about the foci of parasite transmission, their intensity and the feasibility of various methods of control.

4. Methodology

The microscope remains the principal diagnostic tool for the clinical parasitologist. The cultivation of parasites for diagnostic purposes is usually too difficult or too slow, and some parasites have never been grown *in vitro*. Serology is being increasingly used but for most parasitic infections it is of secondary importance compared with the microscope.

Living specimens of the smaller parasites are fascinating objects when viewed microscopically and stained microscopic preparations, especially those of the blood parasites, have considerable aesthetic appeal. It is perhaps not surprising that many of the pioneers of clinical parasitology have been keen natural historians, for the subject can have enormous appeal to those who enjoy field work and whose interests are oriented towards zoology and ecology.

Because human parasites, or their close relatives, are usually relatively safe organisms to manipulate experimentally, and because they can often be maintained in the commoner species of laboratory animal, these infections have been greatly used as biological models. Immunologists, in particular, have in recent years made great use of these biological systems, and our current knowledge of eosinophil function, immune complex disease, cellular immune mechanisms and the dynamics of granuloma formation, is based to a considerable degree upon work using these parasite models.

Parasites have always been of great importance in veterinary medicine, and such species have been intensively studied. The current realisation that medically important parasites are not disappearing, as many had predicted, is rekindling interest in the field. Recent years have witnessed a far greater interchange of ideas between veterinary and medical parasitologists, mainly perhaps to the benefit of the latter.

THE SCOPE OF MEDICAL ZOOLOGY

Medical parasitology deals not only with the clinical aspects of parasitism, the principal subject matter of this book, but also with many other areas of parasitology. This field of enquiry falls fairly naturally into the disciplines of medical protozoology, medical helminthology and medical entomology. Each is concerned with the morphology, physiology, taxonomy, genetics, evolution, behaviour, host-parasite relationships and ecology of the organisms within its domain.

In contrast, medical zoology has an even wider scope for it embraces the biology of parasites, and also the biology of reservoir hosts and those intermediate hosts that are not insects or arachnids. In addition, it is concerned with several categories of free-living animals that cause disease. These will now be briefly reviewed as they provide a number of contrasts when compared with parasites. The first three categories come within the province of toxinology, while the last is generally the concern of the dermatologist and allergist.

1. Venomous animals

For the purpose of offence and defence many animals have evolved specialised venom glands connected to structures that facilitate the injection of venom into their victims. Venom composition is often very complex. Pain and local damage to tissues and blood vessels may be produced by vasoactive amines, proteases, hyaluronidase, and phospholipases. Systemic toxicity occurs when toxins enter the circulation; toxins are nearly all enzyme proteins. Neurotoxins can affect the autonomic system causing cardiovascular collapse and arrhythmias, or neuromuscular blockade can produce bulbar and respiratory paralysis. A haemorrhagic state can be precipitated by defibrination following activation of the fibrinolytic system, or intravascular coagulation consequent upon widespread endothelial damage. Other toxins can cause haemolysis and muscle necrosis.

The structure and origin of the poison apparatus shows great diversity. Among the coelenterates, the tentacles that hang from the floating medusa of jellyfish and 'Portuguese man-of-war' are covered with minute stinging capsules or nematocysts that discharge on contact. The marine cone shells of the genus *Conus* have an extrusible harpoon-like tooth that can penetrate human skin. Among the arthropods, the centipedes (Chilopoda) have horny claw-like fangs that are the modified limbs of the first body segment; venomous spiders have fangs derived from a pair of mouthparts known as chelicerae; the scorpions have the last segment of their tail-like hind body adapted into a hooked sting that is freely articulated with the penultimate segment; while the wasps, bees and ants (Hymenoptera) have an eversible sting, which is a modified ovipositor, at the posterior end of their abdomen. The spiny spicules of many sea-urchins (Echinoidae) have venom glands at their base. Among the venomous fish, those of the genus *Muroena* have venom glands associated with hollow teeth; but a greater number that include the stonefish and the weever-fish have barbed spines in their dorsal fins; while the stingrays have barbed bony spines on the upper surface of their tails. The venom glands of snakes are analogous to the parotid glands of mammals. They are connected to the fangs which are hollow or grooved teeth in the upper jaw; the fangs may be fixed or hinged. The only other venomous reptiles are the 'Gila monster' lizards (*Heloderma*) which have venom secreting submaxillary glands connected to hollow teeth in the lower jaw. Lastly, in the only venomous mammal, the duck-billed platypus, the male has a venom gland in the groin that is connected to a movable grooved spine on the heel of each tarsus. It has been suggested that this structure serves to immobilise the female during copulation, but it is more likely to be used for defence or to overpower other males.

2. Urticating and vesicating animals

Many invertebrates can release irritant substances on contact with a potential predator. Man is quite commonly affected when he handles or otherwise makes contact with these creatures. The haemolymph of several beetles (Coleoptera) contains blister-inducing compounds, and these insects can voluntarily discharge their body fluid through joints of the integument. Intense irritation is caused to the skin and the fluid is easily rubbed into the eye. The responsible substances are cantharidin in the meloidid beetles that include the 'Spanish Fly', and pederin in certain staphylinid or rove beetles (*Paederus*). Both groups are active at night and fly to artificial lights from which they may fall upon their human victims.

A more common mode of defence is provided by rigid hollow hairs on the body surface. These can penetrate the skin of their assailant and discharge poisons secreted by hypodermal cells that lie within or below each hair. Severe dermatitis with urticaria and blistering is produced, especially when the hairs break off. The best known examples are the caterpillars of many butterflies and moths (Lepidoptera); but this same mechanism is used by the 'stinging sea mouse' (Annelida), several corals and sea anemones, and by millipedes (Diplopoda).

3. Poisonous animals

The flesh of animals that are intrinsically poisonous is not likely to be eaten very often. However, under certain circumstances, species that are normally edible may become toxic. Some marine clams and mussels may accumulate a neurotoxin called saxitoxin after feeding upon dinoflagellate protozoans that swarm as a 'red tide' of plankton in certain oceanic conditions. The toxin causes a rapidly progressive flaccid paralysis and sometimes respiratory arrest.

Toxins derived from dinoflagellates may also be concentrated in certain fish. Ciguatera poisoning is a similar condition that can follow the ingestion of several species of carnivorous fish that live near tropical reefs and coastlines; this toxin originates from blue-green algae that enter the food chain when they are consumed by small fish. Another less serious type of fish toxicity is scombroid poisoning which occurs when tuna and other members of the mackerel family are partly decomposed by *Proteus morgani*; histidine is broken down by these bacteria to produce a poison that causes urticaria and autonomic effects.

4. Allergenic animals

Animal proteins include many potent allergens and these frequently induce IgE-mediated immediate hypersensitivity in predisposed persons. Symptoms of sensitivity may be systemic or confined to the skin, nose, lungs or gut. Well-known examples are the animal danders and bird feathers that frequently cause asthma, and gastrointestinal allergies produced by birds' eggs and shellfish.

In addition, however, there are many examples of sensitisation to free-living arthropods. The most widespread of these are the house dust mites *Dermatophagoides pteronyssinus* and *D. farinae*, which can be found in most households, especially in bedding and furniture where they feed upon exfoliated human skin scales. Inhaled particles of these mites and their excreta are among the commonest causes of allergic asthma; but a contact dermatitis can also be produced. Many other kinds of non-parasitic mites can cause allergic dermatitis; exposure is often related to certain occupations. Several species of forage mite can infest stored food products including grain, flour, dried fruit and cheese. Workers handling these substances are repeatedly exposed to the crushed bodies and excreta of these mites. Some examples

are baker's itch caused by the flour mite *Tyroglyphus farinae*, copra itch due to *T. longior* among dockers unloading copra and grocer's itch due to the cereal mite *Glyciphagus* or cheese mite *T. siro*. Another mite, *Pyemotes ventricosus* the grain itch mite, is a predator upon insects infesting straw and hay; it frequently bites agricultural workers and persons sleeping on straw mattresses, causing a severe papular and sometimes petechial rash. Swarms of flying insects can also cause asthma and rhinitis; the main offenders are non-biting midges (Chironomidae), mayflies (Ephemeroptera) and caddis flies (Trichoptera). Swarms are often attracted to lights and houses, especially near lakes and dams; the airborne body fragments, hairs and scales constitute potent inhalent antigens. Inside houses and warehouses, hairs from the bodies of larval carpet beetles (*Dermestes*) may create similar problems.

As is well-known, venomous Hymenoptera can be very serious sensitisers and deaths from wasp and bee stings are nearly always due to anaphylaxis following systemic spread of the venom. With other venomous creatures, repeated exposure is less likely and acquired hypersensitivity is therefore uncommon.

FURTHER READING

Belding, D.L. (1965) *Textbook of Parasitology*, 3rd edition. New York: Appleton-Century-Crofts.

Faust, E.C., Russell, P. and Jung, R.C. (1970) *Craig and Faust's Clinical Parasitology*, 8th edition. Philadelphia: Lea and Febiger.

Frazier, C.A. (1969) *Insect Allergy: Allergic and Toxic Reactions to Insects and other Arthropods*. St. Louis: Warren H. Green.

Garnham, P.C.C. (1971) *Progress in Parasitology*. London: Athlone Press.

Halstead, B.W. (1965–1970) *Poisonous and Venomous Marine Animals of the World* (3 volumes). Washington, D.C.: U.S. Government Printing Office.

Smyth, J.D. (1976) *Introduction to Animal Parasitology*, 2nd edition. London: Hodder and Stoughton.

van der Hoeden, J. (ed.) (1964) *Zoonoses*. Amsterdam: Elsevier.

2

Protozoan parasites

INTRODUCTION

The electron microscope has contributed a great deal to our present understanding of the structure and function of the parasitic protozoa. Some of the more important structures found in the various types of protozoa are shown diagramatically in Figures 2.1, 2.2 and 2.3; many of these structures are common to all animal cells but the figures also show some of the specialised organelles found in these organisms.

The protozoan cell is bounded by a trilaminar unit membrane that is often supported, immediately beneath, by a sheet of fibrils which together with the plasma membrane make up the **pellicle**. The fibrils are contractile and enable the cell to change its shape, or move in a gliding manner. The nucleus is enclosed by a double unit membrane and often contains one or more nucleoli, or alternatively a central body called an **endosome**. A mitotic spindle is formed when the nucleus divides and the chromosome number in most parasitic species is six or less; during mitosis nucleoli disappear but endosomes do not. Between mitoses the chromatin is often distributed partly on the inner surface of the nuclear membrane as the 'peripheral chromatin', and partly as a condensed mass around the nucleoli or central endosome; clear nuclear sap lies between, and this type of nucleus is described as **vesicular**. The cytoplasm is often separated into a more transparent outer part called the **ectoplasm**, which is a colloidal gel that gives the cell some rigidity, and an inner **endoplasm** that is a colloidal sol in which many of the organelles are suspended. Nearly all protozoa have an endoplasmic reticulum and many have mitochondria and a Golgi apparatus; some have contractile vacuoles which act as osmoregulators.

During the active feeding stages of the life cycle the protozoan is called a **trophozoite**. Some nutrients cross the cell membrane by diffusion or by active membrane transport but larger food particles are engulfed by phagocytosis, either through temporary membrane invaginations, or at the site of permanent mouth structures known as **cytostomes**. In addition, minute drops of surrounding medium may be taken up by **pinocytosis**, which is similar to phagocytosis but on a much smaller scale. Ingested food can be seen as membrane-bound vacuoles within the endoplasm, where they may later fuse with enzyme-laden lysosomes. Energy is stored as adenosine triphosphate and is often principally derived from anaerobic glycolysis; but in those species with mitochondria, there is, in addition, aerobic oxidative phosphorylation via the Krebs (tricarboxylic acid) cycle. Many protozoa live in conditions where glucose is freely available. In these circumstances complete oxidation can be dispensed with, and the products of glycolysis are excreted as acetate, succinate and short-chain fatty acids; these metabolites are often available to the host, who completes the oxidative process.

A resistant **cystic stage** is formed by several species and this allows the organism to survive in the external environment. Before the cyst wall is secreted projecting parts of the cell are reabsorbed and certain internal structures de-differentiate. The cysts are relatively inactive metabolically, although nuclear division may occur and food reserves are slowly used up.

Reproduction is usually asexual, and in its commonest form, **binary fission**, two daughter cells are formed by mitosis. Multiple fission occurs among the coccidia, by two processes called **schizogony** and **sporogony**, in which several nuclear divisions are followed by separation of the cytoplasmic mass and cell membrane to surround each nucleus. Sexual processes only occur in the coccidia and the ciliates.

Before considering the individual parasites in their ecological context, it will be useful to look at the main zoological groups into which they are divided. This grouping is based principally on their different means of locomotion. One parasite, *Pneumocystis*, does not fall neatly into this classification and its taxonomic position is still disputed. While it is certainly a unicellular eukaryote, a few authors regard it as a primitive

fungal organism; however, the current consensus is that it is an atypical protozoan; it is sensitive to antiprotozoan drugs. The life cycle of *Pneumocystis*, a lung parasite, will be described at the end of the section on lumen dwellers; it is usually regarded as a sporozoan parasite belonging to the class Haplosporea.

Flagellates (Superclass Mastigophora)

Flagellates move by means of whip-like flagella that extend from the body surface (Figs. 2.1, 2.6, 2.9, 2.16). Each **flagellum** originates from, and is controlled by, a minute body known as a **kinetosome** that is located in the ectoplasm. Kinetosomes

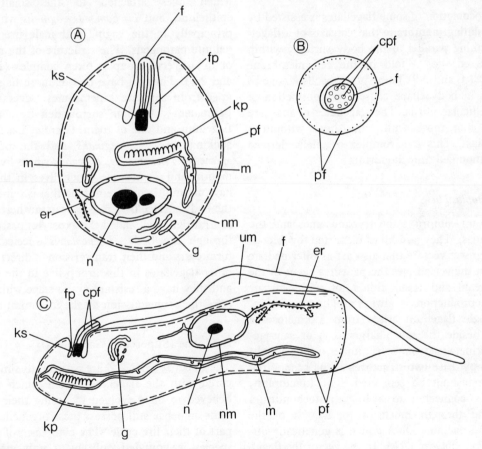

Fig. 2.1 Fine structure of Kinetoplastida (kinetoplast–bearing flagellates)
A. Amastigote (leishmanial form) in sagittal section
B. Anterior end of amastigote in transverse section
C. Trypomastigote (trypanosome) in partial longitudinal section
Abbreviations: cpf — central and peripheral fibrils forming axoneme; er — endoplasmic reticulum; f — flagellum; fp — flagellar pocket; g — Golgi apparatus; kp — kinetoplast; ks — kinetosome; m — mitochondrion; n — nucleolus; nm — nuclear membrane; pf — pellicular fibrils; um — undulating membrane

are believed to be analogous to the centrioles which organise the mitotic spindles of higher organisms. The flagellum itself is composed of a central **axoneme** surrounded by a sheath which is continuous with the cell membrane; the axoneme is made up of a ring of nine fibrils that surround two central fibrils (Fig. 2.1 B). This fibrillar structure is identical to that of the cilia and flagella found throughout the animal kingdom, and also to the bacterial spirochaetes. It has been suggested that all these structures are originally derived from symbiotic spirochaetes that became endoparasites within the eukaryotes. This hypothesis is similar to that which proposes that all mitochondria in eukaryotes are derived from endosymbiotic bacteria.

The locomotion of some flagellates is assisted by an **undulating membrane** that consists of a flagellum running parallel to the body surface, within the free edge of a fold in the cell membrane (Figs. 2.1.C and 2.9) These protozoa also move by changes in body shape caused by contraction of their pellicular fibrils. The flagellates of man are divided into those with, and those without a **kinetoplast**. This is a complex organelle derived from a modified mitochondrium.

A. Kinetoplastida

This group comprises the trypanosomes and the leishmanias. They are all transmitted by blood-feeding insect vectors that also act as intermediate hosts. In the vertebrates the parasites occur in the bloodstream and tissue fluids, or within tissue cells. Reproduction is always by binary fission. The single flagellum arises from a kinetosome located beside the much larger disc or sausage-shaped kinetoplast; however, under ordinary light microscopy these two structures at the base of the flagellum cannot be separated. The kinetoplast, which is connected to a huge mitochondrium extending through much of the length of the organism, contains DNA which is genetically different from nuclear DNA. In the vector the flagellum may act as an attachment organ.

These parasites adopt various body forms during their life cycle and these are illustrated in Figure 2.16. The **trypomastigote** has a posteriorly situated kinetoplast, an undulating membrane and

usually a free flagellum. The **epimastigote** also has an undulating membrane and a free flagellum, but the kinetoplast is anterior to the nucleus. In the **promastigote** the kinetoplast is further forward and there is no undulating membrane. Unlike the other forms, the **amastigote** is spherical or ovoid in shape, and the very short flagellum lies wholly within a **flagellar pocket** (Fig. 2.1.A); under light microscopy only the nucleus and the very large kinetoplast can be seen within the cell.

B. Flagellates without kinetoplastids

Seven human parasites come into this category. However, only two of them, *Giardia lamblia* which lives attached to the small bowel epithelium, and *Trichomonas vaginalis* which lives principally in the vagina and male urethra, are definite pathogens. The structure of the members of this diverse group is often complex (Figs. 2.6 and 2.9). They all have two or more flagella that arise from separate kinetosomes, several have a permanent cytostome surrounded by a modified flagellum and one of them, *Giardia*, has a ventral sucking disc. *T. vaginalis* and the other two species of *Trichomonas*, *T. tenax*, which lives in the mouth, and *T. hominis* which lives in the colon, have an undulating membrane that is reinforced at the body surface by a rod-like **costa**; there is also a central rigid rod, called the **axostyle**, passing right through the body. *Trichomonas* species do not form cysts and their transmission is direct. All the other flagellates in this group live in the intestine and they have a resistant cystic stage which facilitates their transmission by the faeco-oral route.

Amoebae (Superclass Sarcodina)

The amoebae (Fig. 2.2) are structurally simple compared with the flagellates, from which they are believed to have evolved by losing their flagella; some amoebae still possess these organelles during part of their life cycle. The cytoplasm of parasitic species is bounded only by a unit membrane, covered with a mucopolysaccharide 'fuzzy layer'; there are no supporting fibrils. Movement and phagocytosis take place by means of temporary **pseudopodia**. The cytoplasmic colloids can interchange their physical state between that of

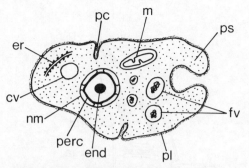

Fig. 2.2 Fine structure of an amoeba
Abbreviations: cv — contractile vacuole; end — endosome; er — endoplasmic reticulum; fv — food vacuoles; m — mitochondrion; nm — nuclear membrane; pc — pinocytotic channel; perc — peripheral chromatin; pl — plasmalemma with fuzzy coat; ps — pseudopodium forming food vacuoles by phagocytosis

an ectoplasmic gel and an endoplasmic sol. The propulsive force is provided by the contractile properties of the ectoplasmic gel. A pseudopodium begins when an area of ectoplasmic gel becomes a sol, endoplasm streams into the defect and lines it with newly formed gel to produce a tube-like extension of the body.

Two very different groups of amoebae infect man:

1. The amoebae of the alimentary tract, which include *Entamoeba histolytica*, are all obligatory parasites that normally live as anaerobic commensals within the gut lumen; they have no mitochondria. *E. histolytica* trophozoites sometimes invade the tissues where they become very active and change their appearance.

2. Soil-living amoebae of the genera *Naegleria* and *Acanthamoeba* may rarely invade human tissues, particularly the meninges, to produce serious and often fatal disease. They are aerobic organisms and can be grown on simple agar plates seeded with a bacterium. They possess numerous mitochondria, and unlike the gut amoebae they have a Golgi complex, contractile vacuoles and a prominent endoplasmic reticulum. Their ability to damage mammalian cells was first noted in 1958 when they were found as cytopathic contaminants of tissue cultures, and shown to be pathogenic to mice after intranasal inoculation. The lytic lesions produced in cell monolayers were initially attributed to an unknown virus; a classical example of failure to use the microscope.

Coccidia (belonging to the subphylum Sporozoa)

The protozoa in this group all live intracellularly for at least part of their life cycle. Because the members of this group all show a structure known as the **'apical complex'** they are now sometimes referred to as the 'Apicomplexa'; this complicated organelle enables the parasites to enter host cells (Figs. 2.3.A and B). The apical complex disappears during parts of the life cycle; it consists of one or more anterior **polar rings** supported by a conical structure, the **conoid**, which is made up of spirally arranged fibres. Several long electron dense bodies, the **rhopteries**, and many smaller tubules, the **micronemes**, run anteriorly to join the cell membrane within the polar ring; these structures are believed to be secretory and to assist host cell penetration following the attachment of the polar ring. The contractile pellicular fibrils, which allow the organisms to move by a twisting or gliding motion, are also attached to the polar rings.

The species of coccidia that infect man fall into three groups: the suborder Eimeriina which includes the causative agent of toxoplasmosis and also the less well known species of *Isospora* and *Sarcocystis*; the family Plasmodidae to which the malarial parasites *Plasmodium* belong; and the family Babesidae which contains the uncommon human parasites of the genus *Babesia*. These coccidian parasites all have a life cycle showing an alternation of sexual and asexual multiplication. The full life cycles of *Toxoplasma* and *Sarcocystis* have only been worked out during the last 10 years, while in the case of *Babesia* the details of the cycle in the tick vector are still the subject of some dispute. For simplicity we will describe the biology of *Babesia* separately, as it has only recently been realised that they are coccidian parasites; formerly they were classified as piroplasms belonging to a separate class of the Sporozoa.

The biology of Isospora, Sarcocystis, Toxoplasma and Plasmodium

The life cycles of these parasites are rather complex but they all involve a similar sequence (Fig. 2.4) which includes two types of asexual reproduction, schizogony and sporogony; and also a sexual process. Schizogony is always intracellular

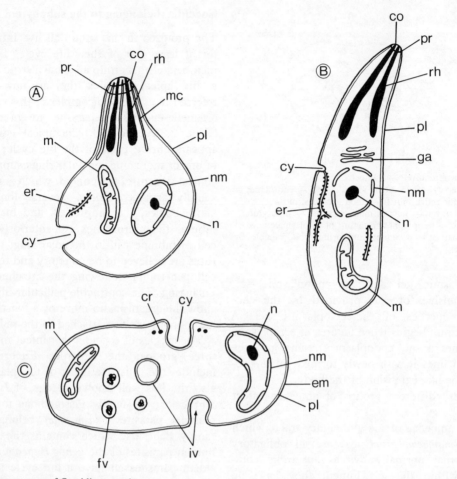

Fig. 2.3 Fine structure of Coccidian parasites
A. Merozoite of *Plasmodium*. B. Tachyzoite (trophozoite) of *Toxoplasma*. C. Trophozoite of *Plasmodium* inside erythrocyte (not shown) in cross-section.
Abbreviations: co — conoid; cr — cytostomal ring; cy — cytostome; em — erythrocytic membrane; er — endoplasmic reticulum; fv — food vacuole containing haemozoin (in Figure C); ga — Golgi apparatus; iv — invagination; m — mitochondrion; mc — micronemes; n — nucleolus; nm — nuclear membrane; pl — plasmalemmal membrane (double in merozoite A and tachyzoite B); pr — polar rings; rh — rhoptery
Note: the pellicular fibrils of the merozoite (A) and tachyzoite (B) are not shown.

and it follows penetration of the host cell by a **sporozoite**; multiple fission produces a large number of daughter cells, the **merozoites**. When the host cell ruptures merozoites are released and these invade further host cells to repeat the schizogonic process. Eventually, some merozoites, instead of dividing, develop into male and female gamete-forming cells called **gametocytes**. The mature male gametocyte undergoes multiple fission to produce many motile flagellated **microgametes** which fertilise the larger, relatively inactive, female **macrogamete**. Fertilisation may occur

extracellularly, or within the host cell in which the female gametocyte developed. The zygote secretes a cyst wall to become an **oocyst,** and within this it divides by multiple fission to produce sporozoites. The first nuclear division of the zygote is meiotic and for the remainder of the life cycle the coccidia have a haploid number of chromosomes. The sporozoan protozoa take their name from the spore-like appearance of the sporozoites within the mature oocyst; the later finally ruptures and releases the sporozoites which initiate schizogony once more. The spore-like oocyst is the resistant

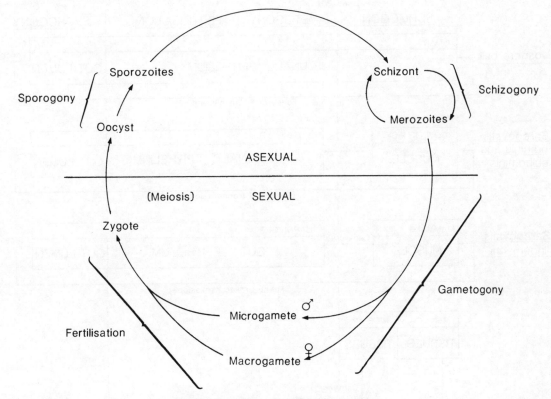

Fig. 2.4 Basic life cycle of Coccidian parasites

infective stage in the life cycle of most coccidian parasites and it must survive in the external environment. The malaria parasite, however, has no need for a resistant 'spore' because the mosquito vector inoculates the infective sporozoites directly into the capillaries of the next host.

The life cycles of these parasites are compared in Figure 2.5. They all involve an entero-epithelial phase, during which there is development within or just beneath their host's gut epithelium. In the simplest cycle, represented by *Isospora belli*, man is the only host and schizogony, gametogony and fertilisation all occur within the jejunal epithelial cells. The immature oocyst is released into the gut lumen and sporogony takes place within the oocyst as it passes down the gut into the faeces. Transmission is faeco-oral and follows the ingestion of mature sporulated oocysts. The life cycle of *Sarcocystis* involves a host alternation between the carnivore definitive host with an entero-epithelial cycle, and a herbivore intermediate host with an asexual cycle in muscle. In *S. hominis* and *S.*

suihominis man is the definitive host and he becomes infected by eating undercooked meat, beef and pork respectively, containing infective trophozoites. In the case of the uncommon infection, *S. lindemanni*, man is an accidental intermediate host and asexual multiplication occurs in skeletal and cardiac muscle; the normal definitive and intermediate hosts are unknown. In toxoplasmosis the entero-epithelial phase occurs only in the cat, the definitive host; man and other mammals are infected by mature oocysts derived from cat faeces, the released sporozoites cross the gut wall and establish asexual cycles in many tissues. Cats are reinfected by carnivorism, principally by eating infected mice whose tissues contain infective trophozoites. Toxoplasmosis normally therefore involves an alternation of hosts; but it may also be maintained for a while, as a one host species infection. Thus, it may persist, at least temporarily, within a population of intermediate hosts, such as mice, by repeated transplacental transmission; or it may persist in cats when they

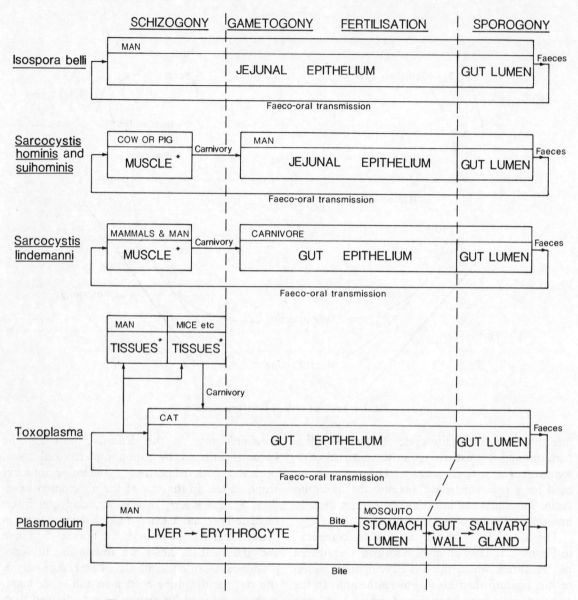

Fig. 2.5 Comparative life cycles of Coccidian parasites of man (excluding *Babesia*)
*Toxoplasma and *Sarcocystis* multiply asexually by internal budding (endodyogeny)

repeatedly infect each other by ingesting the faecal oocysts. Finally in malaria, there is schizogony in the human liver parenchyma and later in erythrocytes. This is followed by gametogony in erythrocytes and fertilisation within the mosquito stomach to form a motile **ookinete**, which penetrates the gut epithelium and develops into an oocyst beneath its basement membrane. The cycle

is completed when sporozoites, from the ruptured oocyst, enter the haemocoel and migrate to the salivary glands from where they are inoculated into another person. It should be mentioned that the asexual multiplication of *Toxoplasma* outside the feline gut epithelium and also *Sarcocystis* within muscle is not by schizogony, but by a process known as **endodyogeny** or **internal budding**.

Two daughter cells are formed within each mother cell; this involves nuclear division and the appearance of two sets of new cell membranes inside the mother cell cytoplasm, which finally ruptures to release the two new organisms. The tissue trophozoites of *Toxoplasma* and *Sarcocystis* have special names and these will be mentioned later.

The appearance of the *Plasmodium* trophozoite inside an erythrocyte (Fig. 2.3.C) is very different from that of the merozoite. The parasite is disc-shaped, its apical complex has gone, and the cell surface is surrounded by two membranes. The inner membrane belongs to the parasite and the outer one to the erythrocyte; the latter is derived from the original membrane invagination produced around the invading merozoite. The membrane-bound vacuole that surrounds intracellular protozoa is described as the **parasitophorous vacuole**. In the case of the *Plasmodium* trophozoite the double membrane is itself invaginated into the organism in places and may be seen in section as an inclusion with a double membrane. True food vacuoles have a single membrane and these are all produced at the cytostome which is reinforced with rings. An important feature of the *Plasmodium* parasite is its ability to partially digest red cell haemoglobin, and the final waste product, **malaria pigment** or **haemozoin**, can be seen inside the food vacuoles. In stained blood films the young malaria trophozoites often collapse in the centre; so that when looked at from above, their cytoplasm appears as a ring.

The biology of Babesia — the 'piroplasms'

Many important veterinary diseases characterised by haemolysis and haemoglobinuria are caused by these pear-shaped intra-erythrocytic parasites. The trophozoites have an apical complex, but this is less evident than in other coccidia. They multiply within vertebrate red cells by binary fission, but form no haemozoin pigment. Human infections with *Babesia* have only been recognised with certainty since 1957, but they are probably more common than is currently realised.

The remainder of the life cycle occurs in the tick vector within whose gut gametocytes form. The fertilised zygote, the ookinete, penetrates the gut epithelial cells where multiple fission occurs, and this is followed by dissemination of the parasites throughout the tissues of the tick, including the salivary glands and the ovaries. In ticks that feed on more than one host in their life, transmission may occur at the next blood meal; however many important vectors are 'one host ticks' that take blood from only one host. These can only transmit the infection because of the phenomenon of **transovarial** transmission in which the infected ovum produces an infected daughter tick which transmits the infection in her saliva. This is an example of vertical transmission between generations and it also occurs in tick-borne rickettsial infections and in tick-borne relapsing fever due to *Borrelia* spirochaetes. In all these examples ticks can form a reservoir of infection, independent of vertebrate hosts, by repeating the process of transovarial transmission.

Ciliates (subphylum Ciliophora)

Most of the ciliated protozoans are free-living, but many are gut commensals of vertebrates and invertebrates. *Balantidium coli* is the only species infecting man (Fig. 2.8); its body surface is covered by rows of cilia that propel the organism forward with a spiral motion. **Cilia** have the structure of a minute flagellum and each arises from a minute kinetosome. Adjoining kinetosomes are connected together within the ectoplasm by fibrils that co-ordinate the ciliary beats in each row. Food is ingested through a large anterior cytostome and waste products are excreted through a posterior **cytopyge**. Inside the organism can be seen several contractile vacuoles and two nuclei, a large **macronucleus** and a minute **micronucleus**. Division is by binary fission. Sometimes two organisms come together and conjugate sexually. Their pellicles fuse, the macronuclei disappear and the micronuclei undergo meiosis to produce haploid pronuclei, and a pair of these are exchanged between the two organisms. The zygote nucleus in each partner gives rise to new macro- and micronuclei. Macronuclei are polyploid and appear very dense; they divide amitotically and are concerned with phenotypic expression. Transmission is by means of resistant cysts.

LUMEN-DWELLING PROTOZOA — COMMENSALS AND PATHOGENS

The cavities of the various hollow structures of the human body which communicate with the external environment provide niches for several parasites. Only the pathogenic ones need be described here in any detail; the main importance of the others is the diagnostic difficulties they can cause (Ch. 13). These parasites share many characteristics and these will be described later.

The mouth

Two species of protozoa are quite common residents in the mouth. One is an amoeba, *Entamoeba gingivalis*, whose trophozoites closely resemble those of *E. histolytica* except that red blood cells are never ingested. The other is a flagellate, *Trichomonas tenax*, which is very similar to *T. vaginalis* except that it is smaller and narrower. Both of these parasites live in periodontal tooth pockets, carious tooth cavities and less commonly in tonsillar crypts. Prevalence rates commonly exceed 25 per cent in persons with poor oral hygiene.

Neither species form cysts and transmission is by kissing and respiratory droplets, or by means of shared drinking vessels, eating utensils and toothbrushes. Both species are probably non-pathogenic although it has been suggested that they may contribute to periodontal disease by causing immunologically-based inflammatory responses.

The small bowel

The flagellate *Giardia lamblia* is the only protozoan that lives in the lumen of the human small bowel; its morphology and life cycle are shown in Figure 2.6. The binucleate trophozoites are unmistakable pear-shaped discs that are pointed posteriorly; the mean dimensions are 15 μm in length, 9 μm in width and 3 μm in thickness. The dorsal surface is convex while the ventral surface is flattened and bears a large adhesive disc anteriorly. Two crescent-shaped median bodies lie centrally and there are four pairs of flagella, the hindmost pair arising from twin axonemes that run medially throughout the length of the organism. The trophozoite normally lives attached, by means of

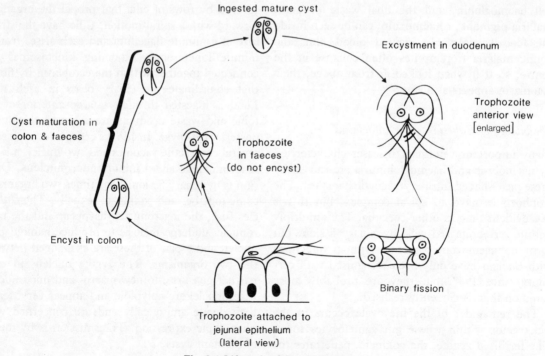

Ingested mature cyst

Excystment in duodenum

Trophozoite anterior view [enlarged]

Cyst maturation in colon & faeces

Trophozoite in faeces (do not encyst)

Encyst in colon

Binary fission

Trophozoite attached to jejunal epithelium (lateral view)

Fig. 2.6 Life cycle of *Giardia lamblia*

its adhesive disc, to the epithelial cells of the villi and crypts of the duodenum and jejunum. It feeds by pinocytosis on the dorsal surface, and also ventrally in the centre of the disc region. The host mucosa is not invaded but the adhesive discs make impressions upon the microvillous surface of the epithelial cells. The trophozoite divides by binary fission perpendicular to its long axis.

Encystment takes place within the ileum and colon. The cysts are ovoid and measure 8–12 μm in length and 7–10 μm in width; the mature cyst has four nuclei and several axonemes can be seen running longitudinally. Sometimes trophozoites can be found in diarrhoeal faeces but these cannot encyst. Under suitable conditions cysts may survive several weeks in the external environment. When swallowed by a new host they excyst in the duodenum to produce two daughter trophozoites.

The colon

The lumen of the colon is a favoured site for parasitic protozoa and the known human parasites comprise four species of flagellate, six species of amoebae and one ciliate. The semiliquid contents and low motility of the caecum make it an especially suitable habitat. These parasites live mostly near to the mucosal surface or actually within the mucus layer that covers the crypt epithelium; they feed as commensals upon bacteria, exfoliated epithelial cells and other debris. Only two of these species, the amoeba *Entamoeba histolytica*, and the ciliate *Balantidium coli*, have definite pathogenic potential, and even these may live as commensals for part, or even the whole, duration of an infection. A few of the other species may have a low pathogenicity.

1. *Entamoeba histolytica*. The life cycle of this species is depicted in Figure 2.7. Immediately after excystment within the small bowel, the four nuclei of the mature cyst divide to produce eight very small uninucleate amoebae. These colonise the caecum and ascending colon where they live adjacent to the mucosa. The commensal forms measure 10–20 μm in diameter and are commonly referred to as the 'minuta' form of the parasite; their food vacuoles contain bacteria and other materials but never host erythrocytes. Binary fission occurs about every eight hours. Encystment takes place within the faecal stream when minuta forms round up, discharge their food vacuoles and secrete a cyst wall. The cysts are almost spherical and measure 10–14 μm in diameter; when immature they are still uninucleate and contain a large glycogen vacuole. As the cyst matures the nucleus divides twice to produce four nuclei, the vacuole disappears and a number of cigar-shaped bodies known as **chromatoids** make their

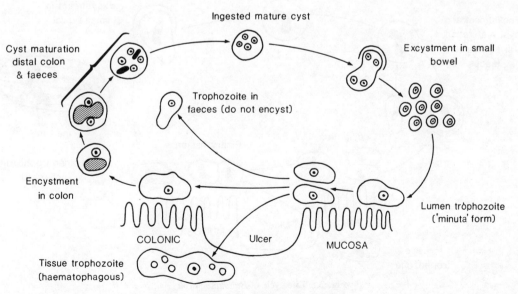

Fig. 2.7 Life cycle of *Entamoeba histolytica*

appearance. The latter are believed to represent a crystalline aggregation of ribosomes; they slowly disappear in old cysts. Sometimes 'minuta' trophozoites are found in diarrhoeal stools, but these cannot encyst.

Under certain circumstances, lumen-dwelling amoebae invade the tissues to become tissue trophozoites that are considerably bigger than the 'minuta' forms. They measure up to 40 μm in diameter and move very actively, often in an apparently purposeful manner in one direction; they are frequently haematophagous and contain host red cells within their food vacuoles; they never encyst. Host cells are destroyed only upon contact with tissue trophozoites. The initial lesion is a mucosal erosion, but eventually there may be extensive ulceration of the mucosa and submucosa. Blood-borne dissemination via the portal vein to the liver is quite common and can result in the formation of a necrotic liver abscess which may then extend into adjacent structures. Occasionally amoebae are carried from a liver abscess, by the blood stream, to distant organs including the brain. In addition, tissue invasion sometimes involves the perianal tissues and genitalia by contamination and sexual transfer; and also colostomy stomas and skin sinuses that communicate with amoebic lesions of the bowel or liver.

The nuclear structure of *E. histolytica*, in all its forms, is characteristic and of diagnostic importance. The peripheral chromatin is fine and evenly distributed around the nuclear membrane; the endosome is small, compact and centrally placed. A related smaller species, *E. hartmanni*, was previously referred to as the small race of *E. histolytica* and was sometimes included with the latter in surveys. However, *E. hartmanni* is never pathogenic or haematophagic, and its cysts have a diameter less than 10 μm, the mean value being 8.5 μm.

2. *Balantidium coli*. The life cycle of this relatively uncommon human parasite is similar in many respects to that of *E. histolytica*, see Figure 2.8. Trophozoites vary considerably in size and may reach 150 μm in length although the usual size is 50–70 μm in length and 40–50 μm in breadth. The large densely staining macronucleus is kidney-shaped and closely associated with the small spherical micronucleus. The trophozoite divides by transverse binary fission and normally lives as a commensal adjacent to the colonic mucosa. Encystment occurs within the host or outside, within the faeces. The cysts are ovoid or spherical and measure 45–65 μm in diameter;

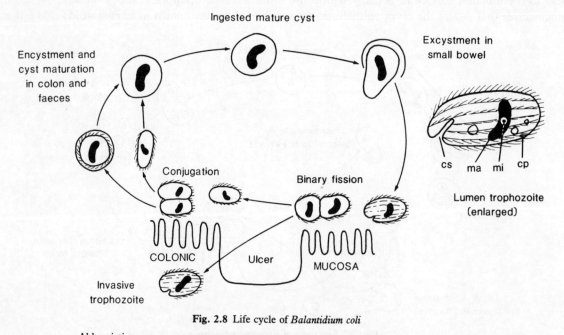

Fig. 2.8 Life cycle of *Balantidium coli*

Abbreviations: cp — cytopyge; cs — cytostome; ma — macronucleus; mi — micronucleus

unstained they appear greenish-yellow in colour. In immature cysts the organism retains its cilia and can rotate within the cyst wall; the cyst nuclei are difficult to see in temporary wet mounts. Within a new host, cysts excyst within the small bowel and soon reach the colon.

Tissue invasion can occur in the colon producing extensive colonic ulceration, sometimes with perforation. Lesions outside the colon are very rare although vaginitis, liver abscess and lung abscess have each been reported on a few occasions. The organism can apparently penetrate healthy mucosa by means of its motility and the release of hyaluronidase. Nests of trophozoites may be found within the colonic wall; tissue trophozoites never encyst. *B. coli* infection is a zoonosis and the principal reservoir hosts are pigs and rats.

3. *Other possibly pathogenic species*. There is now reasonably good evidence that another amoebic species, *Dientamoeba fragilis*, can cause self-limiting diarrhoea in man, although nothing is known of its pathology. Trophozoites of this species, unlike all other parasitic amoebae, are often binucleate, being in a state of arrested telophase; the cytoplasm may also show traces of a flagellar remnant. No cyst is formed and transmission is believed to be direct, or possibly within the eggs of the threadworm *Enterobius*. *Dientamoeba* is closely related to *Histomonas meleagridis*, which lives in the turkey caecum, causing serious disease, and is transmitted within the egg of the roundworm *Heterakis*. Based upon their fine structure and antigenic make-up, both *Dientamoeba* and *Histomonas* should now be classified as amoebo-flagellates, rather than with the true amoebae.

None of the other four colonic flagellates are known pathogens although two of them, *Chilomastix mesnili* and *Trichomonas hominis* are sometimes associated with a transient diarrhoea in man. The relationship may be coincidental, the trophozoites being more readily seen in unformed faeces; but it is perhaps relevant that the related gut parasites *Chilomastix gallinarum* and *Trichomonas gallinae* do cause disease in quails and pigeons respectively. It is worth remembering that 20 years ago the pathogenicity of *Giardia lamblia* was still seriously questioned.

Lower genital tract

In women, *Trichomonas vaginalis* is found principally in the vagina and endocervix but it also occurs quite commonly in the Bartholin glands, the urethra and even the bladder. In men, it is localised mainly in the anterior urethra but it may also be present in the prostate gland and in the preputial sac. There is no cystic stage and transmission is almost exclusively by sexual contact. In males the infection is normally self-limited and in the absence of reinfection, rarely lasts more than four weeks; however, in women it may persist for several years.

The structure of this organism is shown in Figure 2.9. It varies considerably in shape from an elongate ovoid form to spherical; length varies from 7–32 μm and width from 5–12 μm; amoeboid movements may be seen. There are four free anterior flagella and a fifth that runs in the free margin of an undulating membrane, which is supported at its base by a flexible rod, the costa. A rigid tubular structure, the axostyle, which is made up of a sheet of microtubules, runs throughout the length of the organism and protrudes posteriorly. Another inconspicuous structure is the parabasal filament which runs backwards from the kinetosome complex. Prominent cytoplasmic granules can be seen in the vicinity of the costa and the axostyle. This species is closely related to *T. tenax* and *T. hominis*; but it is larger, has more prominent cytoplasmic granules and the undulating membrane is shorter.

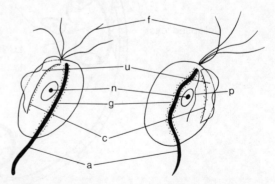

Fig. 2.9 Morphology of *Trichomonas vaginalis* trophozoites
Abbreviations: a — axostyle; c — costa; f — anterior flagella; g — granules; n — nucleus; p — parabasal filament; u — undulating membrane

This species is not invasive but its close contact with the epithelium causes subepithelial inflammatory changes and epithelial shedding; leucocytes migrate across the epithelium in large numbers.

Lung

Pneumocystis carinii lives within the lung alveoli and should therefore be regarded as a luminal parasite. The structure and life cycle of this organism is shown in Figure 2.10. It is normally a commensal that is transmitted by respiratory droplets. Parasites occur in clumps and throughout their life cycle the organisms remain adjacent to the alveolar epithelium, possibly attached by means of pseudopodial extensions that are in contact with lung macrophages. The uninucleate trophozoites have an irregular lobed shape and vary in size between 1 and 5 μm. They divide by binary fission and their cytoplasm contains mitochondria, an endoplastic reticulum, and various granules and vacuoles. Some of the larger trophozoites secrete a cyst wall and this is followed by nuclear and cytoplasmic division, so that the mature cyst which has a very thick wall eventually contains two to eight intracystic bodies, called sporozoites, that each measure 1–2 μm in diameter. The cyst itself may measure up to 10 μm in diameter; its wall eventually collapses and the sporozoites escape through a perforation and establish new cycles of trophozoite multiplication, either in the same host or in another one if they have been spread by coughing. No evidence of phagocytosis or pinocytosis has been detected in the trophozoites, and nutrition is presumably by active membrane transport.

In stained lung sections the infection is recognised by the clumps of nuclei that are lying within the cysts. Infected alveoli are filled with a hyaline or foamy alveolar exudate that contains numerous plasma cells and macrophages, but no

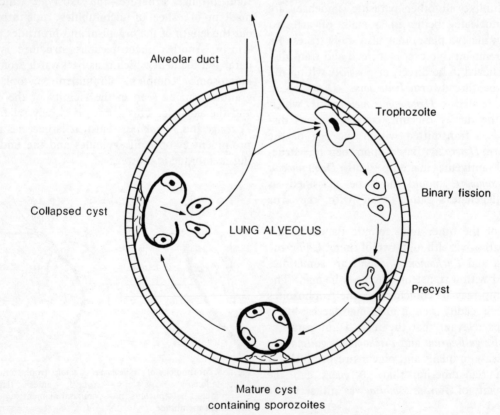

Fig. 2.10 Life cycle of *Pneumocystis carinii*

polymorphs. Serological and histological studies suggest that the prevalence in normal human subjects is between 1 and 10 per cent; however, significant pathology only occurs in debilitated subjects.

General characteristics of lumen-dwelling protozoans

1. Occupation of body cavities is the simplest form of parasitism and the various species have probably been derived more or less directly from free-living forms.

2. These parasites all have simple direct life cycles that involve no intermediate host. The transmissive forms are usually relatively resistant to environmental conditions. These parasites all have a cosmopolitan distribution with high prevalence rates occurring whenever human behaviour favours transmission.

3. All the infections can persist as anthroponoses since none have obligate reservoir hosts. Only two of the species are normally maintained as zoonoses. *Balantidium coli* is primarily a parasite of pigs and rodents, and many human infections are accidental. *Pneumocystis carinii* has been isolated from many domestic and wild mammals, especially rodents, sheep, goats and dogs. It is likely that this parasite is a normal commensal of many host species; there is good evidence that human infection is commonly derived from dogs. Natural infections of primates with several of the human amoebae and flagellates have been recorded and experimental transmission is quite easy. Dogs are sometimes infected with *E. histolytica* and may develop dysentery, but such infections are believed to derive from human sources.

4. With the exception of *P. carinii*, all these parasites lack mitochondria and live as anaerobes, although some can utilise oxygen *in vitro* by poorly understood mechanisms. Because of their selective drug uptake, all the anaerobic species are susceptible to the nitroimidazole compounds that include metronidazole. *P. carinii* is presumed to be aerobic because it contains mitochondria and lives in a well oxygenated environment.

5. These infections are normally diagnosed by the finding of trophozoites or cystic forms in the stools, vagina or mouth. Once again, *P. carinii* is the exception, as this infection is diagnosed by histology or serology.

FACULTATIVE PARASITISM BY SOIL AMOEBAE

Human infections with free-living soil amoebae were first recognised in Australia in 1965, but they have since been reported from many countries. The scanty reports from the tropics suggest that these infections are often overlooked, since in nature the causative amoebae are cosmopolitan. Several species are involved and they live principally in the soil and in muddy water. They proliferate in warm water that is polluted with bacteria, and can survive chlorination; they have even been found in tap water and the humidifier units of air-conditioning systems. The trophozoites form resistant cysts that allow survival in dry conditions, and also air-borne dispersal. The two genera responsible for human disease differ in appearance (Fig. 2.11), clinical effects and epidemiology. In both genera the nuclei have a very large central endosome.

1. *Naegleria*. These amoebae, particularly *N. fowleri* can cause an acute meningoencephalitis which is nearly always fatal. More than 100 cases have now been described. Infection follows swimming and diving in infected water; the amoebae invade the nasal epithelium and pass through the olfactory plate into the meninges. Cases have sometimes occurred in small outbreaks during warm weather. Patients are nearly always previously healthy young adults and children. The organism never forms cysts in the tissue. During its free-living existence, *Naegleria* amoebae sometimes transform into a non-dividing flagellate form; the transformation occurs in hypotonic media and these free-swimming forms are believed to facilitate dispersal.

2. *Acanthamoeba*. The clinical effects of *A. culbertsoni* and related species are much more diverse; the light thick-walled cyst favours air-borne infections and these amoebae are quite commonly isolated from throat swabs taken from healthy persons. They may also be isolated from normal stools, having presumably passed innocently

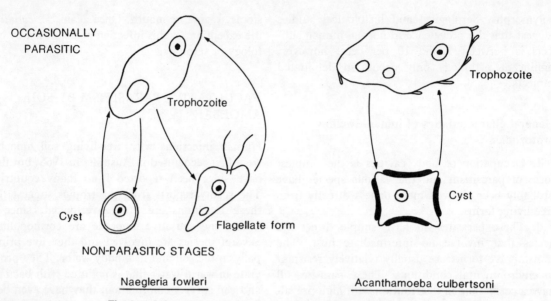

Fig. 2.11 Life cycle forms of soil amoebae potentially pathogenic to man

through the gut as cysts, although trophozoites have been found as well. Clinical presentations include granulomas of the skin, lung, orbit, brain, middle ear and gastric mucosa; but acute mening-oencephalitis and also isolated corneal ulcerations have been described. All of these infections are derived by various means from the environment; sometimes they may follow direct trauma to the skin and orbit. Many of the cerebral and systemic infections have occurred in debilitated persons suffering from other diseases, hence these amoebae are opportunistic as well as facultative parasites. The trophozoites of *Acanthamoeba* are usually covered with characteristic small spiny pseudopodia known as acanthopodia; unlike *Naegleria* and *Entamoeba histolytica*, trophozoites of *Acanthamoeba* may encyst within the tissues.

Infections with *Naegleria* and *Acanthamoeba* are sometimes only diagnosed histologically after death, although the motile trophozoites of the former may be seen in warmed wet mounts of cerebrospinal fluid. Identification in stained sections may be difficult but the large central endosome is often diagnostic; amoebae must be distinguished from degenerating host cells. Sections may also be incubated with specific antisera and counterstained with fluorescein-tagged antiglobulin; this method has been used to confirm several retrospective diagnoses.

Recently amoebae of these two genera have been incriminated as causes of an allergic alveolitis that follows inhalation of amoebic antigens derived from trophozoites growing in the humidifiers of air-conditioning systems. Sera from such patients shows antibody to these amoebae.

TISSUE PROTOZOANS WITHOUT VECTORS

The life cycles of these protozoa, which are all coccidia, have been compared in Figure 2.5. They are all obligatory intracellular parasites during part of their life cycle. Toxoplasmosis is the most important human disease in this group.

Isosporiasis

Infections with *Isospora belli*; a relatively uncommon parasite, are recognised by finding oocysts in the stool. These are ovoid in shape and measure 23–33 μm long and 12–14 μm wide, the cyst wall is translucent and there is a moderate neck-like narrowing at one end (Fig. 2.12.A). Man is the only known host.

Immature cysts are liberated into the lumen of the upper bowel; they contain an undivided spherical mass, which divides into two **sporoblasts** before

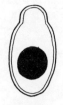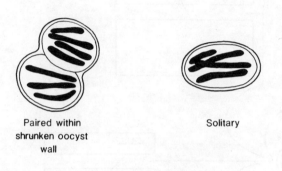

| Immature (not found in faeces) | Pair of sporoblasts | Pair of sporocysts containing sporozoites |

A. Oocysts of <u>Isospora belli</u>

Paired within shrunken oocyst wall   Solitary

B. Sporocysts of <u>Sarcocystis hominis</u>

Fig. 2.12 Coccidian parasites found in human faeces

the oocyst appears in the faeces. Further development usually occurs outside the body; after secreting a cyst wall to form a spherical **sporocyst**, each sporoblast divides into four crescent-shaped sporozoites. Ripe oocysts are very resistant and can survive in the environment for many months. When ingested by a new host the cyst walls rupture and the sporozoites invade the epithelial cells of the duodenum and jejunum, and undergo asexual schizogony to form numerous merozoites. The host cells rupture and merozoites invade neighbouring cells to repeat the schizogonic cycle. Infections may persist for several weeks, months or even years. Some merozoites undergo sexual differentiation to form unicellular female macrogametes or multiple flagellated male microgametes. After the female gamete is fertilised within the epithelial cell, the zygote enlarges and secretes a cyst wall to form an immature oocyst that is finally released into the gut lumen.

The symptoms of this infection result from destruction of parasitised gut epithelial cells, and the associated cellular infiltration and oedema within the lamina propria.

Toxoplasmosis

Many species of vertebrates are infected with *Toxoplasma gondii*, and serological evidence suggests that a total of about half a billion human beings are infected. The pathogenicity of *T. gondii*, the only known member of the genus, is usually low for it is a very successful parasite. In certain circumstances, however, it can cause severe pathology both in man and in domestic animals. The epidemiology and life cycle of this species is complex (Fig. 2.13), but of great importance because man, one of many intermediate hosts, becomes infected in three quite distinct ways.

The only definitive hosts of this coccidian are the domestic cat and certain wild felids including the ocelot, bobcat and Bengal tiger. In the absence of cats the infection does not persist indefinitely in nature. In the cat's small intestine the development is broadly similar to that of *Isospora belli* in man; a complex series of schizogonic cycles are followed by gametogony, fertilisation and sporogony. Immature oocysts are liberated into the gut lumen and appear in the cat faeces in an undivided state; the oocysts measure 12×10 μm and contain a single sporoblast. Outside the body maturation is completed within one to five days to produce an oocyst measuring 13×11 μm, which encloses two ovoid sporocysts; these each measure 8×6 μm and contain four sporozoites. Oocysts and free sporocysts can survive many months and may be found in cat litter boxes, children's sandpits and garden soil.

The principal intermediate hosts are the house mouse, field mouse and rat and these together with the cat normally keep the peridomestic cycle going. Many other rodents and nearly all orders of mammals may be found infected and also certain birds and reptiles; but many of these are dead-end hosts epidemiologically. In all intermediate hosts the cycle is the same; ingested sporocysts rupture in the intestine and the sporozoites penetrate gut epithelial cells; here they divide by internal budding to form **tachyzoites**, which are rapidly dividing trophozoites (Fig. 2.3.B). The host cell ruptures and neighbouring cells are infected; later,

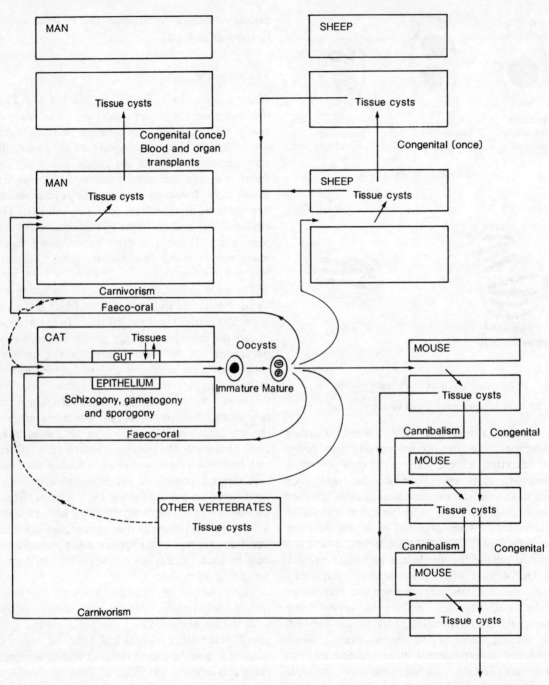

Fig. 2.13 Life cycle of *Toxoplasma gondii* showing relationships between vertical (congenital) and horizontal transmission (faeco–oral and carnivorism)

tachyzoites enter the circulation and infect any type of nucleated host cell. After these cycles have been repeated several times, true **tissue cysts** develop; these are the latent infective form of the parasite and they occur mainly in the brain, eye, skeletal and cardiac muscle. Each cyst may measure up to

100 μm in diameter and is nearly spherical; it may contain several hundred slowly dividing trophozoites known as **bradyzoites**. Cysts may survive for many months or years and it is unlikely that intermediate hosts ever eliminate the infection. If the host's immune competence is depressed, bradyzoites initiate new cycles of tachyzoite proliferation that can lead to acute disease, transplacental transmission or the formation of new cysts.

Cats become infected by ingesting oocysts from other cats, or by eating mice and other hosts that contain either tachyzoites or bradyzoites; the last named are the most efficient mode of transfer, and bradyzoites have been shown to be more resistant to proteolytic enzymes, than tachyzoites. After infection, cats may begin to shed oocysts after nine days and can continue to do so for several months, although excretion is usually soon limited by acquired immunity. In nature, often only about 1 per cent of cats are infective at any one time, but figures as high as 40 per cent have been reported. Reshedding of oocysts may follow new infections or depressed host immunity. Tachyzoite tissue forms occur in the cat and these are believed to initiate new cycles of oocyst formation; chronically infected cats re-shed oocysts when given corticosteroids.

Transplacental transmission can probably occur in all intermediate hosts, but only in mice and other rodents can the process be repeated in more than one litter. In all other hosts, including man, congenital infection can only take place if a primary infection is acquired during pregnancy; infections in early pregnancy may cause abortion. A woman who has infected one foetus cannot infect another during a subsequent pregnancy. Congenitally infected mice can themselves produce congenitally infected offspring and this is one of the ways that infection is maintained in mice; the other is through repeated cannibalism.

Sheep, pigs and rabbits are the commonest intermediate hosts to infect man directly, and the undercooked meat of these species is an important source of infection. Even handling the raw meat can cause infection if the fingers are licked afterwards. Between 10 per cent and 30 per cent of healthy sheep and pigs may be infected, but the rate is much lower in cattle. Toxoplasmosis is an important cause of abortion in sheep; transmission between sheep is entirely congenital and this can only happen once.

Of the three main modes of transmission to man, the congenital route is the least common but causes the greatest morbidity. The relative importance of the other two routes, the faeco-oral transmission of oocysts from the cat, and the ingestion of tissue cysts in meat, is still disputed. Transmission by ordinary blood transfusion is very rare, but it may occur with leucocyte transfusions or organ transplants, especially when the recipient is on immunosuppressive therapy. There is no good evidence that persons with acute disease can transmit the infection directly to others via the respiratory tract, or by sexual contact.

Sarcocystosis

1. *Sarcocystis hominis*. The gut cycle of this parasite is somewhat similar to that of *I. belli* except that there is no preliminary schizogony within the epithelial cells, and the oocysts are much more mature when they appear in the faeces. Man becomes infected by eating undercooked beef containing **sarcocysts** that appear macroscopically as minute greyish-white streaks. Man is the definitive host of this infection and the cow the intermediate host. Infection rates in man are variable but may reach 7 per cent or even 60 per cent where local dietary customs encourage the eating of improperly cooked meat. Symptoms, if any, are very mild, but the infection may be confused with *I. belli*. The faecal forms usually consist of pairs of sporocysts containing sporozoites within the shrunken oocyst wall (Fig. 2.12.B), but commonly separate sporocysts are found; these are oval in shape, and about 14.7 μm long and 9.3 μm wide.

The cycle in the cow is still unknown but it is probably similar to other *Sarcocystis* species. Sporocysts rupture in the gut, sporozoites invade the bowel wall and reach the circulation to enter endothelial cells of blood vessels where they undergo schizogony to produce rapidly dividing tachyzoites, these disseminate to muscles to form non-infectious **mother cells** (**metrocytes**) and, finally, numerous slowly multiplying bradyzoites within a large sarcocyst. Before its true life-cycle was appreciated, this parasite was referred to as *Isospora hominis*. A related parasite infects the pig and has been named *S. suihominis*; its sporocysts are shorter (12.6 μm by 9.3 μm) than those of *S. hominis*; man becomes infected by eating under-cooked pork.

2. *Sarcocystis lindemanni*. The life cycle of this species is probably like that of *S. hominis* with the important difference that man is an intermediate host of *S. lindemanni* and the definitive host is a carnivore whose identity is still unknown. By 1974 only 28 human infections with this muscle parasite had been reported, but it may not be as uncommon as is generally supposed since many of the known cases have been found accidentally in histological sections of striated and cardiac muscle. Similar parasites in domestic herbivores can cause systemic illnesses with myositis and myocarditis, and it is likely that this can happen in man also. The sarcocysts are elongated structures that lie longitudinally within muscle fibres, sometimes reaching a length of 5 cm; in sections many thousands of bradyzoites can be seen lying within the compartmentalised thick-walled cyst, the bradyzoites

closely resemble those of *Toxoplasma*. Man is an accidental host for this species and the infection cannot proceed further; *S. lindemanni* may well be identical with one or more of the many species of *Sarcocystis* species found in domestic herbivores, which have dogs and cats as their definitive hosts.

VECTOR-BORNE TISSUE PROTOZOANS

A. Malaria

The four species of *Plasmodium* infecting man have similar life cycles that follow the typical coccidian sequence (Fig. 2.4). Gamete fertilisation and sporogony take place in mosquitoes of the genus *Anopheles*, which act as vectors, and in man the cycle is continued with schizogony in the liver parenchymal cells, and then further schizogony and finally gamete formation in the erythrocytes.

One of the remarkable features of malaria infections is the tendency for the red cell schizogonic cycles to become synchronised. It is presumed that the cycles are triggered by the human circadian rhythm, for they are usually multiples of 24

Table 2.1 Comparative life cycles of the four species of *Plasmodium* that infect man

	P. vivax	P. falciparum	P. malariae	P. ovale
Sporogony				
Duration of sporogonic cycle in mosquito at 24°C	9 days	11 days	21 days	16 days
Liver schizogony				
Duration of primary exo-erythrocytic cycle	8 days	5–6 days	13–16 days	9 days
Persistence of secondary exo–erythrocytic cycles	5 years	None	None	3 years
Erythrocytic schizogony				
Duration	48 hours	48 hours	72 hours	49–50 hours
Number of merozoites (mean)	12–24	16	6–12	8
Red cells invaded	Reticulocytes	All ages	Older cells	? All ages
Changes in red cell				
1. size and shape	Enlarged	No change	No change	Slightly enlarged, and often distorted
2. inclusions	Schuffner's dots	Maurer's clefts	Ziemann's stippling	Schuffner's dots
Duration of recrudescences	Probably <2 yrs	2 years, usually <1 yr	40 years	Probably <2 yrs
Gametogony				
First appearance of gametocytes after parasite patency	3–5 days	9–11 days	5–21 days	5 days

hours. Malarial illnesses are characterised by more or less regular paroxysms of fever that coincide with the simultaneous rupture of infected erythrocytes at the end of each schizogonic cycle. The periodicities of the three more common infections have given them their vernacular names; the distinct illnesses were recognised long before the discovery of the parasites. Thus the commonest infection in man, benign tertian malaria, is caused by *P. vivax* which has a 48 hour cycle, to produce fever on the first and third day using the Roman system of counting. Quartan malaria is caused by *P. malariae* which has a 72 hour cycle; and malignant tertian or subtertian malaria is caused by *P. falciparum*, the most dangerous species. The name subtertian is used because in *P. falciparum* infections, the cycles are often poorly synchronised and fevers recur at intervals of less than the expected 48 hours. Sometimes, especially in early *P. vivax* infections, there may be daily or quotidian parox-

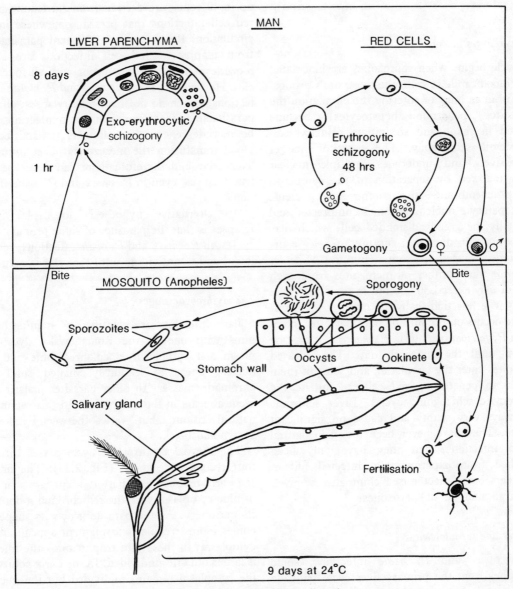

Fig. 2.14 Life cycle of *Plasmodium vivax*

ysms; these occur when two regular independent broods of parasites have overlapping cycles. The rarest infection in man, due to *P. ovale*, was only distinguished from *P. vivax* in 1918. Its schizogonic cycle often slightly exceeds 48 hours; this infection is normally referred to as ovale malaria, but the illness it produces closely resembles benign tertian malaria.

The life cycle of *P. vivax* is shown diagramatically in Figure 2.14 and the differences between the life cycles of the four species are presented in Table 2.1.

The liver stages in man

The cycle begins when sporozoites are inoculated into a blood capillary from the mosquito's proboscis. Within an hour of entering the circulation the sporozoites penetrate hepatocytes, become rounded in shape and so initiate primary exo-erythrocytic schizogony. The parasite enlarges progressively and undergoes multiple nuclear fission followed by separation of the cytoplasm and cell membranes to surround each nucleus. The hepatocyte nucleus becomes compressed and eventually the greatly distended cell, which may reach 60 μm in diameter, ruptures to release the minute pear-shaped merozoites (Fig. 2.3.A). In *P. falciparum* the number of merozoites from each schizont may exceed 30 000 but in the other three species it is less than half this number. Schizont rupture occurs on the fifth or sixth day after infection in *P. falciparum*, but in *P. malariae* it may be delayed until the sixteenth day. The released merozoites enter the circulation and some of them succeed in penetrating red cells to initiate the erythrocytic schizogonic cycles. Liver schizonts are always very scanty and cause no significant damage. They have never been found in natural human infections, and they have only been described from experimentally infected human volunteers or splenectomised chimpanzees, given very large numbers of sporozoites.

Relapses and recrudescences

In *P. vivax* and *P. ovale* infections, some merozoites from the primary liver cycle reinvade other hepatocytes and establish secondary exo-erythrocytic cycles. These two infections can **relapse** if these secondary liver cycles, which are apparently repeated many times, re-establish new erythrocytic infections. In *P. vivax* infections, relapses can recur for up to five years. The secondary liver cycles are not affected by the drugs used to treat acute malaria and to eliminate them an 8-aminoquinoline drug must be used. *P. malariae* was formerly thought to have a similar secondary liver cycle, but it is now believed that the reappearances of this parasite, which may continue for up to 40 years, are derived from extremely scanty red cell infections that persist somewhere in the circulation. Reappearances of patent parasitaemia from inapparent red cell infections are called **recrudescences** and they occur with all four species. However, in *P. falciparum* and *P. malariae* infections, which do not have true relapses, all new parasitaemias that are not due to reinfection must be recrudescences. If malaria is transmitted by blood transfusion the merozoites never initiate a liver cycle and therefore there can never be any true relapses, even in *P. vivax* and *P. ovale* infections.

An alternative hypothesis to explain true relapses is that the parasites of some primary liver cycles, in *P. vivax* and *P. ovale* infections, remain latent and non-dividing until the relapse occurs.

The erythrocytic stages

Malaria infections are identified by staining blood films with one of the Romanowsky dyes; the plasmodial cytoplasm is coloured blue and the nuclei appear as variously shaped solid red chromatin masses. In older parasites malaria pigment appears in the cytoplasm and this retains its natural colour that varies between yellowish brown and black.

The asexual erythrocytic cycle passes through four recognisable stages (Fig. 2.15). The first is the **early trophozoite** that often appears as a ring of blue cytoplasm with the red chromatin dot near its periphery. As the parasite grows its shape becomes more irregular and pigment appears in the cytoplasm; in these **late trophozoites** the nucleus is larger but still undivided. In the **early schizonts** the cytoplasm remains undivided but the nucleus separates into a number of irregular lumps of chromatin. The process continues in the **late schizont** and in these each chromatin mass, the nucleus, becomes surrounded with cytoplasm to form separate merozoites. After the red cell ruptures the residual mass of unused cytoplasm, which contains all the pigment, is ingested by macrophages. In blood films from heavily infected subjects, pigment granules are often seen in blood monocytes and polymorphs.

Gametocytes are first seen several days after asexual parasites become detectable. In their early stages they may be indistinguishable from late trophozoites but the organisms continue to grow until they nearly fill the red cell; the nucleus remains undivided. When mature the male and female gametocytes are clearly distinguishable; the latter are nearly always the more numerous. The male gametocytes have a pale blue cytoplasm and a large, rather pale and diffusely stained nucleus; while the females have a dark blue cytoplasm and a smaller, compact, deeply staining nucleus. Pigment is always prominent in gametocytes, it is more widely distributed in the male cell. The gametocytes of *P. falciparum* require nine days to mature and they can persist in the circulation for up to three weeks; in all the other species maturation is completed within three days and they disappear more quickly.

Stages in the mosquito

Within 15 minutes of entering the mosquito stomach the male gametocyte loses its red cell envelope and produces, at its periphery, six to eight actively motile whiplike gametes; this process is called **exflagellation** and it can quite easily be witnessed *in vitro*. Successful male gametes fertilise the inactive female gametes and the zygote rapidly assumes an elongated motile form that is armed anteriorly with an apical complex. These **ookinetes** penetrate the epithelial cells of the mosquito stomach wall and come to lie just beneath the basement membrane. Before the first cell division, which is meiotic, a cyst wall is secreted; this is followed by sporogony, which involves multiple nuclear fission to produce up to 1000 elongated sporozoites, each armed with an apical complex. The oocysts bulge into the body cavity and may eventually reach 50 μm in diameter. The cyst wall

finally splits and sporozoites enter the haemocoel; many of them reach the salivary glands, which lie in the mosquito thorax, and bore their way through the acinar cells to enter the duct system of the glands. The duration of the mosquito cycle is of critical importance in the epidemiology of malaria, since transmission can obviously only occur if the mosquito lives long enough to inject sporozoites into a new human victim. *P. vivax* has the shortest sporogonic cycle and at 24°C the process is completed in nine days.

Identification of the different malarial species

The four plasmodial species can usually be quite easily identified in thin blood films that have been fixed in methanol before staining; the changes in the host red cells are sometimes of diagnostic importance (Table 2.1 and Figure 2.15). To detect lower levels of parasitaemia, thick blood films are used (Ch. 13), in these the red cells have been lysed before staining, and this makes the recognition and identification of the parasites more difficult. The thin film appearances can be summarised as follows:

Plasmodium vivax. The early trophozoites are nearly always ring-shaped and have a diameter at least one-third that of the red cell. As they mature the shape becomes very irregular, so that they are said to be amoeboid in form. The red cell becomes enlarged and its cytoplasm paler as it is progressively dehaemoglobinised; numerous pinkish granules known as **Schuffner's dots** appear in the red cell cytoplasm. The schizonts nearly fill the red cell and typically produce 16 merozoites. The mature gametocytes are very big and have a diameter greater than a normal erythrocyte. Gametocytes may be quite common, even in early infections. *P. vivax* selectively invades reticulocytes and large ring forms seen in red cells with a polychromatic cytoplasm are likely to be this species. The total proportion of red cells parasitised rarely exceeds 1 per cent.

Plasmodium falciparum. The early trophozoites take the form of small rings that may have a diameter as small as one sixth of the red cell. Two or more rings may be present in one red cell and some are binucleate; sometimes they lie closely apposed to the red cell wall (accolé forms). In this

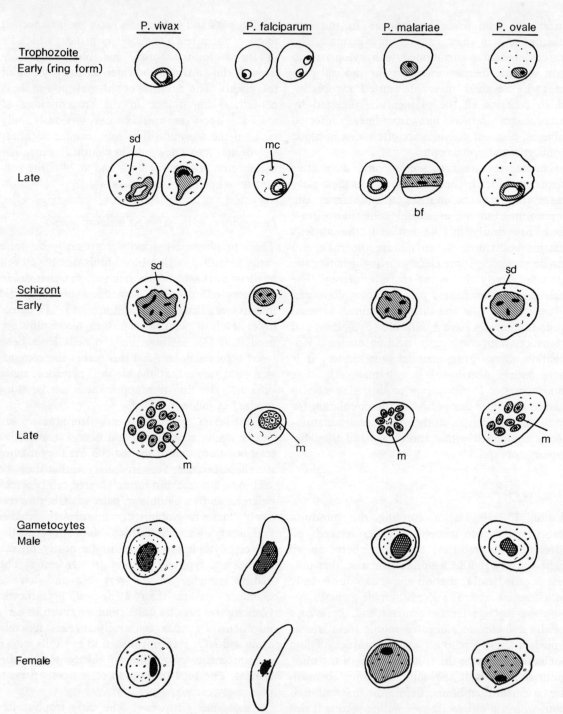

Fig. 2.15 Erythrocytic stages of the four species of *Plasmodium* that infect man.
Abbreviations: bf — band forms; m — merozoites; mc — Maurer's clefts; sd — Schuffner's dots

species the late trophozoites, schizonts and early gametocytes are usually only seen in the blood films from very heavily infected subjects; these stages normally mature outside the general circulation, especially within the capillaries of the spleen, brain and placenta. When late trophozoites and schizonts are seen, the parasites are much smaller and more compact than those of *P. vivax*; the red cell is not enlarged and in well-stained films the cytoplasm may contain a small number of irregular reddish-brown bodies known as **Maurer's clefts**. The mature gametocytes are unmistakable, for they are crescent-shaped and produce gross distortion or even the apparent disappearance of the red cell membrane; the female gametocyte is longer than the male and has more pointed ends. Parasitaemia can reach 10 per cent, or even more, in *P. falciparum* infections.

Plasmodium malariae. The early trophozoites resemble those of *P. vivax* although the cytoplasm is often more deeply stained and the vacuole less evident. The late trophozoites are compact and not amoeboid, the host cell is not enlarged and its cytoplasm contains no inclusions when routinely stained. Only after very prolonged staining can the very fine Ziemann's stippling be seen. In thin films, late trophozoites often appear as **band forms** that extend transversely across the red cell from one side to the other. Schizonts nearly fill the red cell and in their mature state they appear as a rosette of about eight large merozoites that surround a central mass of pigment. Gametocytes are usually scanty and appear relatively late; they nearly fill the normal sized erythrocyte. The percentage of red cells infected by this species rarely exceeds 0.2.

Plasmodium ovale. This parasite somewhat resembles *P. malariae* in that it is small, non-amoeboid and produces about eight merozoites. However, the red cell becomes enlarged, although not as much as in *P. vivax*, and it is easily deformed when the blood film is made. This latter feature gives the species its name; the infected cells are often oval in shape and frequently have crenated margins. Schuffner's dots are prominent in the red cell cytoplasm and appear early; they are fewer in number and more dense than those of *P. vivax*. Levels of parasitaemia may reach about 1 per cent.

B. African trypanosomiasis

The human disease is caused by two subspecies of *Trypanosoma brucei*; *T.b. gambiense* and *T.b. rhodesiense*; they are closely related to a third subspecies, *T.b. brucei*, which causes the economically very important infection of cattle known as nagana. The vectors are several species of tsetse fly, belonging to the genus *Glossina*, which is restricted to tropical Africa.

The life cycle is shown in Figures 2.16 and 2.17. In the vertebrate host the trypanosome exists only in the trypomastigote form, dividing extracellularly by repeated binary fission. After inoculation by the tsetse fly the trypanosomes proliferate at first in the dermis, but they soon extend via the regional lymphatic system to the blood circulation. In chronic infections the central nervous system is involved and trypanosomes can be found in the cerebrospinal fluid and perivascular nervous tissues. When taken up in the blood meal of the tsetse, the trypanosomes pass posteriorly to the midgut (stomach). Then they migrate forwards and multiply rapidly underneath the **peritrophic membrane**, which they later pierce anteriorly, to pass up through the crop, and then via the salivary ducts to the salivary glands; here they transform into epimastigotes. Two to five days later the parasites transform back into trypomastigotes and the fly becomes infective. The total duration of the parasite cycle in the tsetse fly is about 20 days; infective flies can live for many months. Only young flies become infected because when they are older the peritrophic membrane becomes tougher and cannot be pierced by the trypanosomes.

Because *T. brucei* is transmitted by the saliva of the vector it is known as a **salivarian trypanosome**. The tsetse can sometimes transmit the infection mechanically when the vertebrate host has a very heavy parasitaemia; in this circumstance the organisms remain in the pharynx for up to a few hours and the complex stomach and salivary gland cycle is omitted.

The three subspecies of *T. brucei* are morphologically identical. The vertebrate forms vary in length from 14–32 μm, and in width from 1.5–3.5 μm; when blood films are stained with Romanowsky dyes the cytoplasm becomes pale

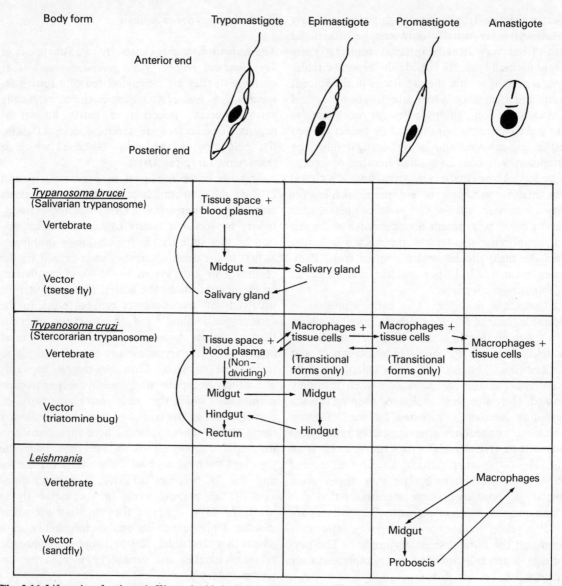

Fig. 2.16 Life cycles of pathogenic Kinetoplastida in their vertebrate hosts and vectors showing the different body forms adopted by the parasites

blue and the nucleus red; the kinetoplast appears as a small dark-red dot.

Gambian sleeping sickness (Trypanosoma b. gambiense)

This infection is found in scattered foci throughout West and Central Africa, between the latitude limits 15°N and 18°S. The northern limit extends from Senegal in the west to Southern Sudan and Uganda in the east, the eastern limits then pass southwards through East Zaire and Angola. About 10 000 new cases are reported each year, nearly half of them in Zaire; however the reported infections are probably a gross underestimate of the true number. The principal vectors are the so-called **riverine flies**, *G. palpalis* and *G. tachinoides*, that live in forest and bush near to permanent sur-

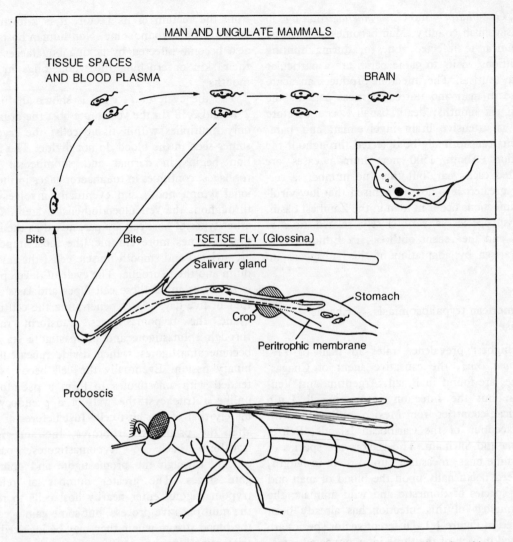

Fig. 2.17 Life cycle of *Trypanosoma brucei* in vertebrate host (inset shows trypomastigote greatly enlarged) and in tsetse fly

face water. Although many mammal species (including wild and domestic ungulates) can be experimentally infected, it is believed that in the natural state the infection is usually limited to man and perhaps the pig. Severe epidemics can occur when conditions favour transmission. The infection is a chronic one and it can persist for up to five years; parasitaemia is intermittent and trypanosomes are rarely found in the blood stream after the first few months. Involvement of the nervous system is a later manifestation and occurs at least several months after the initial

infection; it produces the classical sleeping sickness syndrome.

East African trypanosomiasis (*Trypanosoma b. rhodesiense*)

The distribution of this infection is limited to foci in southwest Ethiopia, Uganda, Kenya, Tanzania, Zambia, Botswana and Zimbabwe. It is normally maintained as a zoonosis in antelopes, warthogs and other game animals, but it also occurs in domestic cattle. The vectors are *G. mor-*

sitans, G. pallidipes, and *G. swynnertoni* that live in open savannah country. Man becomes infected by living near to infected zones or during hunting expeditions; visits to game parks are a particular risk to tourists. The infection produces an acute disease in man and untreated most patients die within six months; death usually occurs before there is extensive brain involvement and parasitaemia can normally be detected throughout the infection. About 1500 new human cases are reported each year, but the true number is certainly greater; it is now recognised that low virulence infections occur in man in the Zambesi basin. This subspecies is very closely related to *T.b. brucei* and the recent outbreak in Ethiopia may have arisen by adaptation of this subspecies to man.

C. American trypanosomiasis — Chagas' Disease

The highest prevalence rates in man of *Trypanosoma cruzi*, the causative agent of Chagas' disease, are found in Brazil, Argentina and Venezuela; but the infection occurs in all Latin American countries from Mexico southwards with the exception of the Caribbean Islands, Belize, Guyana and Surinam. The vectors are species of triatomine bugs, measuring up to 3 cm in length, that feed nocturnally upon the blood of man and many species of domestic and wild animals; the epidemiology of this infection has already been outlined in Figure 1.1. Different vector species are involved in each of the three interconnected infection cycles: the sylvatic zoonosis in wild mammals; the peridomestic zoonosis among dogs, cats and other animals; and the domestic infection in man. The most dangerous vector species to man are *Triatoma infestans* and *Rhodnius prolixus*, which are well-adapted to living in houses; another species, *Panstrongylus megistus*, appears to be in the process of becoming domesticated. Bugs defaecate during or shortly after their blood meal and the trypanosomes from their rectum may then be deposited on the human skin. The trypanosomes can enter the skin through the puncture wound or through mucosal surfaces, particularly the conjunctivae, lips and nose, after being transferred there by the victim's fingers. Because *T. cruzi* is transmitted

from the rectum of its vector, it is known as a **stercorarian trypanosome**. Non-human hosts may also become infected by licking bug faeces from their skin or crushing the whole bugs in their mouths.

The life cycle of *T. cruzi* is shown in Figures 2.16 and 2.18. In the vertebrate host the organism only multiplies within tissue cells; the trypanosomes seen in the blood do not divide. The infection begins in dermal and submucosal macrophages, continues in the macrophages in the regional lymph nodes and eventually involves cells throughout the reticuloendothelial system. Many other types of host cell are parasitised as the infection becomes more chronic; the most important are striated and smooth muscle cells, the myocardium and the neuroglia. The cycle of development is the same in all these cell types and lasts about four or five days. After penetrating the cell membrane the trypomastigotes transform rapidly through epimastigote and promastigote stages to become amastigotes, which divide repeatedly by binary fission. Eventually the cell becomes distended with amastigotes to form a **pseudocyst**; unlike a true cyst the wall of a pseudocyst is merely that of the host cell. Just before, or soon after the pseudocyst ruptures, the amastigotes transform back to trypomastigotes, passing quickly through the promastigote and epimastigote stages. The greater number of released trypomastigotes enter nearby host cells to repeat the multiplicative process, but some gain access to the blood stream where they may be ingested by a triatomine bug.

In the vector, ingested trypomastigotes pass to the midgut (stomach) where they become epimastigotes that divide repeatedly for several days. Later they pass backwards into the hindgut and rectum and revert back to an infective trypomastigote form. The parasite cycle in the bug takes between 10 and 30 days to complete and is entirely extracellular.

In stained blood films, *T. cruzi* averages about 20 μm in length, and is often fixed in a curved posture having the shape of the letter C. When compared with the African parasite, *T. brucei*, the trypanosomes of *T. cruzi* are more slender and have a more acutely pointed posterior end, the kinetoplast is very large and nearly spherical.

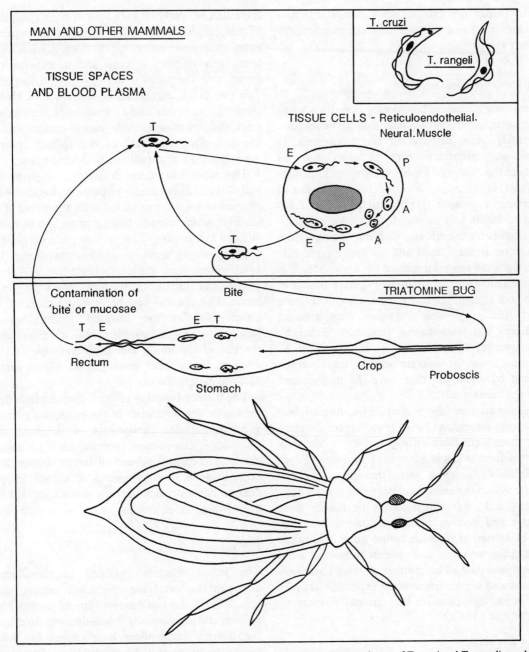

Fig. 2.18 Life cycle of *Trypanosoma cruzi*. At the top of the figure (inset) the trypomastigotes of *T. cruzi* and *T. rangeli* are shown together for comparison.
Abbreviations: A — amastigote; E — epimastigote; P — promastigote; T — trypomastigote

Levels of parasitaemia may be high in early acute infections, but later parasitaemia becomes intermittent and in chronic infections it may be detected only occasionally. Although many chronic infections are symptomless, it is unlikely that spontaneous cure ever occurs; so that patients remain infected for the rest of their lives. The main target organs in late infections are the myocardium, the oesophagus and the colon. It has been estimated that a total of about 35 million human beings are exposed to *T. cruzi* infection and that about one-third of this number actually harbour the parasite.

Other human trypanosomes

Trypanosoma rangeli. This species is quite a common parasite of man, dogs and cats in Venezuela, Colombia, Chile, El Salvador and Guatemala. It causes only transient fever in man and no significant pathology. Since its distribution overlaps that of *T. cruzi*, accurate differentiation is important. *T. rangeli* trypomastigotes (Fig. 2.18) measure 26–36 µm in length and have a prominent undulating membrane with many curves; the kinetoplast is very small and an appreciable distance from the posterior end of the organism. It is likely that this species divides by binary fission in the blood stream, as no tissue stages have been found. *Rhodnius prolixus* and other triatomines act as vectors and transmission can occur either by contamination from the bug's rectum as in *T. cruzi*, or from the salivary glands that become infected by organisms that leave the midgut and cross the haemocoel.

Trypanosomes of South Asia. Five human trypanosome infections have been reported from Asia, three were from different parts of Malaysia and two from a single household in India. Fever and possibly anaemia were the only observed effects. All of the infections were discovered accidentally and more will probably be found; their identity and vectors remain unknown but they may be related to parasites found quite commonly in macaque monkeys and rodents in several parts of southeast Asia. The monkey parasites are stercorarian and can be transmitted experimentally by triatomine bugs, however they are not *T. cruzi*.

D. Leishmaniasis

Parasites of the genus *Leishmania* form a large group of closely related organisms that infect many different vertebrates in various parts of the world. They are all transmitted by sandfly vectors and within their vertebrate hosts they all multiply exclusively as amastigotes within macrophages. Human infections may be caused by several species and subspecies of mammalian *Leishmania*;

these can be grouped into four species complexes (Table 2.2). Classification is based upon antigenic, isoenzyme and other biochemical characterisations, growth rates *in vitro* and in experimental hosts, and the natural ecology of the infection. The two major complexes of the Western Hemisphere, *L. mexicana* and *L. braziliensis*, can be distinguished by their growth rates in culture and the hamster skin; members of the former complex grow much more rapidly in both situations.

The general life cycle is shown in Figures 2.16 and 2.19. The infective process begins when promastigotes are inoculated with the saliva of the sandfly, which usually bites man on the face, ears or limb extremities. The parasites are ingested by dermal macrophages and soon transform into amastigotes that divide repeatedly by binary fission and finally cause most macrophages to burst. The process can be repeated more or less indefinitely, as the released amastigotes are ingested by new macrophages which accumulate at the site of the lesion and proliferate locally. Cell division by infected macrophages allows further parasite dissemination.

The further progress of the lesion depends upon the innate characteristics of the particular parasite, and the immune competence of the host. The situation is complicated because each *Leishmania* taxon may contain several differing strains; however, in general, each species or subspecies produces a fairly predictable outcome which falls into one of three main groups:

1. Cutaneous leishmaniasis

The lesion remains confined to the dermis, although the overlying epidermis usually ulcerates. This is the commonest type of leishmaniasis in man and it is usually a self-limiting disease. In the Eastern hemisphere it is caused by the *L. tropica* complex; and the condition is often known as 'oriental sore'; in the Western hemisphere it is caused by the *L. mexicana* and *L. braziliensis* complexes. Some members of the *L. braziliensis* complex can cause local lymphatic spread. A few persons infected with *L. aethiopica* and certain members of the *L. mexicana* complex develop **diffuse cutaneous leishmaniasis**; because of a specific defect in cellular immunity the amastigotes con-

Table 2.2 *Leishmania* infections in man

Names of species complexes, species and subspecies	Distribution	Reservoir hosts	Type of lesions
L. donovani complex			
L. donovani	Eastern India, Bangladesh, Burma, Central and Eastern Africa	Man in the Indian subcontinent. Rodents and wild carnivores in Africa	Visceral disease, sometimes PKDL
L. infantum	Mediterranean littoral and north African coast. Middle East. Southern USSR. Northern China	Dog. Also fox, jackel and wolf	Visceral disease, common in children
L. chagasi	Latin America from Mexico southwards to Argentina; commonest in N.E. Brazil and Paraguay	Fox. Dog and cat	Visceral disease
L. tropica complex			
L. tropica (= *L.t. minor*)	Mediterranean littoral and north African coast. Middle East. Southern USSR. Afganistan. Western India. Pakistan	Man and perhaps the dog	Dermis. Usually mild, chronic and solitary
L. major	Middle East and Central Asia. Africa — North and in a sub-Saharan belt from Senegal to Sudan	Burrowing rodents. Probably the dog in Senegal	Dermis. Often acute, sometimes severe and multiple
L. aethiopica	Mountains of Ethiopia, northern Kenya and South Yemen	Rock hyraxes	Dermis. Usually mild, but may cause DCL
L. mexicana complex			
L.m. mexicana	Yucatan. Mexico. Belize. Guatemala	Forest rodents	Dermis. Mild = 'chiclero's ulcer'
L.m. amazonensis	Amazon Basin	Rodents and marsupials	Dermis. Usually mild, sometimes DCL
L.m. pifanoi	Amazon Basin and Mato Grosso. Venezuela	Forest rodents	Rare. Dermis with DCL
L. braziliensis complex			
L.b. braziliensis	Brazil. Peru. Ecuador. Bolivia. Paraguay. Colombia	Forest rodents	Dermis. Single or multiple. Spread to nasopharynx in up to 85%
L.b. guyanensis	Guyanas. Northern Amazonas	Unknown	Dermis with lymphatic spread giving multiple ulcers
L.b. panamensis	Central America, especially Panama and Columbia	Forest rodents. Monkeys. Sloths	Dermis. Mild, occasional lymphatic spread
L. peruviana	Western Peruvian Andes	Dog	Dermis, mild — 'uta'

PKDL — post-kala–azar dermal leishmaniasis (in up to 20% patients in Indian subcontinent and 2% in Africa)
DCL — diffuse cutaneous leishmaniasis

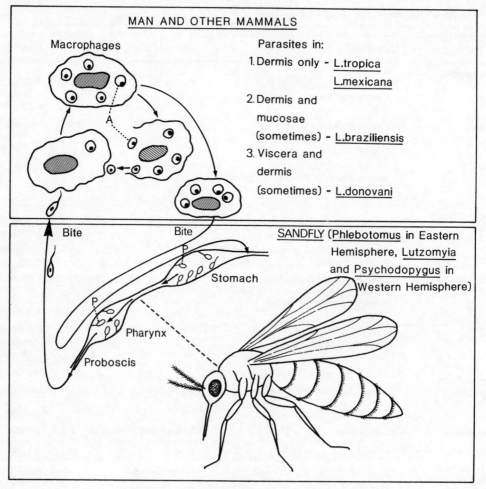

Fig. 2.19 Life cycle of *Leishmania*
Abbreviations: A — amastigote; P — promastigote

tinue to proliferate and the overlying epidermis does not ulcerate.

2. *Mucocutaneous leishmaniasis*

Parasites of the subspecies, *L.b. braziliensis* can spread in blood-borne macrophages to the nose, mouth and palate, where they multiply in macrophages within cartilage or connective tissues, producing destructive lesions often known as espundia. The process may extend to the pharynx and larynx; and occasionally the external genitalia are affected. The frequency of this serious and sometimes fatal complication depends upon the strain of parasite and varies between 5 and 85 per cent; strains in Southern Brazil and in Paraguay

have particularly high rates of spread. Metastatic lesions may appear before the primary lesion has healed or they may be delayed for as long as 20 years after healing. Reports of mucosal lesions with *L.b. guyanensis* and *L.b. panamensis* may be due to misidentification; if they are not, the complication must be very rare with these subspecies.

3. *Visceral leishmaniasis*

Members of the *L. donovani* complex produce a systemic disease often known as kala-azar. Usually, there is no evident primary skin lesion and the disease presents some months or years later as a systemic infection with hepatosplenomegaly; in East Africa, however, a primary lesion is sometimes noted. Parasites multiply within the macrophages of the spleen, liver, bone marrow and other organs; they may sometimes be seen in blood monocytes, particularly in India. Untreated, the infection is usually fatal. With some strains of *L. donovani*, parasites may reappear in the skin after apparently successful treatment with antimonial drugs. This complication is known as **post-kala-azar dermal leishmanoid** and its appearance may be delayed for up to five years or even more after treatment. There is no relapse within visceral tissues, but the skin becomes infiltrated with infected macrophages. Post-kala-azar dermal leishmanoid is very important epidemiologically because the heavily infected dermis is a potent source of infection to feeding sandflies; in India up to 20 per cent of patients may develop this complication, but it is much less common in East Africa.

With the exception of *L. donovani* infections in the Indian subcontinent, and *L. tropica*, all the *Leishmania* infections of man are zoonoses. Sandflies become infected when they feed upon the dermal tissues of infected reservoir hosts. The lesions, which usually take the form of infiltrated nodules, are most common on the ears, nose or perianal regions, or at the base of the tail; these are the preferred vector feeding sites on the reservoir hosts. In Indian *L. donovani* infections, sandflies become infected from blood macrophages, or from dermal macrophages particularly in the lesions of post-kala-azar dermal leishmanoid. In *L. tropica* infections, sandflies must feed very near to the lesion if they are to become infected.

Development within the sandfly takes at least 10 days. In the midgut (stomach), the parasites escape from the macrophages and transform into promastigotes which divide by binary fission. The parasites then extend forward through the crop into the pharynx where they produce a partial blockage of the insect's foregut. When the fly feeds again and it attempts to pump saliva down the proboscis, the parasites are inoculated into the new host.

E. Babesiosis

Babesia trophozoites are usually seen in pairs within red cells, they may quite easily be mistaken for *Plasmodium falciparum*; repeated binary division finally destroys the erythrocyte. The trophozoites measure 2–3 µm in diameter and when stained with Romanowsky dyes they show an irregularly shaped blue cytoplasm and a red nucleus; they may appear as ring, binucleate or quadrinucleate forms.

By 1979 at least 21 cases of symptomatic human babesiosis had been reported. Parasitaemia may be prolonged and in the fulminating cases up to 10 per cent of erythrocytes have shown parasties. Five patients had previously been splenectomised, and four of these died; two of these patients were from Yugoslavia, and one each from Ireland, Scotland and California, USA. A further 16 patients with generally milder infections came from Nantucket Island, off the coast of Massachusetts, USA, and from the neighbouring Martha's Vineyard Islands and the tip of Long Island. A serological survey of 133 persons on Nantucket Island, giving a history of tick bite, showed 10 with significant antibody titres. A survey of 101 healthy subjects in rural Mexico showed 38 seroreactors and *Babesia* were isolated by hamster inoculation from three of these symptomless persons, a smaller study in Mexico City revealed no seroreactors; another symptomless patient has recently been found in Georgia, USA. The cases from the Nantucket area and probably also those from Mexico were caused by *B. microti*, a rodent species that is highly prevalent in local field mice; four of the infections in splenectomised patients have been attributed to the cattle parasite *B. bovis*; and one to the horse parasite, *B. equi*. It is of great interest that in 1904, during an outbreak of the tick-borne rickettsial disease Rocky Mountain spotted fever in Montana, USA, a number of human blood films were found to contain intraerythrocytic parasites resembling the piroplasms of cattle.

The species of *Babesia* are numerous and widespread. Rural populations, agricultural workers, campers and others are probably often exposed to these zoonotic infections when fed upon by ticks. While splenectomised persons are at special risk, it is now evident that subjects with spleens can become infected as well, and a few of these develop severe disease. It is certain that many more cases will be reported in man.

FURTHER READING

Baker, J.R. (1969) *Parasitic Protozoa*. London: Hutchinson.

CIBA Foundation Symposium (1974) No. 20 Trypanosomiasis and Leishmaniasis with Special Reference to Chagas' Disease. Amsterdam: Associated Scientific Publishers.

Garnham, P.C.C. (1966) *Malaria Parasites and Other Haemosporidia*. Oxford: Blackwell Scientific Publications.

Kean, B.H., Mott, K.E. and Russell, A.J. (1978) *Tropical Medicine and Parasitology, classic investigations*, Vol 1. London: Cornell University Press.

Mulligan, H.W. and Potts, W.H. (eds) (1970) *The African Trypanosomiases*. London: Allen and Unwin.

3

Helminthic parasites

INTRODUCTION

Platyhelminthes (Trematodes and Cestodes)

Flukes and tapeworms appear superficially to be very different creatures and yet they belong to the same zoological phylum. Perhaps their most obvious shared characteristic is that the adults are usually dorsoventrally flattened. Adult flukes however are unsegmented and generally lanceolate or leaf-shaped, while the adult tapeworm consists of a ribbon of loosely connected 'segments' extending backwards from a minute holdfast organ at the anterior end. Platyhelminths are bilaterally symmetrical and their tissues are derived from three embryonic layers, ectoderm, mesoderm and endoderm. There is no coelom and the internal organs which include a nervous system, lie in a loose cellular mesenchyme which is itself enclosed by layers of circular and longitudinal muscle. The body surface has no cuticle but is covered by a metabolically active **tegument** which performs vital absorptive functions, especially in the tapeworms which have no gut (Fig. 3.1.A). Nutrients are taken up by active transport or by pinocytosis across the tegument which consists of a non-nucleated cytoplasmic syncitium formed by the fusion of processes that extend outwards from tegumentary cells lying beneath the muscle layer; the tegument may contain secretory vacuoles and mitochondria. Excretion is by means of a complex system of branched collecting tubules at the origin of which are situated **flame cells** whose cilia lie within the tubule lumen (Fig. 3.1.B). The rhythmic movements of these cilia, which can be seen in living specimens, have been likened to a flickering candle.

The reproductive systems are very complex but conform to a basic plan. All the tapeworms are hermaphroditic, as are all the flukes infecting man apart from the blood flukes or schistosomes that have separate sexes. The male reproductive organs include the **testes**, a duct system with associated glands and an eversible muscular **cirrus** which serves as an intromittent organ. The female structures (Fig. 3.1.C) include a simple **ovary** from which an **oviduct** leads to an **ootype** where the manufacture of eggs is completed. A complex system of branched **vitelline glands** release vitelline cells into the oviduct; these collect around the ovum as yolk cells within the ootype. Surrounding the ootype is the **Mehlis gland** whose secretions are believed to stimulate vitelline cells to secrete egg shell material. It is the structure of the ootype that determines the shapes of different platyhelminth eggs; from the ootype eggs pass on into the **uterus**. Connected to the ootype is a **seminal receptacle** and from this leads a duct to the external surface; in the flukes this duct forms **Laurer's canal** which may or may not be open externally, in the tapeworms it forms the **vagina**.

Parasitic platyhelminths are remarkable for their complex life cycles. The larval forms often being structurally very different from the adults, their biological connection has sometimes been recognised long after the two forms were originally described and given independent zoological names. A few platyhelminths are free-living; the planarians are aquatic scavengers and predators. Unlike adult parasitic forms, planarians are covered by a ciliated epithelium, and this feature also appears in the larvae of some parasitic forms.

A.

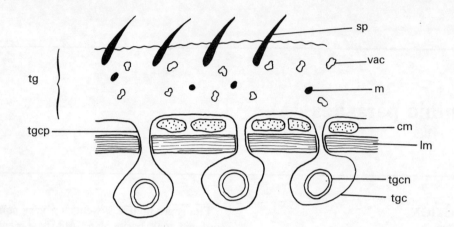

B.

C.

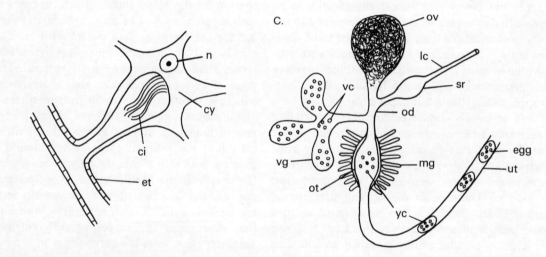

Fig. 3.1 Some details of platyhelminth structure
A. Fine structure of body wall (longitudinal section of a trematode)
Abbreviations: cm — circular muscle; lm — longitudinal muscle; m — mitochondrion; sp — spine; tg — tegument; tgc — tegumentary cell; tgcn — tegumentary cell nucleus; tgcp — cytoplasmic process of tegumentary cell; vac — vacuole
B. Fine structure of flame cell (highly magnified)
Abbreviations : ci — ciliary flame; cy — cytoplasm of flame cell; et — excretory tubule; n — nucleus of flame cell
C. Female genital structures
Abbreviations: lc — Laurer's canal (or vagina); mg — Mehlis gland; od — oviduct; ot — ootype; ov — ovary; sr — seminal receptacle; ut — uterus; vc — vitelline cells; vg — vitelline gland; yc — yolk cells surrounding ovum

Trematodes or Flukes

Adult fluke species range in length from 1 to 75 mm; they are usually greyish or white in colour, or sometimes pinkish. All the human parasites have snail intermediate hosts; these are usually aquatic or less commonly amphibious species.

Only *Dicrocoelium* has a terrestrial snail host. The structure and life cycle of *Fasciolopsis buski*, the giant intestinal fluke, a typical hermaphroditic species, is shown in Figure 3.2; all the hermaphroditic flukes are lumen dwellers. Figure 3.3 shows the structure and life cycle of *Schistosoma mansoni*; the schistosomes are the only flukes with

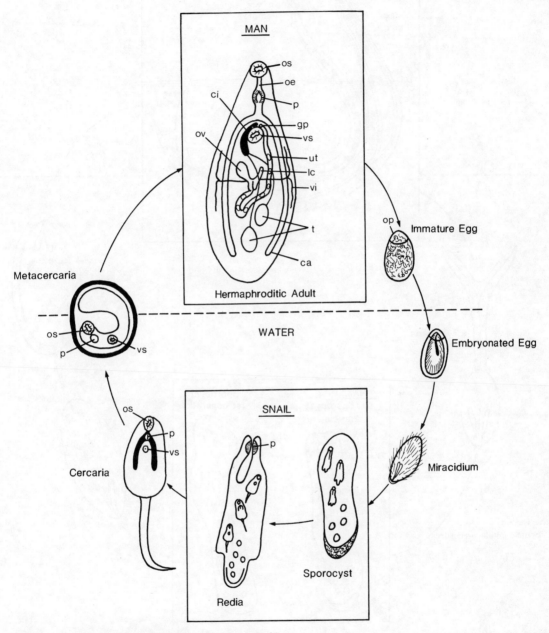

Fig. 3.2 Life cycle of a hermaphroditic fluke (*Fasciolopsis buski*)
Abbreviations: ca — caecum; ci — cirrus; gp — genital pore; lc — Laurer's canal; oe — oesophagus; op — egg operculum; os — oral sucker; ov —ovary; p —pharynx; t — testis; ut — uterus; vi — vitelline glands; vs — ventral sucker

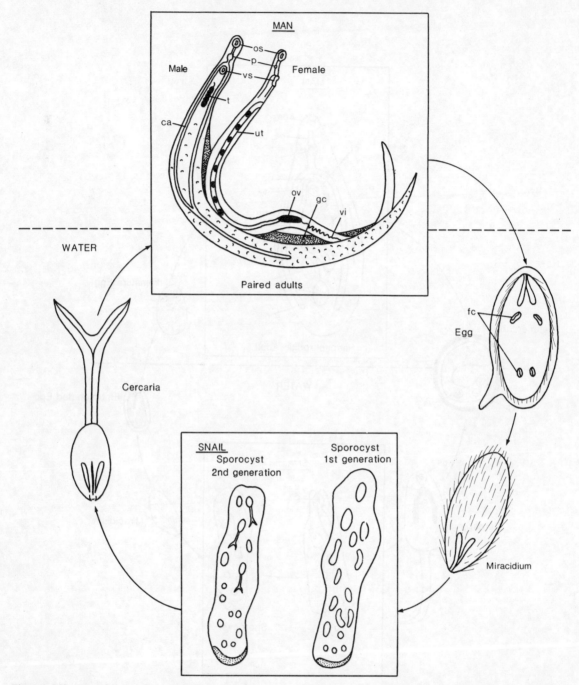

Fig. 3.3 Life cycle of *Schistosoma mansoni*
Abbreviations: ca — caecum; fc — flame cell; gc — gynaecophoric canal; os — oral sucker; ov — ovary; p — pharynx; t — testis; ut — uterus; vi — vitelline glands; vs — ventral sucker;

separate sexes, they live in the venous system surrounding the gut and urinary tract, *Schistosoma mansoni* lives in the inferior mesenteric veins.

The alimentary system comprises a mouth surrounded by an **oral sucker**, an **oesophagus**, a **muscular pharynx**, and two long **caeca** that run posteriorly and end blindly; there is no anus. In the schistosomes the caeca fuse in the posterior half of the body to form a single tube. A **ventral sucker**, used for attachment to the host, is situated behind the gut bifurcation. The tegument is often covered with small spines, papillae or tubercles. In the hermaphroditic flukes the intromittent cirrus and the uterus reach the body surface within a common ventral **genital pore**, adjacent to the ventral sucker. Self-fertilisation is common but these flukes can also be inseminated through the dorsal opening of Laurer's canal, when this is patent. The sex life of the schistosomes is unique; the nearly cylindrical female worms live more or less permanently within a long channel, the **gynaecophoric canal**, formed by the folded ventral surface of the male. Repeated insemination occurs, and the females only leave the gynaecophoric canal during egg laying, which occurs in the fine radicles of the venous system.

Eggs leaving the definitive host may be either immature, as in some hermaphroditic species, or fully embryonated, as in the schistosomes and the remaining hermaphroditic species. The eggs of hermaphroditic flukes have a detachable lid or **operculum** at one end. When the mature egg hatches a motile larva, the **miracidium**, escapes and penetrates the tissues of the molluscan host; in some hermaphroditic species the eggs are eaten by snails and hatch within the intermediate host. The miracidium is armed anteriorly with penetration glands and covered with a ciliated epithelium. Within the mollusc tissues the epithelium is lost and the organism de-differentiates into a sac-like **sporocyst** which comes to lie in the hepatopancreas of the snail. The elongate sporocyst has no recognisable organs but some cells proliferate into germ balls that lie within the lumen of the sac; these differentiate either into a second generation of sporocysts, as in the schistosomes, or into more complex larva known as **redia** that differ from sporocysts by having a pharynx and a short undivided caecum; in some species the redia cycle is repeated. The next stage of the life cycle, the tailed free-swimming **cercariae**, are formed within redia, or in the case of schistosomes within second generation sporocysts. The cercariae of the schistosomes have a forked tail and they directly penetrate the skin of the definitive host; those of the

hermaphroditic flukes have an undivided tail of variable structure and they encyst, as more or less spherical **metacercariae**, upon aquatic vegetation or within the tissues of another host. The total number of cercariae produced in a snail by one miracidium can exceed half a million in some species; the sporocyst and redia cycles are completed in about three weeks but an infected snail may shed cercariae for several weeks or even months. Sometimes the parasite kills the snail. Trematode multiplication within the snail is by polyembryony and new sporocysts and redia are formed from cells of the germinal line derived directly from the zygote; the same cell line eventually forms the testes and ovaries of the adult worms.

The resistant metacercariae of hermaphroditic flukes can survive several months; only when eaten by a suitable definitive host do they escape from the cyst and develop further (Fig. 3.4). Some species remain within the gut of the definitive hosts, while others ascend the bile ducts, and some penetrate the gut wall and enter the liver or lung. Schistosome cercariae lose their tail on entering their host's skin; the larval worms, known as **schistosomulae**, reach the lungs via the lymphatic or venous system and are then carried in the systemic circulation to the portal vein.

Cestodes or Tapeworms

Tapeworms have no alimentary tract and all nutrients must cross the tegument. The adults live within the small intestine of their host anchored to the mucosa by means of a holdfast organ, the **scolex**. The rest of the worm is called the **strobila** and consists of a ribbon of flat 'segments' known as **proglottids** whose principal contents are the reproductive structures of both sexes. During life the strobila lies in intimate contact with the host's gut epithelium; the absorptive surface of the worm's tegument is greatly increased by the minute microvilli which cover its surface. New proglottids are continuously being formed just behind the scolex, while the hindermost ones are shed or disintegrate. Sexual maturation occurs as the proglottids slowly pass backwards along the length of the worm; the male structures mature first, followed by the female ones. The most mature proglottids

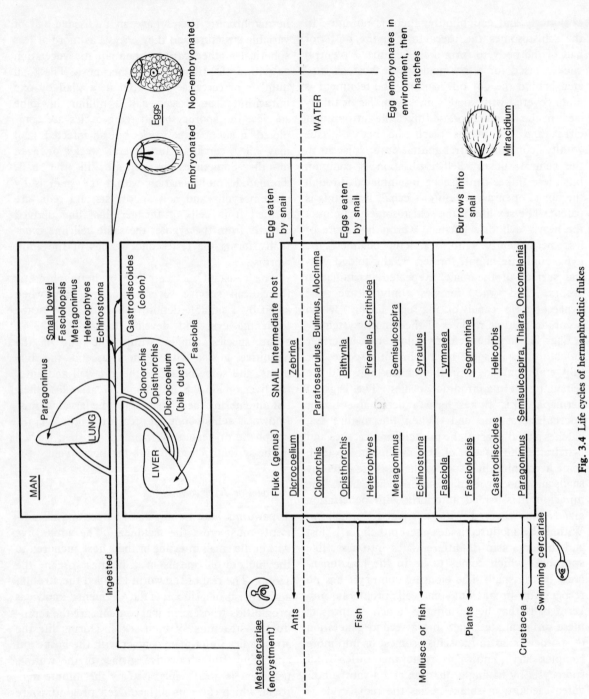

Fig. 3.4 Life cycles of hermaphroditic flukes

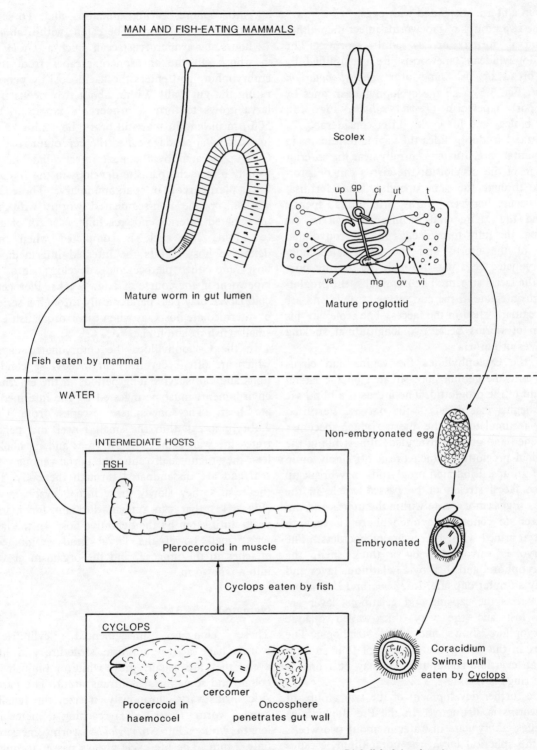

Fig. 3.5 Life cycle of pseudophyllidean tapeworm (*Diphyllobothrium latum*)
Abbreviations: see Figure 3.6

contain a uterus distended with eggs.

The two groups of tapeworms infect man either as larval forms, or as adult worms. The pseudophyllidean tapeworms are exemplified by the broad or fish tapeworm (*Diphyllobothrium latum*, Fig. 3.5), and the cyclophyllidean ones by the pork tapeworm (*Taenia solium*, Fig. 3.6); their biology and life cycles differ considerably.

In the Pseudophyllidea the vagina terminates in the genital pore situated centrally near the anterior margin of the proglottid; the cirrus can be protruded through the same opening. Cross fertilisation occurs between nearby proglottids, sperms ascend the vagina and fertilise the ova in the ootype; the fully formed eggs fill the convoluted coils of the uterus and the operculated non-embryonated eggs pass through the **uterine pore** into the faecal stream. The terminal spent proglottids disintegrate at the end of the strobila and are not regularly shed in the faeces. The scolex in this group of worms bears two longitudinal **sucking grooves** or **bothria**.

In the Cyclophyllidea the vagina and cirrus open into the genital pore situated on the lateral margin of the proglottid. The uterus is a blind sac that begins just distal to the ootype. Fertilised eggs accumulate in the uterus which becomes branched and greatly distended, almost filling the terminal proglottids which break off singly or in small groups. Liberated proglottids may break up in the faecal stream or be passed whole in the faeces. Eggs embryonate within the uterus and can be seen to contain the **oncosphere** (**hexacanth** embryo armed with three pairs of hooklets). The embryo is surrounded by a thick shell, the **embryophore**, and then by a **gelatinous layer** and finally an **outer capsule**. In *Taenia* and *Echinococcus* species the capsule and gelatinous layer are soon lost and the very thick-walled opaque embryophore shows fine radial striations. The scolex in this group bears a ring of four **suckers** and an eversible **rostellum** that may bear one or more rings of hooklets.

The further development of the two groups of tapeworms is distinctive. In the Pseudophyllidea the eggs embryonate in water in about two weeks and the spherical larva, the **coracidium**, escapes through the operculum. The coracidium contains an oncosphere with six hooklets, surrounded by an embryophore bearing numerous cilia. To survive the coracidium must be eaten, within about 12 hours, by a microcrustacean, such as *Cyclops*, in whose gut the oncosphere escapes from the embryophore and enters the haemocoel by penetrating the gut wall. Within about two weeks the larva grows to form a **procercoid** larva, up to 500 μm in length, that still bears the six hooklets in a caudal appendage called the **cercomer**. If the *Cyclops* is eaten by the next intermediate host, usually a fish, the parasite develops in the tissues into a **plerocercoid** or **sparganum** larva. These are whitish opaque non-segmented worms with an invaginated anterior end, reaching a length of up to 6 mm. The cycle is completed when the definitive host ingests the infected intermediate host and the plerocercoid develops into a tapeworm in the course of a few weeks. Plerocercoid larvae may pass paratenically through a series of intermediate hosts, as when carnivorous fish eat smaller fish or amphibia.

In the Cyclophyllidea the embryonated eggs, which are often very resistant to adverse conditions and can survive long periods in the external environment, must be ingested by the intermediate host. The oncosphere escapes from the embryophore within the small bowel and penetrates the wall using lytic enzymes and its hooklets; they then usually enter the portal venous system and are disseminated through the body. In the tissues they slowly grow into a cystic larva (Fig. 3.13) that can remain dormant for many years until eaten by the definitive host. In the latter's small bowel the larval head evaginates, attaches to the mucosa, and the organism grows into a tapeworm.

Nematodes

These elongate, unsegmented, cylindrical worms have a very uniform structure and life cycle; they are usually grey, white or pinkish in colour and sometimes semitransparent. The parasitic forms vary enormously in size, the female guinea worm (*Dracunculus*) reaching a meter in length while adult *Strongyloides* worms measure only 2 mm. The life cycle always passes through the sequence of egg, four larval stages and adult; the sexes are always separate and the adults are

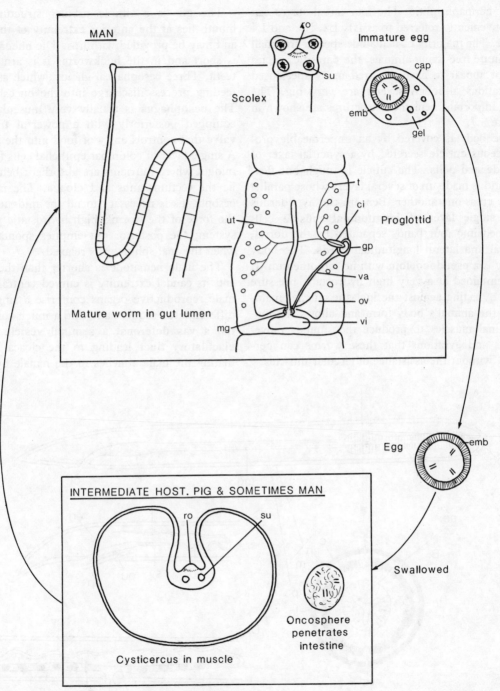

Fig. 3.6 Life cycle of cyclophyllidean tapeworm (*Taenia solium*)
Abbreviations: cap — egg capsule; ci — cirrus; emb — embryophore containing oncosphere; gel — gelatinous layer of egg; gp — genital pore; mg — Mehlis gland; ov — ovary; ro — rostellum; su — sucker; t — testis; up — uterine pore; ut — uterus; va — vagina; vi — vitelline glands

never hermaphroditic. The four larval stages can be conveniently referred to as L1, L2, L3, and L4 larvae. The majority of nematode species are small or minute free-living animals, the parasitic species do not appear to have acquired many specialised adaptations although several are very big. The more important nematode structures are shown in Figure 3.7.

The body is covered by an impermeable proteinaceous **cuticle** secreted by a syncitial layer of **hypodermal cells**. The cuticle is tough but flexible and is made up of several layers whose parallel fibres cross one another. Beneath the hypodermis is a single layer of **longitudinal muscle** cells grouped into four bands separated by the dorsal, ventral and lateral longitudinal **cords**. The body cavity is a **pseudocoelom** with no mesothelium. It is maintained at a very high hydrostatic pressure that, by acting against the inelastic cuticle, maintains the animal's body form and allows the longitudinal muscles to produce the sinuous movements and gyrations that these worms can perform, without the assistance of circular muscles.

The gut is a simple tubular structure. The mouth lies at the anterior extremity of the worm and may be provided with lips. The **buccal cavity** is short and in the hookworms it is armed with teeth. Three oesophageal glands, which assist the feeding process discharge into the buccal cavity. The **oesophagus** is usually very muscular, it is equipped posteriorly with a powerful **triradiate valve** that controls entry of food into the **midgut**. A single layer of columnar epithelial cells form the midgut where nutrients are absorbed; behind this lie the rectum, anus and **cloaca**. The muscular oesophagus is necessary to fill the midgut against the force of the worm's high hydrostatic pressure system; the posterior gut empties spontaneously when the anal sphincter is relaxed.

The male nematode is shorter than the female and its caudal extremity is curved ventrally. The male reproductive organs comprise a single tube differentiated sequentially into a much coiled **testis**, a **vas deferens**, a **seminal vesicle** and an **ejaculatory duct** leading to the cloaca. During mating the male attaches to the female by means

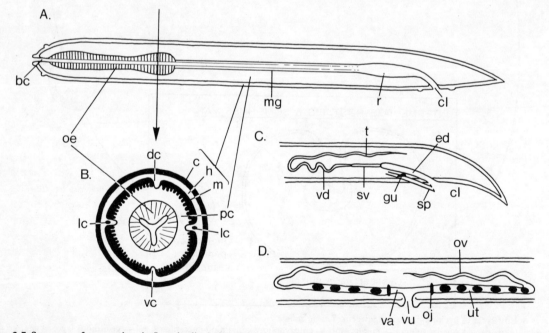

Fig. 3.7 Structure of nematodes. A. Longitudinal view showing gut B. Cross–section across worm at level of posterior oesophagus to show triradiate structure. C. Male genital structures D. Female genital structures

Abbreviations: bc — buccal cavity; c — cuticle; cl — cloaca; dc — dorsal cord; ed — ejaculatory duct; gu — gubernaculum; h — hypodermis; lc — lateral cord; m — longitudinal muscle; mg — midgut; oe — oesophagus; oj — ovijector; ov — ovary; pc — pseudocoelom; r — rectum; sp — spicule; sv — seminal vesicle; t — testis; ut — uterus; va — vagina; vc — ventral cord; vd — vas deferens; vu — vulva

of cement glands and also by one or two long **spicules** that can be inserted into the vulva, a structure known as the **gubernaculum** controls the movements of the spicules through the cloaca. The males of some species, including the hookworms, have an expanded cuticular process, reinforced with ribs, at their caudal extremity. This is known as the **copulatory bursa** and assists anchorage to the female during mating. The female reproductive organs comprise a single or double tubular system opening on the body surface as the vulva which is usually situated anteriorly on the ventral surface of the worm. Each genital tube is differentiated into a coiled thread-like **ovary** leading into the **oviduct, seminal receptacle, uterus, ovijector** and **vagina**. Ova are fertilised in the seminal receptacle and acquire their shell in the proximal uterus; the egg shell comprises three layers, the **chorionic membrane** and the true **chitinous shell** produced endogenously by the fertilised ovum; and the outer **albuminous covering** secreted by the uterus. The albuminous layer becomes yellow or brown due to a tanning process, and the eggs of species lacking this layer, such as the hookworms, are uncoloured. The ovijector is a muscular sphincter controlling the release of eggs from the uterus. The uterus of most adult worms is normally filled by a line of eggs. The daily egg output reaches its maximum in *Ascaris lumbricoides* which produces 200 000 each day. Some nematodes (*Trichinella, Dranunculus*) are viviparous and discharge first stage larvae from the uterus. Filarial worms produce **microfilariae** which are young embryos that may be surrounded by a sheath derived from the egg shell.

Nematodes possess quite complex excretory and nervous systems. The cuticle has sensory papillae around the mouth, cloaca and caudal extremity. **Amphids** are cuticular pits with secretory and sensory functions situated near the mouth, and many species have similar cuticular pouches called **phasmids** at their posterior end. Larvae must moult four times to reach maturity; moulting is probably triggered by the nervous system causing the hypodermal cells to secrete a moulting fluid whose enzymes digest the inner cuticle. Escape of moulting fluid into the host's tissues during exsheathment can be a potent antigenic stimulus.

It is frequently the third stage larva that is the infective stage of the parasite.

LUMEN-DWELLING HELMINTHS

Many helminth species use the body lumens of the gut, biliary, urinary and respiratory tract as the normal location for their adult forms. This allows a relatively easy exit route for their eggs and larvae, and also gives some protection from the host's immune defences. They will be considered here under the headings of trematodes, cestodes and nematodes. The eggs and larvae of these parasites are illustrated in Figures 13.3, 13.4 and 13.5.

1. Trematodes

All the hermaphroditic flukes of man are lumen dwellers. An outline of their life cycle is shown in Figure 3.4, which gives the generic names of the snail intermediate hosts.

A. *Flukes of the biliary tract*

Clonorchis sinensis, the Chinese liver fluke, infects man in Japan, Korea, Taiwan, China and Vietnam. While man is usually the principal host many other fish-eating carnivores are infected; the dog is the most important non-human source of infection. Metacercariae encyst beneath the scales of many fresh-water fish of the carp family (Cyprinidae) and cause infection when these are eaten raw; the sticky metacercariae may easily be transferred to the fingers or cooking utensils when fish are being prepared for the table. Young flukes ascend the bile ducts from the duodenum and adult worms, which measure up to 20 mm in length and 4.5 mm in width are found attached to the more proximal parts of the biliary epithelium; they may live for 15 years or more. The eggs are embryonated when they appear in the faeces and can survive three months in water, they hatch when eaten by the appropriate snail. The snail intermediate hosts may be abundant in fish ponds that are often deliberately treated with, or at least contaminated by, human faeces. The cercariae penetrate beneath fish scales and encyst in connective tissue and muscle.

Opisthorchis viverrini is an important related species found in Thailand and Laos, where the civet cat is an important reservoir. Another species *O. felineus* occurs in Siberia, Ukraine and Poland and mainly infects the cat in addition to man.

Fasciola hepatica is the most widespread and largest fluke infecting the human liver but the primary host is the sheep and, much less commonly, other domestic herbivores. 'Liver rot', caused by this species is economically important in most sheep-raising parts of the world where pastures are low lying and wet; the snail intermediate host *Lymnaea* is partly amphibious. Metacercariae encyst upon all types of emergent vegetation but man normally becomes infected by eating watercress gathered in the wild or commercially grown in watercourses contaminated by sheep faeces. Outbreaks of human infection have been reported mainly in Europe, including Britain and Ireland, the Middle East and Latin America. Larval worms penetrate the duodenal wall, traverse the peritoneum and enter the liver through its capsule; finally coming to lie in the bile ducts or adjacent liver tissue. Not all larval flukes reach the liver and these may enter the abdominal wall or cross the diaphragm into the lungs. Adult flukes measure up to 30 mm in length and 13 mm in width. Occasionally when raw infected sheep liver is eaten small flukes may attach to the human pharynx and cause a condition called halzoun. Eggs are not embryonated when they are passed in the stool and at least three weeks maturation is required before the miracidium hatches out to seek its snail host. A related but larger species, *F. gigantica*, sometimes infects man in tropical Africa, Asia and Hawaii, but its normal host is the cow.

Dicrocoelium dentriticum is a rare infection in man although it has a worldwide distribution in sheep and other herbivores. Embryonated eggs passed in the faeces are eaten by terrestrial snails and the cercariae later appear in slime balls secreted by the snails. Ants of the genus *Formica* eat the slime balls, and mammals become infected by eating the ants, whose tissues contain the metacercariae, when feeding upon vegetation. The flukes ascend the bile ducts and when mature measure up to 15 mm in length and 2.5 mm in width. Spurious infections are quite common in man

since after eating infected sheep liver, eggs may be passed in the faeces for several days. True human infections with a related species, *D. hospes*, have recently been reported from Sierre Leone.

B. Flukes of the intestine

Fasciolopsis buski (Fig. 3.2) is the largest trematode infecting man. Adult worms measure up to 70 mm in length and 20 mm in width, and live attached to the small bowel mucosa. The infection occurs in foci throughout East and Southeast Asia and in parts of the Indian subcontinent; pigs are also commonly infected. Metacercariae are found on fresh-water plants, particularly the fruits and tubers of the water calthrop. Infections occur when these are eaten raw or peeled with the teeth; this plant is a great delicacy and is grown in fish ponds fertilised with human and pig faeces.

Gastrodiscoides hominis has a focal distribution similar to the previous species; pigs, rats and monkeys act as reservoir hosts. Adult flukes live attached to the wall of the caecum and ascending colon and measure up to 8 mm in length and 5 mm in width; the anterior end is pointed and posteriorly there is a large sucking disc called the acetabulum. As in the previous species miracidia hatch from the egg and penetrate the snail host; the metacercariae encyst on various water plants including the water calthrop.

Several smaller species of fluke can also infect the human small bowel; man is usually an accidental host, the principal reservoirs being fish-eating mammals or birds. Species of *Echinostoma* occur in East and Southeast Asia; the adult worms measure up to 6 mm in length and have a collar of spines behind the oral sucker; encysted metacercaria occur in fish and fresh-water molluscs. *Heterophyes heterophyes* is quite common in man in the Eastern Mediterranean and Far East; adult worms measure only 1–2 mm in length and metacercariae occur in estuarine fish such as the mullet, or fresh-water fish including tilapia. This species is of interest because it, and some related fluke species, superficially invade the gut mucosa and their eggs may be carried via the lymphatics or portal vein to ectopic sites such as the myocardium, brain and spinal cord. Sometimes the minute worms themselves are carried embolically to these sites. *Metagonimus yokogawa* is present in the Far East and measures 2.5 mm in length; the metacercariae occur in a variety of fresh-water fish.

C. Fluke infection of the lung

Several species of the genus *Paragonimus* may infect man; the most important being *P. westermani* that occurs in Korea, parts of China and Japan, Taiwan and locally in parts of India and Southeast Asia. *P. africanus* and *P. uterobilateralis* are two species that have fairly recently been described from man in Cameroun, Liberia, Eastern Nigeria and Zaire. Several others may rarely infect man in South and Central America and in Southeast Asia but these do not usually complete their development in man. Pairs of adult worms measuring up to 16 mm in length and 8 mm in width live in cystic cavities adjacent to the bronchi, for up to five years. The non-embryonated eggs are coughed up in the sputum, and then sometimes swallowed to appear in the faeces. After maturation the eggs hatch and the miracidia penetrate the snail host. The cercariae have no tail but they penetrate the tissues of fresh-water crabs and crayfish to form metacercariae in the gills or muscles. Fish-eating mammals including wild and domestic cats, and mongooses act as definitive hosts, but man is the principal host of *P. westermani* throughout much of its range. Metacercariae hatch in the small intestine of the vertebrate host and the larval flukes penetrate the gut wall, cross the peritoneum and enter the lungs by penetrating the diaphragm. In man most worms reach their destination in the lungs but some, especially species other than *P. westermani*, may be found in ectopic sites including the abdominal cavity, subcutaneous tissues and brain.

2. Cestodes

Adult cestodes of the gut

These live in the small bowel lumen attached to the mucosa by their scolex. The life cycles of the six important species described here are compared in Figure 3.8; one (*Diphyllobothrium latum*) is a pseudophyllidean tapeworm, the others are cyclophyllidean. Occasionally other species, from both groups are described in man but these are all accidental infections. Tapeworm species are distinguished by the structure of their scolices, the reproductive organs in the mature proglottids (Fig. 3.9), and their eggs. Infections with the three large species (*D. latum*, *Taenia saginata* and *T. solium*) frequently involve only one mature worm.

Diphyllobothrium latum — Broad or fish tapeworm. The largest tapeworm in man, it may reach 10 metres in length and comprise up to 4000 proglottids. It is maintained in nature partly by man, and partly as a zoonosis in the dog and other fish-eating mammals; the cycle involves freshwater fish and *Cyclops* (Fig. 3.5); carnivorous fish sometimes act as paratenic hosts. Human infections occur mainly in Finland and other parts of Scandinavia, U.S.S.R. and Siberia, Central and Eastern Europe, Japan, the Great Lakes region of North America, Chile and Argentina. They are acquired by eating raw or semicooked pike, perch, burbot and other fish containing the plerocercoid larvae. Worms mature in three to five weeks and can live for up to 25 years. The scolex has two sucking grooves or bothria. Mature proglottids measure 10–12 mm in width by 2–4 mm in length; the much-coiled uterus is full of darkbrown eggs and occupies the central portion of the proglottid. The eggs are passed through the uterine pore into the faeces, they much resemble those of hermaphroditic flukes. Spent proglottids disintegrate at the end of the strobila and are not often seen in the stool.

Taenia saginata — Beef tapeworm. Man is the only definitive host for this species and cattle are the principal intermediate hosts. The adult worms may reach 5–15 metres in length and contain up to 2000 proglottids. This species has a worldwide distribution and occurs nearly everywhere that beef is eaten. Worms mature in six to eight weeks after ingestion of raw or improperly cooked beef containing the white cystic **cysticerci** that measure 8 by 5 mm; the worms may live in man for up to 25 years. The scolex has four suckers, but no hooks on the rostellum. The laterally placed genital pores alternate to left and right on adjacent proglottids (Fig. 3.9.B); when fully gravid the proglottids measure 5–7 mm in width by 16–20 mm in length and are filled with a branched

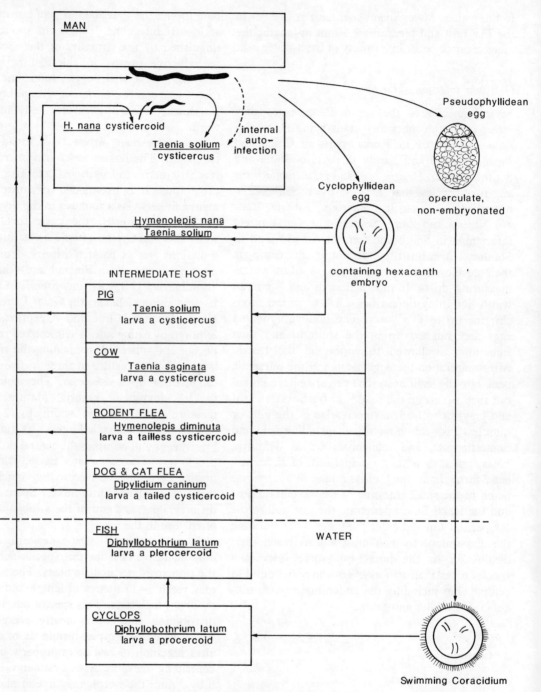

Fig. 3.8 Life cycles of tapeworms whose adults infect man

uterus, with at least 15 branches on each side, containing a total of up to 100 000 eggs. Each day one or more gravid proglottids usually break free from the end of the strobila and appear in the faeces, or more commonly migrate actively out of the anus; in the external environment proglottids remain motile for several hours and can move a metre or more. The eggs are very resistant and can

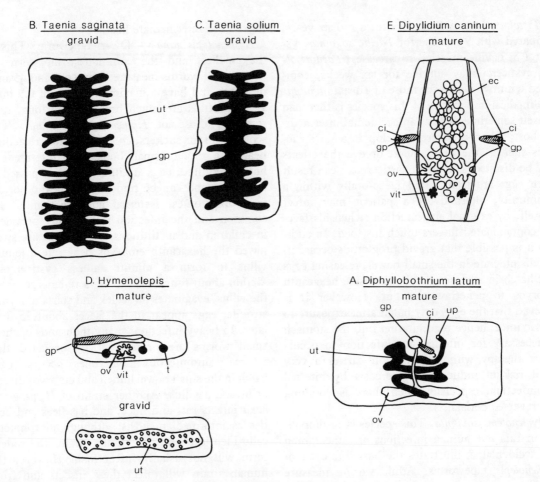

B. Taenia saginata
gravid

C. Taenia solium
gravid

E. Dipylidium caninum
mature

D. Hymenolepis
mature

gravid

A. Diphyllobothrium latum
mature

Fig. 3.9 Tapeworm proglottids of different species, mature or gravid (not drawn to scale)
Abbreviations: ci — cirrus; ec — egg capsules within uterus; gp — genital pore; ov — ovary; t — testis; up — uterine pore; ut — uterus; vit — vitelline glands

survive many months, they can withstand most forms of sewage treatment and may be dispersed to agricultural land when sewage sludge is applied; another dispersal method is by seagulls which ingest proglottids at sewage outfalls into the sea, and then fly inland to disperse intact worm eggs in their own faeces.

Although the pathogenic effects of this worm in man is slight, its economic impact is great because beef carcasses containing cysticerci are unmarketable. Developing countries suffer most because control measures are more difficult to supervise.

Taenia solium — Pork tapeworm (Fig. 3.6). As with the previous species man is the only definitive host; the pig and wild boar are the principal intermediate hosts. Worms may reach 4

metres in length and contain up to 1000 proglottids. Distribution is fairly limited and the species occurs mainly in Eastern Europe, Central and South America, Southern Africa, India, China and Indonesia. It has recently spread eastwards into Irian Jaya (Western New Guinea) as an epidemic among highland peoples whose association with pigs is very close. The scolex has four suckers and the rostellum is armed with two rows of hooks. Gravid proglottids contain about 50 000 eggs and measure about 12 mm in length, being twice as long as wide; they may be distinguished from *Taenia saginata* by having only 7–13 lateral branches to the uterus (Fig. 3.9.C). Proglottids are not very active and rarely migrate actively out of the anus or move much on the soil. In pig muscle *T. solium* cysticerci can live for up to six years, compared with 9 months for *Taenia saginata* cysticerci in bovine muscle; in carcasses, *Taenia solium* cysticerci may survive for six weeks, compared with two weeks for those of *Taenia saginata*. The medical importance of this species is that man himself sometimes acts as an accidental intermediate host; when cysticerci develop in vital structures such as the brain, heart or eye the effects may be disastrous. Human cysticercosis can result when eggs are transmitted faeco-orally within a community; alternatively a patient may infect himself, by external autoinfection, when his faecally contaminated fingers touch his food. In addition it is possible that gravid proglottids occasionally disintegrate in the small bowel, releasing eggs that hatch locally, so allowing invasive hexacanth embryos to penetrate the gut. However it is believed that the eggs only hatch after exposure to gastric juice, hence regurgitation into the stomach is necessary for internal autoinfection to occur. Chemotherapy without purgation carries a very small risk of inducing cysticercosis by internal autoinfection, especially when there is vomiting and reversed peristalsis.

Hymenolepis diminuta. This species is cosmopolitan in rats but human infections are uncommon and accidental; it illustrates the basic life cycle of *Hymenolepis* tapeworms. Adult worms measure 10–60 cm in length and have a maximum width of 2–4 mm. Up to 1000 proglottids may be present; they are all much wider than long (Fig. 3.9.D). The mature ones are 0.75 mm in length, and each contains three prominent testes. The scolex has four small suckers and a small unarmed rostellum. The terminal gravid proglottids are nearly filled with eggs, which are not released until the terminal proglottids break free and rapidly disintegrate in the gut; hence eggs are found in the faeces. Eggs in rat faeces are normally eaten by larval fleas, beetles (*Tribolium*), cockroaches and other scavenging insects. Within the intermediate host the hexacanth embryo penetrates the gut to enter the haemocoel where it develops into a minute larva called a **cysticercoid** (Fig. 3.13.F). These contain an invaginated scolex, as a cysticercus does, but the amount of cyst fluid is minimal, the larva has a small tail-piece. The cycle is completed when a rodent, or rarely man, ingests the intermediate host.

Hymenolepis nana — Dwarf tapeworm. This is the smallest and the commonest tapeworm in man. Adult worms measure between 5 and 45 mm in length and have a maximum width of 0.9 mm; all proglottids are much broader than long, they resemble those of *Hymenolepis diminuta*. The scolex has four suckers, and an eversible rostellum bearing a ring of small hooks. No intermediate host is required; eggs are infective when passed in the faeces and can be transmitted via the normal faeco-oral routes. External autoinfection is also common and the infection is especially prevalent in children and institutions. When eggs are swallowed the hexacanth embryos penetrate a jejunal villus to form a minute tailless cysticercoid. Within about four days the larva re-emerges from the villus, evaginates its scolex and starts to form a strobila; eggs appear in the faeces about 25 days later. In heavy infections many thousands of these small worms are present. It is suspected that internal autoinfection sometimes occurs; eggs hatch in the small bowel lumen and embryos directly invade a villus. Another strain of *Hymenolepis nana* infects rats and mice, and has fleas and beetles as intermediate hosts; although morphologically identical with the human strain, the rodent form will not usually infect man. However the human strain will infect these insects and from them mice can be infected; so it is possible that rodents could act as a subsidiary reservoir of infection.

Dipylidium caninum — Dog tapeworm. A common cosmopolitan infection in dogs and cats but accidental and relatively uncommon in man. The strobila consists of up to 150 relatively narrow elliptical proglottids and reaches a total length of 15–70 cm. The scolex is armed with four prominent suckers and up to seven rows of minute hooks on the eversible rostellum. Gravid proglottids reach 3.5 mm in width and 12 mm in length (Fig. 3.9.E). The uterus contains eggs in groups of 8–20 enclosed, as egg capsules, within a shared embryonic membrane. Proglottids are very motile and are normally passed intact in the faeces but sometimes egg capsules may be found if disintegration has occurred. Each proglottid has two independent sets of reproductive structures that open through separate genital pores on each side. Eggs are eaten by larval dog or cat fleas (*Ctenocephalides*) and tailed cysticercoids develop in the body cavity; the latter survive insect metamorphosis and the cycle is completed when adult fleas are eaten by dogs or cats, and sometimes man.

3. Nematodes

Nematodes of the gut

The nematodes that complete their development in man and live as adults within the gut lumen or its surface mucosa are all, with a single exception (*Capillaria philippinensis*), dependent to some degree upon the soil for their transmission from host to host. These 'soil-transmitted helminths' may be exclusively human parasites, or zoonoses that accidentally infect man.

A. Non-zoonotic soil-transmitted gut nematodes. As a group these are the most important helminths that infect man. Their life cycles are shown in Figure 3.10; they form a biological sequence in their degree of dependence upon the soil. They will be described here in order of descending soil dependence; the five-membered sequence shows a progressive simplification of the life cycle. In Figure 3.10 the sequence proceeds in an anticlockwise order as they leave the human body; thus *Strongyloides* is the most dependent upon soil conditions, and *Enterobius* the least dependent.

1. *Strongyloides stercoralis*. This species is unique among human helminths in having a free-living cycle that can persist in the soil, feeding upon soil bacteria, for several generations. The parasitic adults are almost all parthenogenetic females, measuring 2 mm in length; they live embedded in the jejunal mucosa for a life span of three to four months. Their eggs hatch near to or at the mucosal surface to produce first stage larvae (L1), these are known as **rhabditiform** larvae because they have a relatively short muscular oesophagus with an enlarged posterior bulb (Fig. 13.5), and so resemble the free-living nematode *Rhabditis;* they measure 0.25 mm in length. These larvae pass out in the faeces and reach the soil where they either moult twice to form non-feeding infective **filariform** third stage larvae (L3), or develop through four moults into free-living male and

female adults, measuring respectively 0.8 mm and 1 mm in length. The eggs of free-living adults, whose oesophagi have posterior bulbs, hatch to form rhabditiform larvae (L1) that either produce another generation of free-living adults or proceed to infective filariform larvae. Unlike rhabditiform (L1) larvae, filariform larvae (Fig. 13.5) have a long oesophagus of uniform width; the tip of their tail is finely triradiate and their total length is 0.55 mm. Filariform larvae, which live for up to 12 days, penetrate the skin, usually at the sides of the feet or between the toes, and reach the heart via the venous circulation or the lymphatics. From the heart they are carried to the lungs where they penetrate the alveoli and moult twice to become young adult worms; these ascend the respiratory tract epithelium to the pharynx to be swallowed and so reach their final destination, the jejunum, where they burrow into the mucosa and mature in 17 days. The parasitic female worm has a long filiform oesophagus.

The life cycle of this species is further complicated by the phenomenon of autoinfection which explains the persistence of this infection for up to 30 years in persons leaving some endemic areas. The commonest type of autoinfection is externally on the perianal skin; some L1 larvae mature into filariform larvae (L3) by the time they reach the faeces or more commonly this maturation occurs on faecally-soiled perianal skin. In either case filariform larvae penetrate the skin and after wandering in the dermis for a day or two, enter the lymphatic or venous system to complete the cycle in the usual manner; the dermal wanderings of L3 *Strongyloides stercoralis* larvae constitute one form of the condition known as **cutaneous larva migrans**. The other type of autoinfection occurs internally and is much more serious, because in immunodeficient hosts, enormous worm populations may build up to produce a frequently fatal disease. In internal autoinfection filariform larvae (L3) mature in the lumen of the small or large bowel, and penetrate the gut wall to reach the liver via the portal vein; after traversing the liver they reach the heart and so complete the cycle.

Because of its very close relationship with the soil, *Strongyloides stercoralis* is limited to warm humid climates whose soils support the cycle.

2. *Hookworm*. Two species of hookworm regular-

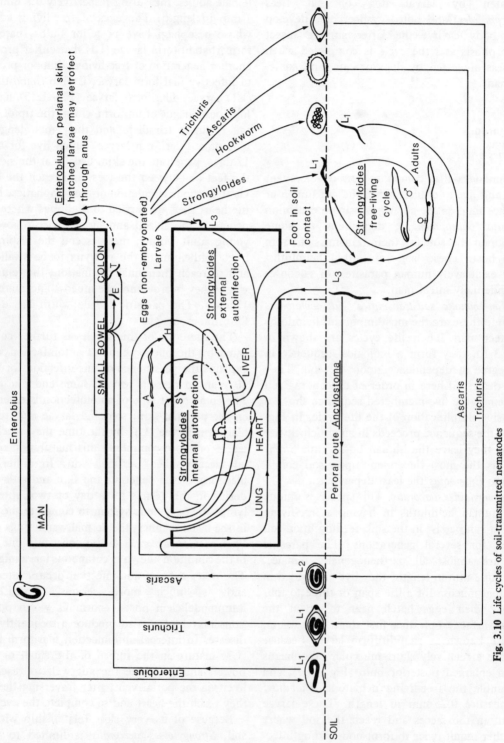

Fig. 3.10 Life cycles of soil-transmitted nematodes
Abbreviations: A — *Ascaris*; E — *Enterobius*; H — hookworm; L_1, L_2, L_3 — first, second and third stage larvae; S — *Strongyloides*; T — *Trichuris*

ly infect man, *Ancylostoma duodenale* and *Necator americanus*; they were originally referred to as the Old World and New World hookworms respectively, but their distributions are now so mixed that these terms are no longer appropriate. However, in general *Ancylostoma duodenale* is adapted to more temperate climates with seasonal transmission, and *Necator americanus* to more tropical climates with perennial transmission. *Necator americanus* was originally an African species, which was transported to the New World by the Atlantic slave trade. *Ancylostoma duodenale* is the larger species, the adult females being 10–13 mm in length and the males 8–11 mm. In *Necator americanus* the respective lengths are 9–11 mm and 5–9 mm. Both species are blood-feeding parasites and live attached by their buccal cavities to the jejunal and duodenal mucosa. The buccal cavity of *Ancylostoma duodenale* has two pairs of sharp ventrally placed teeth, while that of *Necator americanus* is armed with two ventral cutting plates. The males of both species have a prominent copulatory bursa posteriorly. *Ancylostoma duodenale* is a considerably thicker worm and ingests about 0.15 ml of blood daily, the female produces about 25 000 eggs daily. *Necator americanus* produces about one-third this number of eggs and its daily blood meal is about 0.05 ml. Most hookworm adults probably live for one to three years, but a few may survive for up to eight years. Eggs are passed in the faeces, usually at the four, eight or 16 cell morula stage, and hatch in the soil within 48 hours. The rhabditiform larvae (L1) feed on bacteria and in warm soil (26°C) moult twice on days three and five to form infective filariform larvae (L3) whose tails form a simple sharp point; depending upon the degree of soil abrasion the cuticle of L2 may or may not be retained around the filariform larvae, which are non-feeding and may live for up to five weeks. Skin penetration and migration is generally similar to that of *Strongyloides stercoralis*; the third moult may occur in the trachea, or in the jejunum where the last moult takes place. After attachment to the mucosa the worms mature and in the case of *Necator americanus* eggs first appear about six weeks after larvae penetrate the skin. In *Ancylostoma duodenale* there is commonly a period of arrested development, probably an adaptation to seasonal transmission in temperate climes, and most females start laying after a delay of six or eight months following skin penetration.

At least in the case of *Ancylostoma duodenale* there is good evidence that filariform larvae may infect man perorally, usually on contaminated vegetables. Larvae may penetrate the buccal cavity and reach the venous circulation to complete their development via the lungs; or they may be swallowed and complete their development in the jejunum without a tissue migration phase.

Hookworm larvae survive best, as do those of *Strongyloides stercoralis*, in shaded sandy soils where they live in the capillary film of water surrounding the soil particles. They are capable of considerable vertical migration in the soil but not much lateral dispersion, unless this is passive in surface rain water. Most transmission occurs at sites of promiscuous defaecation or in the vicinity of poorly maintained latrines. Filariform larvae lie in wait for their victims with their heads waving in the air and they frequently ascend surface vegetation in the capillary water film. Hookworm infections are usually heaviest in adult persons, especially males.

3. *Ascaris lumbricoides* — the 'roundworm'. The adults of this relatively huge worm live within the small bowel lumen, principally the ileum. Females measure between 20 and 40 cm in length and the males are about two-thirds this size; the worms taper gradually at both ends and maintain their position by 'bridging' across the gut lumen in a sinuous curve. They live for between six and 18 months and each female has the prodigious egg output of 200 000 each day; when passed in the faeces each egg contains an unsegmented ovum. In the soil further development cannot continue below 18°C. However eggs can survive for many years, for they are extremely resistant to adverse conditions. At 20°C maturation proceeds through the sequence embryo, first stage larva and second stage larva (L2) in 15 days; at 26°C this process is completed in 10 days. Eggs containing L2 larvae are infective and are often ingested by man on vegetables, especially when human faeces ('night soil') are used as fertiliser. Children frequently become infected when the sticky eggs contaminate their fingers during play; this process is facilitated by the promiscuous defaecation of children within

the peridomestic environment. Children between one and five years usually carry the heaviest *Ascaris* worm loads.

When swallowed infective eggs hatch in the duodenum and the larvae penetrate the gut wall. They enter the portal vein to traverse the liver and reach the lungs in about four days. Here they moult twice, penetrate the alveoli and ascend the respiratory epithelium to be swallowed. Upon re-entering the small bowel they mature into adult worms. Eggs first appear in the faeces eight to 10 weeks after infective eggs are ingested. The apparently purposeless tissue migration of this species derives from the fact that it has evolved from parasites having an intermediate host, in which larval development is arrested in the tissues. Here they remain dormant until this host is eaten by the definitive host in whose gut the cycle is completed. Some zoonotic worms with this type of life cycle can infect man (*Toxocara and Anisakis*, see p. 75); they, like *Ascaris lumbricoides*, belong to the order Ascaridida.

Eggs of *Ascaris* survive best in clay soils that retain moisture, and are killed by dessication. The distribution of this species is worldwide and it can be common in temperate climates when standards of hygiene are poor.

4. *Trichuris trichiura* — the whipworm. The adults of both sexes in this species measure between 30 and 50 mm in length; the anterior three-fifths of the worm is very narrow and thread-like and its posterior part becomes abruptly wider to give the worm a whip-like shape. The adults live in the colon, principally the caecum, but in heavy infections they extend down to the rectum. They live with their heads embedded in the mucosa to a depth of 1–2 mm, and have a lifespan of up to five or 10 years; female worms produce about 5000 eggs per day. The species is not a blood feeder but bleeding can occur at the sites of attachment. The eggs contain an unsegmented ovum when they are passed in the faeces. Development cannot proceed below 15°C but at this temperature it proceeds slowly within the egg to the infective first larval stage (L1) over four to six months; at 26°C eggs become infective within three weeks. The modes of infection are identical to those of *Ascaris*, children once again acquiring the heaviest worm loads; however the subsequent life cycle is much simpler. Eggs hatch in the small intestine and larvae (L1) temporarily enter the mucosa of the terminal ileum and caecum; after two months, these attach to the colonic mucosa and grow into adult worms. Eggs first appear in the faeces about 12 weeks after the ingestion of infective eggs.

The eggs of this species are much less tolerant to dessication, heat and putrefaction than those of *Ascaris*; for this reason and also the much slower development at lower temperatures this species is commonest in the wetter tropics. However the greater longevity of the adult worms means that the infection can persist in a human population through a series of years where soil conditions are arid; hence it may be found in near-desert environments where the occasional wet season allows transmission.

5. *Enterobius vermicularis* — the threadworm or pinworm. The adults of this species live within the lumen of the caecum loosely attached to the mucosa by their mouthparts. They are fusiform in shape and pointed at both ends. The males measure only 2–5 mm in length, but the females reach 8–13 mm and when mature are greatly distended with up to 10 000 eggs. The oesophagus has a prominent posterior bulb and the head bears three longitudinal cuticular expansions known as **cervical alae**. After copulation the males are passed in the faeces. When aged between two and seven weeks the gravid female makes her migration to the rectum and from here she emerges, at night, to lay her sticky eggs upon the perianal skin. After egg laying she frequently dies or is crushed by the scratching activities of the host; however quite often she re-enters the anal canal, or even enters the vagina. When laid the eggs are partly embryonated, and the maturation process to the infective egg containing the first stage larva (L1), proceeds rapidly over a period of four to seven hours at 35°C. Although female worms are commonly seen on the surface of a stool, having been passively expelled from the rectum, eggs are uncommon in the faeces for they are nearly all deposited by the females directly upon the perianal skin.

The modes of transfer of infective eggs to the mouth are various and include direct transfer on fingers, or transfer from fingers onto food, toys or doorhandles. Alternatively they may fall from bedclothes and undergarments onto the floor or soil and from thence be picked up by children; they may also be inhaled in dust from the floor or shaken bedding, and carried up the respiratory tract by ciliary movements, and then swallowed. Eggs can remain viable in cool moist conditions for up to two weeks. After ingestion eggs hatch in the ileum and gain access to the crypts in its terminal part where they undergo four moults and then enter the caecum and mature. It has also been shown that eggs may hatch on the perianal skin and the larvae migrate into the anus, a phenomenon known as **retrofection**.

Enterobius infections often persist for several months or years but this can only occur by repeated autoinfection because the worm has such a short lifespan. The complete life cycle can be completed in three weeks. The infection is much less common in the tropics; the reasons being that less clothing, particularly tight undergarments, are worn, fewer layers of bedding are used, and the eggs are more susceptible to dessication at higher temperatures.

This species represents the end of the sequence of soil-transmitted nematodes for it has a simple direct life cycle and has gained considerable independence from soil conditions.

B. Zoonotic soil-transmitted gut nematodes. The first three parasites to be considered here have eggs that closely resemble those of hookworm; they belong to the order Strongylida and their males have copulatory bursae. *Strongyloides fuelleborni* closely resembles *Strongyloides stercoralis*, while *Capillaria philippinensis* belongs to the same group as *Trichuris trichiura*.

Trichostrongylus. Many species of this genus infect domestic herbivores particularly sheep, donkeys, goats and camels; about nine species can infect man. Human infections are commonest in the Middle East, especially Iran, North Africa and the Far East. The adults measure 5–10 mm in length and although attached to the small bowel mucosa do not suck blood. Their pathogenicity is low. Infective larvae (L3) are ingested on vegetables, grass and contaminated fingers; development is direct and there is no tissue phase except when larvae occasionally penetrate the skin.

Ternidens deminutus. This is a parasite of monkeys and infects man quite commonly in Central and Southern Africa. Infective larva (L3) occur in the soil but the mode of transmission to man is uncertain. The worms develop within the mucosa of the proximal colon within which, at least in monkeys, they become encapsulated in small nodules; the worms measure up to 16 mm in length. In man the eggs of this species are frequently mistaken for those of hookworm. Apart from causing mild blood loss the pathogenicity of this species to man appears to be low.

Oesophagostomium. At least two species of this genus infect monkeys and apes in tropical Africa, Indonesia and the Philippines. Following the ingestion of larvae on contaminated vegetables third stage larvae invade the mucosa of the caecum and proximal colon setting up large granulomatous lesions; the latter may perforate the bowel wall or extend to the mesenteric lymph nodes. Mature worms leave the nodules and attach to the colonic mucosa causing some blood loss. Although uncommon in man, these parasites can cause serious morbidity in humans, similar to that produced in monkeys.

Strongyloides fuelleborni. This parasite infects man in tropical Africa where it is a common parasite of monkeys and baboons, and also in Papua New Guinea where no animal reservoir is yet known. Infection rates are sometimes high; in Papua New Guinea children are primarily infected. The life cycle is similar to that of *Strongyloides stercoralis* with the important difference that eggs, passed in the stool, are fully embryonated and contain a first stage larva. The morphology of the free-living adults and the parasitic females differs slightly from *Strongyloides stercoralis*. Transmammary transmission of larvae can occur in this species.

Capillaria philippinensis. Originally described from man in the Philippines in 1963 this parasite also occurs in Thailand and may be found elsewhere. Man acquires infection by eating certain fresh-water and marine fish that contain infective larvae (L1). The worms mature and live, like those of *Strongyloides*, deeply embedded within the jejunal mucosa. The adult worms of both sexes measure 2.5–4 mm in length; the females are sometimes larviparous and these give rise to internal autoinfection, or they may produce eggs, somewhat resembling those of *Trichuris*, that appear in the faeces 22–96 days after infected fish are eaten. The relevant fish species can be infected with eggs from human faeces but the normal definitive host is unknown, and may be a marine mammal.

Two aberrant zoonotic nematodes of the upper respiratory tract and renal pelvis.

Syngamus laryngeus. This is normally a parasite of cattle, water buffaloes and goats. The adults live in a state of permanent copulation, attached to the mucosa of the trachea, larynx and larger bronchi; the females measure 20 mm in length and the males 4 mm. They cause paroxysms of coughing and eggs are expelled onto the ground, embryonate and are then ingested on vegetation; they hatch in the intestine and larvae migrate to the lungs via the blood stream. Quite a number of infections have been reported in man, especially in the West Indies, and result presumably from eating contaminated salad vegetables; symptoms are similar to those in the normal hosts. Eggs may be found in the sputum; or sometimes the adult worms themselves.

Dioctophyma renale — Giant kidney worm. The life cycle of this species is still incompletely known but a number of human infections are reported from various parts of the world. The adults are reddish in colour and live in the renal parenchyma and renal pelvis; the females reach a length of 20–100 cm and a width of 5–12 mm. The eggs, which resemble those of *Trichuris* in having a bipolar plug, embryonate in water and the cycle probably involves fresh water annelids and then a fish. The natural definitive hosts are carnivores including the dog and the mink.

THE SCHISTOSOMES — PARALUMINAL HELMINTHS

Four species of *Schistosoma* or blood fluke reach maturity in man and three of them are serious pathogens. The adults live in pairs within the small venous radicles of the gut or urinary tract and their eggs pass through the wall of the viscus to be expelled from its lumen into the external world. These worms take up nutrients across their tegument. However they also ingest blood and the final degradation product, schistosomal pigment, is regurgitated from the mouth; this pigment may be deposited in the tissues. Chemically it is similar to malarial haemozoin being derived mainly from haemoglobin. By using a body lumen for egg dispersal without living within it, these flukes can be termed paraluminal parasites. Their general life cycle has already been briefly described and is illustrated in Figure 3.3. The eggs of the different species are shown in Figure 13.3.

After leaving the snail intermediate host the phototactic cercariae come to lie, swimming tail uppermost, beneath the water surface; here they remain viable for up to eight hours. If the skin of a host is penetrated the tails are lost and the larval schistosomulae reach the lungs within four to seven days via the lymphatics and venous system. Within two weeks they take up residence within the proximal portal vein, which is reached via the systemic circulation. After maturation and pairing the worms move peripherally down the portal vein. The mature worms are similar in size in all four species; the males being about 8–15 mm in length and 0.5–1 mm in width, and the females 10–25 mm in length and 0.15–0.3 mm in diameter. While the life span of these worms can exceptionally reach 20 years, it is likely that most die within two to four years. Eggs are deposited by the females in the walls of the small venules; they are fully embryonated and contain a miracidium with two pairs of active flame cells. Egg passage through the viscus wall occurs with the egg spine directed backwards; it is assisted by lytic enzymes secreted through pores in the egg shell, and takes two or three days causing little pathology. However about one third of all eggs never complete the passage and these set up local inflammatory reactions; in addition a number of eggs never enter the wall of the venule and these are carried passively in the venous blood flow to cause distant pathology.

Schistosoma mansoni. The adults of this species live in the mesenteric venous radicles of the colon. Female worms lay about 100–300 eggs daily, and these bear a prominent lateral spine posteriorly. The male worm is covered with coarse tuberculations and the female uterus contains only one or two eggs at any one time. Eggs first appear in the faeces 25–28 days after cercarial penetration. This species is widely distributed in Africa and also occurs in Malagasy, Brazil, Venezuela, Surinam and several Caribbean Islands, Saudi Arabia and the Yemen. Strains of parasite differ in pathogenicity and this species is of greatest public health importance in Egypt and Brazil. The intermediate hosts are flattened planorbid snails of the genus *Biomphalaria*. Baboons constitute occasional animal hosts but nearly all infections are from human sources.

Schistosoma japonicum. The venous radicles of both the ileum and the colon are occupied by the adult pairs of this species. Female worms lay up to 3500 eggs daily, these are ovoid in shape and bear only a small knob postero-laterally. The surface of the male worm is smooth and the female uterus may contain 100 or more eggs at any one time. As with the previous species eggs appear in the faeces 25–28 days after cercarial penetration. Probably because of its very high egg output this is the most pathogenic human schistosome. It is widely distributed in China, parts of the Philippines and Sulawesi; foci of infection occur in Southern Japan, Vietnam and the Mekong region. In Taiwan a strain occurs that is non-infective to man. The intermediate hosts are small amphibious conical snails of the genus *Oncomelania*, which bear an operculum. Control of this species of schistosome by chemotherapy alone is impossible for it exists as an extensive zoonosis in rodents, dogs, water buffaloes and pigs.

Schistosoma haematobium. Adult pairs of this species descend the inferior mesenteric veins and then cross through anastomoses to the venous plexuses surrounding the bladder and ureters and less commonly those of the seminal vesicles, prostate, urethra and fallopian tubes. Females lay about 20–300 eggs daily and these pass mainly into the urinary stream. Although the eggs take two or three days to reach the urine about 80 per cent of the eggs leaving the body are found in urine passed during a four hour period centered about noon; the reason for this is unknown. Eggs may be found in rectal biopsies, but these have usually died *in situ* and are not often passed live in the faeces. The eggs of this species bear a prominent posterior terminal spine, and first appear in the urine 54–84 days after cercarial penetration.

The surface of the male worm bears very fine tubercles and the female uterus contains 10–50 eggs at any one time. This species is widely distributed throughout Africa including Libya, Tunisia, Algeria and Morocco, and also in Malagasy, Saudi Arabia, Yemen, Iraq, Iran, Syria, Lebanon and Turkey. The intermediate hosts are turreted snails of the genus *Bulinus*; several species in this genus can aestivate when their aquatic habitat dries up and for this reason transmission of this schistosome species can occur in seasonal rain-fed pools. No animal reservoir for *S. haematobium* is known.

Schistosoma intercalatum. This is the rarest and least pathogenic schistosome that matures in man. Its known distribution is confined to Cameroun, Central African Republic, Gabon and Zaire, but foci may exist in Upper Volta and Chad. Several rodents have been found to be infected and these may be the normal hosts, although in most human foci transmission appears to be non-zoonotic. Adult worms live in the venous radicles of the colon and eggs appear 50–60 days after cercarial penetration. The eggs are terminal spined, like those of *S. haematobium*, but they are much more narrowed anteriorly and are passed exclusively in the faeces. The male flukes bear fine tubercles on their surface and the female uterus contains 5–60 eggs at any one time, the daily egg output being about 300. The intermediate hosts belong to the genus *Bulinus*.

TISSUE HELMINTHS WITH ARTHROPOD VECTORS OR INTERMEDIATE HOSTS

A. Filarial worms

Seven species of filarial worm complete their life cycle in man. Although the pathology produced by these worms differs greatly their basic biology is similar (Fig. 3.11). The adult worms are long and filiform, the females being much longer than the males; they live in human tissues for many years. Throughout their long reproductive life the viviparous females continuously release active elongate embryos, measuring between 180 and 300 μm in length and between 3 and 9 μm in diameter. These embryos are young stage one larvae and they are known as microfilariae; some

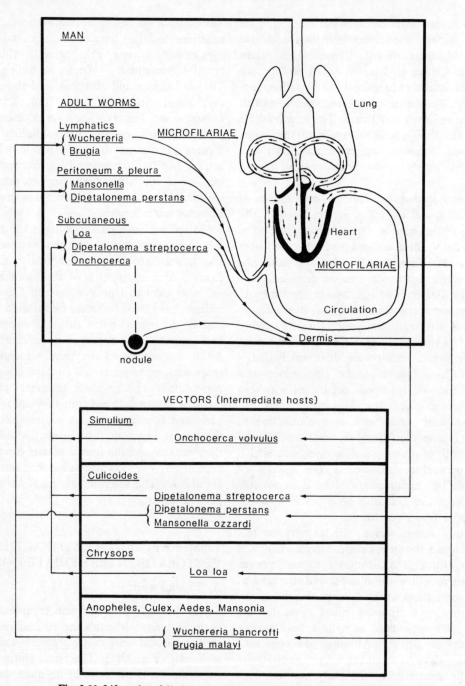

Fig. 3.11 Life cycles of filarial worms that complete their development in man

remain ensheathed by the greatly stretched egg shell (Fig. 13.1.A). The microfilariae themselves can live for several months and depending upon the species they either circulate in the bloodstream or live in the upper dermis. In either situation the cycle can only continue if they are picked up by the appropriate blood-feeding insect intermediate hosts which act as vectors. Several species with blood-dwelling microfilariae show **microfilarial periodicity** with regular changes in the counts during the 24 hour daily cycle. During their absence from the blood, periodic microfilariae are temporarily sequestered within the pulmonary capillaries. The fact that blood microfilaria counts are highest at the time when the specific vectors take their blood meals, suggests that the worms have adapted their life cycles by natural selection.

After being picked up by the vector the microfilariae penetrate the stomach wall and migrate to the thoracic muscles, except in the case of *Loa loa* which migrates to the fat body. During the process of further development the larvae initially shorten and thicken to form inactive sausage-shaped larvae which grow steadily in size. After the second moult they become extremely active filiform infective larvae (L3) measuring 500 μm or more in length, which migrate forwards in the haemocoel. When the vector next feeds some infective larvae escape from its mouth-parts and come to lie on the host's skin in a small pool of haemocoelic fluid; successful larvae then enter the puncture wound made by the vector. Larval development in the vector takes at least six days and often 14 or more; it is temperature dependent. The great majority of ingested microfilariae never enter a new definitive host; many never escape from the stomach, others die in the insect tissues or are unable to escape during a blood meal, while some deposited on the host's skin never enter the puncture wound. However the greatest source of loss is death of the short-lived vector before larval development is completed. In addition infective larvae are wasted when vectors feed upon the wrong host species.

Infective larvae entering the definitive hosts undergo two moults and mature into adult worms in the appropriate tissues where they mate; these stages of development take many months. Filarial infections in man are usually diagnosed by their clinical features and by finding microfilariae, whose morphology is characteristic (Fig. 13.1.B), in blood specimens or skin snips. The structure of the adult worms will not be described here in any detail.

Onchocerca volvulus. This species causes the disease onchocerciasis or river blindness. Its focal distribution is limited by that of the black fly vector species of the genus *Simulium*, which breed only in fast flowing, well oxygenated streams and rivers. Foci are found throughout tropical Africa from Senegal in the North to Angola in the South, the distribution extends northwards into the Sudan and there is a focus in Yemen. In the Western hemisphere foci exist in Mexico, Guatemala, Colombia, Venezuela and Brazil. The worms mature very slowly in man and the unsheathed microfilariae, which themselves may live for up to two years, do not appear in the upper dermis until 18 months after infection. The adult worms, which may live for up to 18 years, live in the subcutaneous tissue and fascial planes, the majority being located in fibrous subcutaneous **nodules**, measuring up to 3 cm or even more in diameter, that may contain a dozen or more tangled worms of both sexes. When disentangled the females measure up to 50 cm in length and their cuticle shows regular annular thickenings. Microfilariae migrate extensively in the dermis and frequently enter the eye causing great damage. Within the *Simulium* vector development is completed in six to 12 days depending upon ambient temperature; there is no development below 18°C.

Dipetalonema streptocerca. The distribution of this species is limited to the rain forests of Ghana, Nigeria, Cameroun and Zaire. Adult worms live in subcutaneous tissue but are very rarely found and complete specimens are unknown in man. The principal medical importance of this relatively non-pathogenic species is that its unsheathed microfilaria live in the dermis and can easily be confused with those of *O. volvulus*; however their tail shows a prominent hook. Larval development in the midge *Culicoides* takes eight days. Gorillas and chimpanzees are also infected by this parasite.

Dipetalonema perstans. This species has an extensive distribution throughout tropical Africa with the exception of coastal East Africa; in the Western hemisphere it extends throughout the eastern parts of South America from Venezuela in the north to Argentina in the south. Adult worms live principally in the retroperitoneal tissues and mesentery; female worms reach a length of 8 cm. The unsheathed microfilariae occur in the blood and are non-periodic. Larval development in *Culicoides* takes about eight days; the vector midges are closely associated with banana plantations where they breed.

Mansonella ozzardi. A Western hemisphere

species found in Mexico, Panama, the Southern Caribbean islands, northern Argentina and extensive areas of northern and central South America, especially Brazil. Adult worms live retroperitoneally and females reach 8 cm in length. The unsheathed blood microfilariae are non-periodic. While *Culicoides* midges are the principal vectors, in Brazil species of *Simulium* are involved.

Loa loa. The distribution of this species is limited to the rain forests of West and Central Africa from Sierre Leone to Western Uganda; southwards it extends into Angola. The adult worms wander continuously through the subcutaneous tissues and may become visible beneath the dermis or more dramatically when they cross beneath the bulbar conjunctiva. Female worms reach 7 cm in length and the cuticle is covered with minute bosses. The worms mature in about six months and can live for 15 years. The sheathed microfilariae occur in the blood and show a prominent diurnal periodicity. The vectors are large day-biting mango flies (*Chrysops*); larval development takes place in the fat body and is completed in 10–12 days. A related strain of this parasite occurs in monkeys, its periodicity is nocturnal and its vector species of *Chrysops* are night biters.

Wuchereria bancrofti. This is by far the most widely distributed filarial worm in man. It occurs throughout Africa between latitude 20°N and 20°S and also in Egypt and Malagasy, extensively in the Indian subcontinent, Southeast Asia and the Western Pacific, in China, Korea and South Japan, on several islands in the Caribbean, and in much of northern and north-eastern South America. In Polynesia and New Caledonia there is a distinct strain, var. *pacifica*, whose epidemiology is different. Worms mature in the lymph nodes; mainly those of the groin, axillae and epitrochlear regions where they live in the afferent lymph vessels entering the node; maturation is completed in about six months and females may reach a length of 10 cm. Some worms mature in other sites especially the lymphatics of the spermatic cords and epididymis. The average life span is perhaps three or four years but a few will survive for up to 12 years. The sheathed microfilariae live in the blood stream where they are usually nocturnally periodic; however var. *pacifica* is diurnally **subperiodic**, that is the microfilariae are continuously

present with higher counts during the day. Larval development in the vector takes 11 to 14 days. Throughout most of Asia, much of South America and on the East African coast the principal vector, especially in urban areas, is the mosquito *Culex fatigans*; elsewhere and especially throughout most of tropical Africa species of *Anopheles* are vectors. Day biting species of *Aedes* transmit var. *pacifica* No animal reservoirs are known.

Brugia malayi. The life cycle and development of this species is similar to that of *W. bancrofti*. The sheathed microfilariae live in the blood. The species is distributed widely in Southeast Asia, especially in Malaysia, Indonesia and Borneo, but it also occurs in southern and eastern India, China and Korea. Two forms exist, the commonest having nocturnally periodic microfilariae and no animal reservoir, and the other being nocturnally subperiodic and occurring as a zoonosis in monkeys, dogs and cats. The periodic form is transmitted mainly by night-biting mosquitoes of the genus *Mansonia* which breed in rice paddies and open swamps. The subperiodic form occurs locally in Western Malaysia, Borneo, Indonesia, the Southern Philippines and the Palawan islands, Vietnam and Thailand; its vectors are *Mansonia* species that breed in forest swamps and feed by day and by night.

B. The Guinea worm (Dracunculus medinensis)

This tissue parasite has a life cycle unlike that of any other human helminth (Fig. 3.12). There is no significant animal reservoir, although dogs are infected in southern Russia where human infections no longer occur. The parasite is widely distributed in foci throughout Tropical Africa, especially its western parts, in many parts of the Middle East, in Iran and Pakistan and extensively throughout India. It formerly occurred in Brazil, having been transported there by African slaves, but it is now extinct in the Western hemisphere.

Man becomes infected by drinking water containing the microcrustacean *Cyclops*, in whose haemocoel the infective larval worm (L3) has matured. Larvae escape in the duodenum to cross its wall, and traverse the mesenteries and the body walls of the abdomen and thorax to reach the subcutaneous tissues after about 100 days; it is here

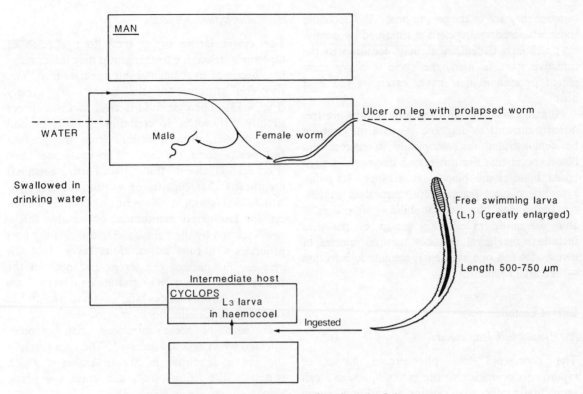

Fig. 3.12 Life cycle of *Dracunculus medinensis* — the Guinea worm

that mating occurs. The fertilised females slowly migrate within connective tissues and fascial planes, and most finally reach the dermis of the lower limbs, mainly below the knee. Male worms die in the tissues and sometimes become calcified, as do females unable to complete their migrations. Mature female worms reach a length of 50–100 cm and have a diameter of 1–2 mm. A blister forms when the female reaches the upper dermis and when this ruptures the free anterior end of the worm lies in a shallow ulcer. The body of the worm is filled by the anterior and posterior branches of the enormous uterus containing up to three million embryos. The vulva lies in the middle of the body but the larvae are expelled from the anterior end of the uterus when this ruptures through the body wall or mouth of the worm. When a guinea worm ulcer is immersed in water the worm contracts expelling the larvae in a white milky stream. The larvae measure 500–750 µm in length and have a narrow pointed tail and a striated cuticle. They swim actively and can live in fresh water for up to seven days; here they are swal-

lowed by the carnivorous *Cyclops* whose gut they perforate. Development in the intermediate host involves two moults and is completed in about two weeks.

The whole cycle takes nearly one year and this is a perfect adaptation to a short transmission season. In consequence infected persons are affected more or less simultaneously each year, as the female worms reach the skin surface. The invalidism, which can last several weeks, has important economic effects when many people are affected in an agricultural society.

TISSUE HELMINTHS WITH NO DISPERSAL IN MAN

Included under this heading are a number of parasites that accidentally infect man. They are all zoonoses. While some are rare or of only local interest, others are important human pathogens. They fall into two groups, firstly those that are unable to complete their development in man because they are in the wrong host. And secondly those whose normal cycle is maintained by carnivory; although development may continue to the infective stage in man, the cycle is never completed because man is never eaten by the next host.

Human infections with these helminths are frequently difficult to diagnose because they cannot be demonstrated microscopically in excreta and blood specimens. For this reason diagnosis is often based upon tissue biopsy or serology. In many cases the clinical features are themselves suggestive and a high blood eosinophilia is often a valuable diagnostic clue. This group of parasites include some larval cestodes, several species of nematodes and one accidental trematode infection — cercarial dermatitis.

Larval cestodes

A. Pseudophyllidean species

The procercoid and plerocercoid larvae of tapeworms belonging to the genus *Spirometra* can accidentally infect man causing a condition known as **sparganosis**. Although uncommon it has been described from most parts of the world. Pathology is caused by wandering plerocercoid larvae that are using man as a paratenic host; they appear as ivory-white unsegmented ribbons reaching several centimeters in length. Most larvae are found in subcutaneous tissues but occasionally other organs are affected; exceptionally the larva proliferates by forming lateral branches producing a tumour-like mass known as **sparganum proliferum**. The definitive hosts of *Spirometra* are dogs, cats and other carnivores. The first intermediate host is *Cyclops* but the second and paratenic hosts include amphibia, reptiles such as snakes, birds, rodents and other mammals; fish are not involved in the cycle. Man may become infected in three ways:

1. Drinking water containing *Cyclops* infected with procercoid larvae.

2. By applying the flesh of frogs containing plerocercoid larvae to ulcers and infected eyes; this is quite a common medicinal custom in some Far Eastern countries.

3. Eating the uncooked meat of mammals, snakes or birds, that contains plerocercoid larvae.

B. Cyclophyllidean species

The cystic larvae of at least four species of tapeworm belonging to this group may infect man, who becomes an accidental intermediate host. The size and structure of the larvae vary greatly (Fig. 3.13). The cyst fluid is clear and sometimes slightly yellowish, it contains electrolytes and some protein derived mainly from the parasite but partly from the host. The cysts are lined (Fig. 3.13.D) by a thin (10–25 µm) **germinal membrane** that consists of a multinucleate syncitium. Surrounding the germinal layer is a noncellular **laminated membrane**, of variable thickness secreted by the parasite. Around this the host produces a **fibrous adventitious layer**. Into the cyst are invaginated the scolex and neck of the future adult worm; the structures so formed are known as **protoscolices** and in them the future suckers and rostellar hooks may be seen.

In each of these infections man becomes infected when eggs are ingested. The eggs hatch in the gut and release hexacanth embryos which penetrate the jejunal wall, and enter the portal vein.

1. *Taenia solium* — Cysticercosis. Although man is the normal definitive host for this species he can accidently become an intermediate host when infective eggs are swallowed, or rarely when proglottids disintegrate in the small bowel and are regurgitated into the stomach. In man, the **cysticerci** (Fig. 3.13.A), which reach 1 cm in length, localise particularly in striated muscle, tongue, heart, subcutaneous tissue, brain and eyes. They remain alive for several years, but when they die calcification occurs, initially in the scolex and later in the cyst wall.

2. *Multiceps* spp. — Coenurus infection. *M. multiceps* is a widespread natural parasite of the dog in which the adult worms reach a length of 50 cm. Sheep and other ruminants are the normal intermediate hosts. The larval cyst (Fig. 3.13.B), known as a **coenurus**, may grow to a diameter of 3 cm and bear up to 100 small invaginated protoscolices on its inner surface; the cysts only mature in the brain and spinal cord. The posterior fossa of the skull is the classic location and in sheep cerebellar damage causes ataxia, giving the disease its name 'staggers'. In Africa other species of *Mul-*

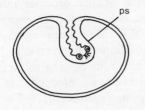

A. CYSTICERCUS Taenia solium

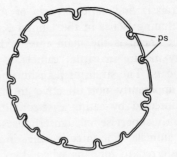

B. COENURUS Multiceps spp

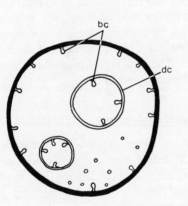

C. HYDATID Echinococcus granulosus

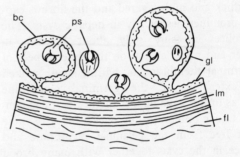

D. Section of wall of hydatid cyst
(highly magnified)

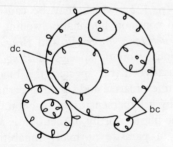

E. ALVEOLAR HYDATID
Echinococcus multilocularis

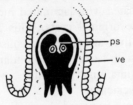

F. CYSTICERCOID (cross section of villus)
Hymenolepis nana (highly magnified)

Fig. 3.13 Larval Cyclophyllidean cestodes in man (not drawn to scale)
Abbreviations: bc — brood capsule; dc — daughter cyst; fl — fibrous adventitious layer; gl — germinal layer; lm — laminated membrane; ps — protoscolex; ve — villous epithelium (destroyed distally)

ticeps can produce subcutaneous or orbital cysts in man. Coenurus cysts in man, an abnormal host, sometimes show no protoscolices making histological diagnosis difficult.

3. *Echinococcus granulosus* — Hydatid disease. The definitive hosts of this species are the dog and other carnivores; the adult worms measure 3–8 mm in length and have only three to five proglottids. This parasite has a worldwide distribution, and occurs wherever sheep husbandry is practised. Human infection occurs especially in North and East Africa, the Middle East, South

America, Australasia and various parts of Asia, and Europe including Wales in the United Kingdom. While the sheep is the main intermediate host, cysts may mature in cattle, camels, water buffaloes and goats. The strain of parasite infecting horses is apparently not infective to man. Dogs become infected by eating cyst-containing raw offal in poorly supervised slaughterhouses, or by eating dead animals. The infective eggs in dog faeces are transferred to humans when dogs are fondled, and live in close relationship with man.

Human hydatid cysts (Fig. 3.13. C and D) grow slowly over a five or 10 year period; most occur in the liver or lungs but almost any organ can be affected. The size of mature cysts ranges from 2 to 30 cm in diameter. The laminated membrane is 1 mm thick and multilayered and the fibrous capsule is prominent especially in hepatic cysts. The protoscolices measure only about 0.1 mm in diameter and may develop on the inner aspect of the germinal membrane or within small stalked cystic extensions of the germinal membrane known as **brood capsules**. A mature cyst can contain up to one million protoscolices; many of these become free from the germinal membrane and float free in the cysts together with many brood capsules, to form the 'hydatid sand'. If a cyst ruptures into the tissues or circulation the spilled protoscolices may form **secondary cysts**. Sometimes **daughter cysts**, coated with laminated membrane develop within the original cysts. This happens particularly in the liver and may be a consequence of partial rupture with leakage or secondary infection; hydatids containing daughter cysts are described as **multivesicular.**

When hydatids are removed surgically a plane of cleavage can be obtained between the laminated membrane and the fibrous adventitious layer.

4. *Echinococcus multilocularis* — Alveolar hydatid. This is a much less common infection in man than the ordinary hydatid but the disease it produces can be very serious. The parasite occurs in Central and Eastern Europe, across Russia and Siberia and in Alaska and Canada. It is normally maintained as a feral zoonosis in foxes, the definitive hosts, and various field rodents and insectivores, particularly voles, lemmings and shrews; much less commonly a domestic cycle between dogs, cats and house mice becomes established. Man usually becomes infected by eating vegetables, salads, or fruit picked up from the ground, that have been contaminated by fox faeces; in addition hunters may become infected when skinning fur-bearing wild canids.

In man nearly all infections are in the liver and the cysts are **multilocular**. The parasite (Fig. 3.13E) grows like a malignant tumour, as a proliferating mass of vesicles, within a fibrous stroma. The laminated membrane is extremely thin and the germinal epithelium is hyperplastic budding externally as well as internally to form daughter cysts on both its outer and inner aspects. In man the cysts are often sterile and form no protoscolices. The local tissue responses include necrosis, inflammation and fibrosis.

Nematode infections

The more common zoonotic nematodes that accidentally infect man are shown in Tables 3.1 and 3.2, which give their distribution, modes of infection and the cycles of development in man and their normal hosts.

Another condition which might have been added to this list is 'tropical pulmonary eosinophilia' (p. 122), which may be caused either by the two common lymphatic-dwelling human filarids, *Wuchereria brancrofti* and *Brugia malayi*, or by various zoonotic species of *Brugia*. Whatever the causative filarid species, the blood is always free of microfilariae and the lung pathology is produced by a hypersensitivity reaction. One further zoonotic filarid worthy of mention is *Meningonema peruzzi*, a parasite normally inhabiting the leptomeninges of African monkeys (*Cercopithecus*); its microfilariae closely resemble those of *Dipetalonema perstans*. Patients with neurological symptoms have recently been described from Zimbabwe in whom this microfilaria was found in cerebrospinal fluid. The clinical importance of this finding remains uncertain. However it is ironically of historical interest because Patrick Manson believed at one time that *D. perstans* was the cause of African sleeping sickness, because microfilariae had been found in the cerebrospinal fluid of some patients.

Two nematodes mentioned in the tables merit further description because of their cosmopolitan

Table 3.1 Zoonotic tissue nematodes (orders *Strongylida* and *Ascaridida*) with no dispersal in man

Parasite	Distribution	Cycle in normal host	Mode of human infection	Cycle in man, final destination (italics)
Angiostrongylus cantonensis	Pacific, S.E. Asia	Rat { Lung (Ad) → faeces (L₁) → snail (L₃) eaten; Meninges (L₄) ← eaten ← crustacea, planarians (L₃) (paratenic hosts)	Ingested L₃ in snails and paratenic hosts, or on contaminated salad	Gut → muscle; *Meninges* ⇌ *peripheral nerve*
Morerastrongylus costaricensis	Central America	Cotton rat (Ad in mesenteric arteries) → egg in faeces → slug (L₃); eaten	Ingested L₃ in slugs, or on contaminated salad	Gut → peritoneum; *Radicles of mesenteric arteries*
Ancylostoma braziliense	Warm temperate and tropical countries	Dog { Gut (Ad) → egg in faeces → soil; L₃ → L₁; Skin (L₃) ← penetration	Skin contact with L₃ in sand and soil	Migration in *dermis*
Toxocara canis	Cosmopolitan	Dog { Gut (Ad) → egg in faeces; Tissues L₂; transplacental, transmammary → Puppy gut (Ad) → egg in faeces; soil	Ingested eggs (L₂) from soil, contaminated fingers	Gut → *tissues* (L₂) (especially liver and lung)
Anisakis spp.	Japan, W. Europe etc	Marine mammal eg porpoise, gut (Ad) → egg in faeces → plankton; eaten ← Herring, mackerel squid, etc (L₃); eaten	Ingested larvae (L₃) in herrings etc	Gut → *wall of stomach and small bowel*

Abbreviations: Ad — adult worm; L₁, L₂, L₃, L₄ — larval stages

Table 3.2 Zoonotic tissue nematodes (order *Spirurida* and superfamily *Trichuroidea*) with no dispersal in man

Parasite	Distribution	Cycle in normal host	Mode of human infection	Cycle in man, final destination (italics)
Gnathostoma spingerum	S.E. Asia Far East	Fish eating mammals, dog, cat. Stomach wall (AD) → egg in faeces; L₁ eaten — Cyclops (L₂); Fish and fish eating paratenic hosts (L₃) ← eaten	Ingested larvae in fish and paratenic hosts (L₃)	Gut → tissues (L₃) especially *dermis, viscera and brain*
Dirofilaria immitis	Warm climates	Dog: Blood (L₁ = microfilariae), Pulmonary artery (Ad) — bite → Mosquito (L₁ → L₃) — bite	Mosquito bite, L₃ on skin	Dermis → heart, *pulmonary artery*
Dirofilaria tenuis and *D. repens*	Warm climates	Dog: Dermis and blood (L₁ = microfilariae), Skin and conjunctiva (Ad) — bite → Mosquito L₁ → L₃ — bite	Mosquito bite, L₃ on skin	Partial maturation in *dermis and conjunctiva*
Trichinella spiralis	Cosmopolitan	Mammal {Muscle (L₁), Gut (Ad)} — eaten → Gut (Ad) — eaten → Muscle (L₁) } Mammal	Ingested larvae (L₁) in meat	Gut mucosa → blood → *muscle*
Capillaria hepatica	Warm climates	Rat (larvae, adults and eggs in liver tissue) — eaten by carnivore (eggs in faeces) — Eggs in soil; death of host → Eggs in soil — ingested	Ingested eggs in soil, or in rodent liver	Gut → *liver parenchyma*

Abbreviations: Ad — adult worm; L₁, L₂, L₃, L₄ — larval stages

distribution and clinical importance.

Trichinella spiralis — Trichinosis. While primarily a pig parasite this species can complete its life cycle in many species, including man. Transmission is based upon carnivory and the cycle of development is the same in all hosts.

The infective stage is a coiled L1 larva, enclosed in an ovoid fibrous capsule, measuring 400 by 250 μm, lying longitudinally between muscle fibres. When ingested by the next host the larva is released in the jejunum and burrows into the mucosa where it rapidly develops through a series of moults into an adult worm. The female worms reach a length of 2.5–3.5 mm and the males 1.1 mm; after mating in the gut lumen the females re-enter the mucosa and start releasing larvae by the fifth day after infection. The viviparous females have a single ovary and uterus which extends forwards to the vulva situated one-fifth of the distance down the length of the worm. Female worms live for up to five weeks and during this time release a total of between 1000 and 2000 larvae; these enter the lacteals of the villi and from thence are carried via the thoracic duct to the circulation. Deposition in muscles begins six to nine days after infection, and the new larvae become infective three weeks later; they remain viable for many years and although the fibrous capsule becomes calcified in about two years, the larva within lives on. In man the larval counts are highest in the following muscles: diaphragm, intercostals, pectoral girdle, cervical, masseters and extra-ocular. Diagnostic muscle biopsies are usually taken from the deltoid. Larvae reaching other organs such as the brain, myocardium and eye do not develop but as they die *in situ*, severe inflammatory reactions are set up.

Trichinosis is still widespread in North America, Europe and Russia but is becoming less common because of control measures. It remains an important infection in the Arctic, in Central and South America, in tropical Africa, and in the Far East and the Pacific. In temperate countries a domestic cycle is maintained in pigs and to a lesser extent in rats, uncooked pig feed ('swill') containing garbage with scraps of pork being the main vehicle of transmission. Rats also eat the swill, and being cannibals can infect one another; pigs can be infected when rats are eaten by them. Man becomes infected by eating undercooked pork, hamburgers or sausages. A temperate feral cycle is maintained in wild boar, rodents, and various carnivores. In the Arctic, the cycle is maintained by walruses, seals, polar bears, foxes, wolves and husky dogs; the infection is particularly important among Eskimos who eat several of these hosts. In Africa man becomes infected by eating warthogs and bushpigs; the carnivore hosts being leopards, lions, hyaenas and jackals.

Toxocara canis — Toxocariasis. This parasite is the common roundworm of the dog; the adult worms reach a length of 15 cm and much resemble *Ascaris* worms in man, to which they are related. The infection particularly affects puppies, since older animals become partially immune so that when eggs are ingested the larvae (L2) become arrested in the tissues in a dormant state. In pregnant bitches the larvae become active again and are transmitted transplacentally or by the transmammary route to the puppies. Young or non-immune dogs develop patent infections by ingesting eggs, in which case the cycle of development resembles that of *Ascaris* in man.

Man, especially children, becomes infected by ingesting the resistant, sticky embryonated eggs from soil contaminated by dog faeces. In the human, development proceeds no further than the second stage larvae, which migrate through many organs of the body for many months (**visceral larva migrans**) causing damage to the liver and lungs, and more importantly to the retina and brain. Being thinner than *Ascaris* larvae, it is possible that *Toxocara* larvae are not filtered out by the lungs, as are the larvae of the human parasite.

Two similar parasites, *Toxocara cati* in cats and *Toxascaris leonina* in dogs, may also, less commonly, cause pathology in man. These species employ mice, earthworms and cockroaches as intermediate hosts, a type of life cycle which is apparently unimportant in *T. canis*.

Trematode infections

Cercarial dermatitis

The schistosome flukes of many mammals and birds can accidentally infect man when their cercariae penetrate human skin. The schistosomulae only survive for a few days in the human dermis but they set up a pruritic skin eruption known as 'swimmers itch' or cercarial dermatitis. The condition usually follows fresh water bathing but some seabird parasites can cause the condition during marine bathing. The distribution of these parasites is worldwide and outbreaks have occurred in Britain. The principal avian parasites belong to the genera *Trichobilharzia* and *Ornithobilharzia*. In South East Asia this condition can be disabling among workers in rice paddy fields, where the offending species is usually *Schistosoma spindale*, a parasite of water buffaloes.

Cercariae enter the skin, as do those of the human species, as the surface film of water dries. A prickling sensation is followed by pruritic papules and local urticarial lesions which may last several days.

FURTHER READING

Beaver, P.C. (1969) The nature of visceral larva migrans. *J. Parasitol.*, 55, 3–12.

Crofton, H.D. (1966) *Nematodes*. London: Hutchinson.

Heyneman, D. (1966) The life cycles of the nematodes parasitic in man: an evolutionary sequence. *Med. J. Malaya*, 20, 249–263.

Jordan, P. and Webbe, G. (1969) *Human Schistosomiasis*. London: Heinemann Medical Books Ltd.

Kean, B.H., Mott, K.E. and Russell, A.J. (1978) *Tropical Medicine and Parasitology, classic investigations*, Vol 2. London: Cornell University Press.

Muller, R. (1975) *Worms and Disease. A Manual of Medical Helminthology*. London: William Heinemann Medical Books Ltd.

Sasa, M. (1976) *Human Filariasis*. Baltimore: University Park Press.

World Health Organization (1964) Soil-transmitted helminths. *Tech. Rep. Series* no. 277. Geneva: WHO.

Wright, C.A. (1971) *Flukes and Snails*. London: Allen and Unwin.

4

Other Metazoan Parasites

The metazoan parasites included here are more advanced biologically than the helminths. Most of them belong to biological groups that contain many free-living members. Because of their zoological diversity they form a rather miscellaneous assemblage of organisms; no attempt will be made to describe their structure in detail. Included here are several orders of insects, the mites and ticks belonging to the order Acarina which is one of the seven orders of the class Arachnida, the pentastomes which are an aberrant group of parasitic crustaceans, and lastly the worm-like leeches belonging to the phylum Annelida. Ecologically the relationship of these organisms to man takes several forms.

BLOOD-FEEDING ECTOPARASITES

The medical importance of this group relates to the pain and local allergic reactions that their bites cause, the secondary bacterial infections of the damaged skin, and their ability to act as vectors of disease. In addition their nuisance potential is considerable, while the presence of some species carries an undeserved social stigma. They can be grouped according to their intimacy with man, giving a spectrum ranging from the almost free-living mosquito to the head louse which resides permanently upon its host. The justification for regarding the mosquito as a parasite rather than a 'micropredator' is firstly that it is ecologically and behaviourally dependent upon its favoured hosts and secondly that its repeated assaults upon the host evoke specific immunological responses that cause tissue damage mediated by hypersensitivity.

1. Winged insects

a. Diptera (two-winged flies)

With one exception only the adult flies are blood feeders. In most species the female requires a blood meal before the next batch of eggs will develop fully in the ovaries. The males are usually free-living, the exceptions being male tsetse flies and male stable flies which do take blood meals. Most bites will be caused by the following groups:

Mosquitoes (Culicidae). At least in warmer climates these 'blood-feeding gnats' will usually be the most numerous assailants. The slender proboscis of the female can be inserted directly into a blood capillary; all other human blood-feeding ectoparasites, except triatomine bugs, are 'pool feeders' and ingest blood from the small accumulations of extravasated blood within the damaged dermis, or even from blebs of blood on the skin surface at the puncture site. Many mosquito species feed nocturnally and others are crepuscular, feeding at dusk and dawn. The larvae are always aquatic, obtaining oxygen by means of a breathing siphon whose tip attaches to the surface meniscus; in one group, *Mansonia*, the siphon is thrust into the air cells of water plants. Breeding occurs in all sorts of aquatic habitats ranging from lakes and rivers, marshes, temporary rain pools, rockpools, tree and crab holes, to the water within the leaf axils of tropical plantains and bromeliads.

Midges (Culicoides). Minute delicate flies that bite viciously at dusk when the wind dies down. The worm-like larvae are aquatic, being equipped with caudal gills; they live in a variety of wet habitats including moist leaf litter. Midges are common in temperate climates.

Black flies or buffalo gnats (Simulium). Small black humpbacked flies with clear unspotted wings; they feed diurnally, sometimes in large swarms. The larvae live totally submerged in well-oxygenated running water attached to the substratum or vegetation by a disc at the posterior end of the body; the mature larvae spin a silken coccoon and the pupa bears prominent external breathing tubes.

Sandflies (Phlebotomus etc.). Small delicate grey or brownish insects with hairy bodies and wings, and prominent black eyes. Restricted to warm climates. They are weak fliers and normally proceed in a series of long 'hops'; the flight range is often less than 100 metres. They feed nocturnally and at dusk, and rest during the day in moist dark microclimates. The larvae bear bristles on each segment, the caudal ones being very long; they are not aquatic and live in mud and rock crevices, tree holes and cracks in old masonry. The larvae feed upon decaying organic matter including the faeces of rodents, lizards and bats.

Horse flies, mango flies etc. (Tabanidae). Relatively large aggressive diurnal feeders giving a painful bite. The cylindrical carnivorous larvae live in mud and sand beneath or in close proximity to water; eggs are often laid on vegetation above the water surface and after hatching these larvae drop into the water and reach the substratum below.

Stable fly (Stomoxys calcitrans). This muscid fly is a close relative of the house fly, and is almost the only blood feeder in the group. Larvae breed in decaying organic matter, especially horse manure and decaying seaweed on the shoreline.

Tsetse fly (Glossina). Restricted to tropical Africa. Aggressive diurnal feeders that may live for up to six months. Reproduction is remarkable because there is no free-living larval stage. The larva is nourished and grows to maturity within the uterus of the female; it is then deposited singly in shaded soil into which it burrows and pupates to form a black ovoid structure with two spiracular lobes at one end; the adult emerges one month later.

b. Triatomine bugs (Reduviidae, Hemiptera)

The medically important reduviids are restricted to South and Central America. These large insects feed upon their victims at night; during the day they rest in cracks of daub and wattle walls and thatched roofs of simply constructed houses. Flight is used for dispersal but not to approach the sleeping host. These insects are hemimetabolous and the larvae and nymphs resemble the winged adults; all stages are blood feeders. Bites are usually painless and occur often on the face and near the lips, the latter site earning them the title 'kissing bugs'.

2. Wingless ectoparasites

a. Leeches (Hirudinea)

These dorsoventrally flattened annelids have a ventral sucker at each end of the body. In the blood-feeding species the buccal cavity is connected to the oral sucker which is armed with a pair of eversible 'jaws' covered with minute teeth that lacerate the host's skin. Feeding can take half an hour or more and is often painless, bleeding may continue because of locally injected anticoagulant. Land leeches (*Haemadipsa*) live in the humid tropics, especially the rainforests of Southeast Asia, where they await their victims on the ground or low vegetation. Vibrations cause them to 'stand' erect upon their posterior sucker ready for attachment, man is usually bitten on the lower legs and feet. Aquatic leeches swim towards their victim in response to water disturbance; the genera that freqently attack man are the medicinal leech (*Hirudo*), the buffalo leech (*Poicilobdella*) and the nasal leeches (*Dinobdella* and *Limnatis*). Aquatic leeches may attach to or enter any part of the external human anatomy including the urethra, vagina, anus and eye. Of greatest medical importance is entry into the nose or mouth, this can occur during swimming or bathing, or small leeches may be ingested inadvertently in drinking water. Attachment to the nasal and buccal mucosa, pharynx or larynx may cause serious bleeding or obstructive symptoms (p. 151).

b. Congo floor maggot (Auchmeromyia)

Larvae of this dipteran fly (*A. luteola*) live under bedding, and in the soil and sand on the floor of native huts in tropical Africa. At night they attack their human victims sleeping on the floor, the larvae feeding upon blood exuding from wounds made by their oral hooklets. The adult insects are free-living and resemble a large house fly.

c. Bedbugs (Cimex)

The nymphal stages and adults live in crevices and cracks in the walls and furniture of human habitations. These insects are blood feeders throughout their life cycle; they approach their sleeping victims at night, usually just before dawn. The bugs are very rarely found in beds but their plentiful brown or black faecal marks on sheets and walls betray their presence. Bedbug species whose natural hosts are pigeons, martins or bats, may also attack man.

d. Fleas (Siphonaptera)

Most adult fleas are laterally compressed leaping creatures that live in the fur or feathers of their mammalian or avian hosts. The legless maggot-like larvae live in the burrows and nests of their natural hosts, feeding upon the organic debris their hosts provide and also the blood passed per anum by the feeding adult fleas. The now rare human flea (Pulex irritans) lives in the bedrooms of dirty damp houses; adults and larvae live in unwashed blankets and bedding; this species is also found in pigstyes. More commonly man is attacked by fleas from domestic cats and dogs (Ctenocephalides), or poultry and pigeons (Ceratophyllus). Rodent fleas (Xenopsylla, Nosopsyllus), the notorious vectors of plague, only bite man when their natural hosts are not available.

e. Mites and ticks (Acarina)

The life cycle of all acarines passes through the stages of egg, larva, one or several nymphal instars and adult. The body is divided into a capitulum bearing the mouthparts, and a fused thorax and abdomen; the larvae have three pairs of legs and the nymphs and adults four pairs. Ticks are larger than mites and their feeding siphon, the **hypostome**, is armed with many small teeth; in the mites this structure is a simple tube.

Mites. The ectoparasitic species are yellow, orange or red in colour. The most important group are the harvest mites or chiggers (*Trombicula, Leptotrombidium* etc.) with representatives all over the world. The larvae are initially vegetarian but a blood meal is required for them to mature further; they climb to the tips of vegetation and attach to passing mammals. On man they usually crawl up the leg to the groin where feeding commences; their saliva digests the skin to form a hardened tube, the **stylostome**, through which the mites ingest lymph. When replete the larvae drop to the ground and for the rest of the life cycle, through the nymphal and adult stages, these mites are free-living carnivores. Sensitivity to these mites is sometimes known as 'scrub itch'. Other mites may attack man and take a blood meal when the opportunity arises, examples are the red poultry mite (*Dermanyssus gallinae*) and the tropical rat mite (*Ornithonyssus bacoti*); unlike the harvest mites, the nymphs and adults of these mites also take blood meals.

Hard ticks (Ixodidae). These have a hard shield on the upper surface. All stages are blood feeders, taking one prolonged blood meal and remaining attached to their hosts for long periods; however most species must leave their host for each moult. They may live for several years and can survive long periods without a blood meal. It is often difficult to remove them from their host without breaking off the mouth parts. Some Ixodid ticks (*Ixodes and Dermacentor*) are unique among human ectoparasites in that they secrete a systemically acting toxin that can produce, over a period of several days, an ascending flaccid paralysis — 'tick paralysis'; removal of the tick, which may be hidden in the hair, produces rapid improvement.

Soft ticks (Argasidae). These have a rough folded cuticle and no dorsal shield. Usually all stages are blood feeders. Unlike hard ticks they are rapid nocturnal feeders and each stage takes several feeds, often on different hosts. Many species attacking man feed normally on dogs, cats, poultry and pigeons, but some (*Ornithodorus*) are closely associated with man and live permanently within simply constructed human dwellings.

f. Lice (Anoplura)

Three kinds of lice parasitise man: the squat pubic or crab louse (*Phthirus pubis*) lives firmly attached to pubic hairs or more rarely those of the axilla, beard area, eyebrows and eyelashes; the body louse (*Pediculus humanus humanus*) lives on unwashed and infrequently changed clothing in close contact with the body surface; and the head louse (*P. humanus capitis*) which lives among scalp hair. The head and body lice are both subspecies of *P. humanus* but they are biologically quite distinct. Lice lay their eggs or 'nits' on hair shafts or, in the case of the body louse, on underclothing. The larvae mature in about seven days through a sequence of three moults, all stages take several blood meals each day. Transmission from person to person is by close contact; in the case of the pubic louse this is usually sexual. Body lice are common in cool climates where hygiene is poor but they are uncommon in the tropics except at high altitudes. Head lice are common everywhere and pubic lice usually indicate promiscuity.

Ectoparasites as disease vectors

Blood-feeding animals are able to transfer pathogens from the blood or dermis of one host to another; in so doing they act as vectors. With the exception of rabies transmission by vampire bats, all vectors of human pathogens are either acarines, or adult or nymphal insects. Sometimes the transfer results simply from contamination of the mouthparts of a frequently feeding arthropod; this is known as **mechanical vector transmission** but is a relatively rare phenomenon in man, examples include the transmission of anthrax, tularaemia (*Francisella tularensis*) and possibly trypanosomes by tabanid flies; and the transmission of hepatitis B virus by bedbugs.

In true **biological vectors** the pathogen must multiply or develop within the vector host. The vector is therefore not immediately infective and this non-infective period is known as the **extrinsic incubation period**. The blood-feeding ectoparasites which act as true vectors of human disease are shown in Table 4.1. To succeed as a vector an arthropod must feed at least twice and have a life span exceeding the extrinsic incubation period. Some host specificity by the vector is essential if infection is to be maintained in a reservoir host species, but man often becomes infected by zoon-

oses because the vectors are not completely host-specific. Pathogens are always taken up by the mouthparts of the vector and usually they are in the blood, tissue parasites (*Leishmania*, *Onchocerca* and *Dipetalonema streptocerca*) can only be taken up when the vector is a 'pool' feeder. Reinoculation of the pathogen is usually in the saliva but may be from the faeces (*Trypanosoma cruzi* in reduviid bugs, *Rickettsia prowazekii* in lice and *R. typhi* in fleas), haemocoelic fluid (*Borrelia recurrentis* from the crushed louse, or in coxal fluid *Borrelia duttoni* in soft ticks). In filariasis the infective larva escapes from the mouthparts during the feeding process and enters the puncture wound. In acarines the pathogen can persist from one instar to the next and can often be passed from the ovary of the adult female to the offspring of the next generation (**transovarial transmission**); in this manner acarines act as reservoirs of infection as well as vectors. Without transovarial transmission trombiculid mites could never transmit scrub typhus, for they only feed on blood once in each generation. Transovarial transmission does not occur in insects, nor do microbial or protozoan infections persist from larva to adult in holometabolous insects; however in the hemimetabolous reduviid bug, *T. cruzi* infection can persist between nymphal instars and from nymph to adult.

EPIDERMAL PARASITES

1. Scabies mite (*Sarcoptes scabiei*)

The newly fertilised female mite makes her burrow in the epidermis with her biting mouthparts, using as anchors the adhesive suckers on the anterior two pairs of legs. She can live in her burrow for up to two months laying about two eggs each day. Eggs hatch in the burrow which the larvae leave to shelter in hair follicles, here they moult to form nymphs and later adults; the complete cycle from egg to adult takes about 14 days. The adults of both sexes make burrows but those of the male are short and he soon leaves it in search of a female. Person-to-person transmission probably nearly always occurs during close bodily contact, when newly fertilised females are transferred. The adult female mites measure 350 μm

Table 4.1 Blood-feeding ectoparasites that act as biological vectors of human disease

Vector		Disease	Pathogen
Insects			
Anoplura (lice)	*Pediculus humanus*	Epidemic relapsing fever (B)	*Borrelia recurrentis*
	humanus (body louse)	Epidemic typhus (R)	*Rickettsia prowazekii*
		Trench fever (R)	*Rochalimaea quintana*
Hemiptera (bugs)	*Panstrongylus, Triatoma*	American trypanosomiasis (P)	*T. cruzi*
	and *Rhodnius* (reduviid		
	bugs)		
Diptera (two-winged			
flies)			
Sandflies	*Phlebotomus*	Leishmaniasis (Old World) (P)	*L. donovani, L. tropica*
		Arboviruses (very few) (V)	Sandfly fever
	Lutzomyia, Psychodopygus	Leishmaniasis (New World) (P)	*L. mexicana, L. braziliensis,*
			L. donovani
		Carrion's disease (B)	*Bartonella bacilliformis*
Mosquitoes	*Anopheles*	Malaria (P)	*Plasmodium* spp
		Lymphatic filariasis (H)	*Wuchereria, Brugia*
		Arboviruses (very few) (V)	O'nyong nyong fever, etc.
	Aedes, Mansonia, Culex etc	Arboviruses (numerous) (V)	Yellow fever, dengue etc.
		Lymphatic filariasis (H)	*Wuchereria, Brugia*
Midges	*Culicoides*	Filariasis (H)	*Dipetalonema, Mansonella*
Black flies	*Simulium*	Filariasis (H)	*Onchocerca, Mansonella*
Deer and mango flies	*Chrysops*	Filariasis (H)	*Loa loa*
		Tularaemia (B)	*Francisella tularensis*
Tsetse flies	*Glossina*	African trypanosomiasis (P)	*T. brucei*
Siphonaptera (fleas)	*Xenopsylla, Nosopsyllus*	Plague (B)	*Yersinia pestis*
	(rodent fleas)	Endemic typhus (R)	*Rickettsia typhi*
Acarines			
Ixodidae (hard ticks)	*Ixodes, Amblyomma,*	Tick typhus (R)	*Rickettsia conori* and *R. rickettsii*
	Dermacentor and	Arboviruses (many) (V)	Encephalitis, some
	Haemophysalis		haemorrhagic
			fevers, etc.
		Babesiosis (P)	*Babesia* spp
		Tularaemia (B)	*Francisella tularensis*
Argasidae (soft ticks)	*Ornithodorus*	Endemic relapsing fever (B)	*Borrelia duttoni*
Trombiculidae	*Leptotrombidium*	Scrub typhus (R)	*Rickettsia tsutsugamushi*
Dermanyssidae } (mites)	*Allodermanyssus*	Rickettsial pox (R)	*Rickettsia akari*
	sanguineus		
	(house mouse mite)		

Pathogens: B — bacterial; H — helminthic; P — protozoan; R — rickettsial; V — viral

in length and 250 μm in width, the males are smaller.

Initially the infection is symptomless although the dark wavy lines of the burrows may be seen at the sites of election and sometimes the female acarus at its termination. Burrows may be a centimeter or more in length and contain faecal pellets and eggs that measure 150 by 100 μm. After three to four weeks the host becomes sensitised producing intense itching, especially at night. The rash occurs not only near the burrows, but also in areas of skin far removed from the parasite. Scratching, secondary infection, and probably the immune reactions themselves, limit the mite populations so that even in persons with extensive rashes the number of mites may be small; their typical burrows must be very carefully searched for. When removed from the burrow with a pin the mite appears as a tiny white speck with dark mouthparts. Species of scabies mites from dogs and rarely cats may attack man but do not form burrows.

2. Follicle mite (*Demodex folliculorum*)

This worm-like mite reaches a length of 400 μm;

they live head down in pilosebaceous follicles around the face, neck and shoulders. The mites may commonly be found in the debris of comedones expressed from these areas. In most people the mite is non-pathogenic but in others it appears to be associated with facial erythema and papules, somewhat resembling rosacea. A related species in dogs sometimes causes demodectic mange.

3. Jigger or chigoe flea (*Tunga penetrans*)

This parasite originated in South and Central America but has now spread throughout tropical Africa and is beginning to enter Asia. Larval fleas develop in sandy soil, hence the name sandflea sometimes given to this species, to produce very active but minute adults in about three weeks. The fertilised female fleas attach themselves to the feet of man and other large mammals including the pig. They rapidly burrow into the soft skin between the toes and under the toe nails to lie wholly within the epidermis. They are blood feeders and expand during a period of 10 days to form a nearly spherical creature 5 mm in diameter, with only the tip of the abdomen protruding from the burrow. Several thousand eggs are produced over a period of several weeks; those falling on sandy ground can continue the cycle. Sepsis is a common sequel when the parasite dies.

TISSUE INVADERS

1. Myiasis

Many species of dipterous fly larvae can invade human tissues to produce the disease myiasis. Some species are obligatory parasites while others are facultative ones that also feed on carrion; others are accidental parasites that do not invade living tissue but can use rotting flesh as a pabulum. Clinically the condition can be divided into three groups:

(1) Cutaneous myiasis involving healthy skin
(2) Atrial myiasis involving the nose and paranasal sinuses, orbit, ear, urethra and vagina
(3) Wound myiasis
The obligatory and facultative species belong to three families (Oestridae, Calliphoridae and Sarcophagidae); none are specifically human parasites but some are quite common and their importance is underestimated. Some myiasis-producing flies are larviparous (see appendix).

A. Obligatory parasites

1. Cutaneous

(a) Warble flies — the eggs of *Hypoderma* species are laid on the host's skin, usually that of cattle or deer. Larvae penetrate the skin and wander throughout the body tissues for about a year, eventually returning to a subcutaneous site from which the larva bursts out, falls to the ground and pupates. Although uncommon in man serious harm may be done as the larvae can enter the skull, or perforate the intestines. Mature warbles in man may appear as faruncles under the scalp or about the shoulders.

(b) Bot flies — the larvae of these species do not migrate but develop *in situ* within the dermis producing large painful faruncular lesions from which the mature larva eventually emerges and falls to the ground. In tropical and Southern Africa the tumbu fly (*Cordylobia anthropophaga*) is usually responsible; eggs are laid on sandy soil near human habitations or on clothes drying in the sun. Skin penetration is painless and the larvae mature in about nine days. In tropical America *Dermatobia hominis* produces similar lesions; the eggs are laid upon the bodies of mosquitoes captured by the female fly, and when the released mosquito feeds again the warmth of the host stimulates the eggs to hatch and the larvae penetrate the skin, where they mature during a period of up to 12 weeks. Other bot flies include *Cuterebra*, a rabbit parasite that occurs in temperate climes.

(c) *Gastrophilus* — These are stomach parasites of horses; the eggs are laid singly upon hairs and larvae are transferred to the horse's mouth by the tongue. They invade buccal tissues and later the stomach and intestine; when mature, after about 12 months, the larvae are passed in the faeces and pupate in the soil. Human infections occur during close contact with horses; presumably it is the larvae which are transferred. They penetrate human skin but cannot mature, and wander in the dermis for several weeks producing sinuous red tracks.

2. Atrial parasites. Two parasites that normally

infect the nasal and paranasal cavities of mammals may attack man; they are *Oestrus ovis* of sheep, and *Rhinoestrus purpureus* of horses. In man larvae may be deposited directly on the conjunctiva so that the dangerous condition of orbital myiasis can arise directly, otherwise it is by upward extension of nasal involvement.

3. *Wound myiasis.* Obligatory parasites infecting wounds are known as screw worms; the initial wound is usually suppurating but it may be very small, even an infected insect bite. Screw worms burrow into healthy tissue and mature in a few days. Infected nasal cavities, ears, perirectal tissue and even the umbilical stump of newborn babies are favoured sites. In the Western hemisphere the principal species is *Cochliomyia hominovorax* and in the Eastern hemisphere it is *Chrysomyia bezziana*; another species extending throughout the Palaeoarctic region is *Wohlfahrtia magnifica*, which deposits living larvae directly into the wound.

B. Facultative parasites

These infect wound and body cavities when they are bacterially infected or have other pathology. Unlike screw worm species these flies prefer deeply ulcerated and necrotic tissues, but their feeding activities do extend into living tissue. The principal genera are *Calliphora* and *Lucilia* (blow flies), and *Sarcophaga* (flesh flies).

C. Accidental parasites

Grossly contaminated wounds may be attractive to many non-parasitic flies. Their maggots sometimes have a beneficial effect by cleaning the wound, for they do not invade living tissues; some apparently secrete antibacterial substances. Muscid flies are often involved, including the house fly *Musca domestica* and related species. In addition certain species from genera containing facultative parasites may be responsible.

2. Pentastomiasis (tissue)

Man may act as an accidental intermediate host for the pentastome *Armillifer armillatus* and this infection is quite common in parts of tropical Africa and Southeast Asia. The definitive hosts are pythons and certain vipers in which the worm-like adults live in the respiratory passages, discharging their eggs in respiratory mucus. The adults show external pseudosegmentation and two pairs of clawed appendages are situated near the mouth. The normal intermediate hosts are rodents and other small mammals and in these ingested eggs hatch in the intestine, penetrate the gut wall and encyst as larvae and later as nymphs in various tissues. The cycle is completed when a snake eats the intermediate host. Man may become infected by handling or eating snakes but eggs remain viable in water and soil for several months so that ingestion in drinking water could be the commonest route. Complete development to encysted nymph takes several months. In man they usually develop only as far as the third larval stage which bears characteristic annulations and measures up to 25 mm in length, they are found most commonly on the liver surface, mesentery, gut wall and lung. The coiled or horseshoe – shaped larvae eventually calcify producing characteristic radiological shadows about 1 cm across; routine radiology and autopsies have revealed prevalences of 20 per cent or more in parts of Zaire and Malaysia. Usually no symptoms result but some patients experience abdominal pain and the parasites can occasionally cause intestinal obstruction, or compress bile ducts and bronchi. Neurological damage has been reported and also larvae within the eye and beneath the conjunctiva.

LUMEN PARASITES

1. Leeches

The ability of various aquatic leeches to enter body cavities, especially the nasopharynx, has already been mentioned (p. 80).

2. Myiasis

(a) *Urinary.* Facultative or accidental myiasis parasites can ascend the urethra to the bladder or reach it by other routes; some maturation occurs in the bladder and their eventual passage down the urethra is very painful. The usual species are the lesser house fly *Fannia canicularis* and the latrine fly *F. scalaris*; both of these are accidental parasites and presumably when eggs are laid near the urethral orifice ascent into the bladder is quite simple. Vaginal myiasis is apparently very rare and larvae do not mature in this site.

(b) *Intestinal*. Various dipterous larvae and eggs may be ingested accidentally. Some larvae survive the journey through the gut and cause transient colic, diarrhoea or even bloody stools. The commonest offender is perhaps the rat-tailed maggot *Eristalis tenax* (Syrphidae) ingested in contaminated water. Dung-breeding fly larvae rarely enter the anus when eggs are laid in this region; transient tenesmus and diarrhoea can result. Similarly larvae of dung beetles (*Onthophagus*) can enter the anus and become temporary accidental parasites of the lower bowel.

3. Pentastomiasis (luminal)

Man may ingest nymphal pentastomes of the species *Linguatula serrata* when he eats raw sheep or goat liver, a common practice in some Middle Eastern countries. The normal definitive hosts of this parasite are dogs and wolves, in which the adults, living in the nasal passages, may reach a length of 10 cm. Eggs are discharged in nasal secretions onto vegetation to be ingested by herbivorous mammals. Man acts as an accidental definitive host; the nymphs ascend the oesophagus from the stomach and attach to the pharyngeal and nasal mucosae causing irritative and obstructive symptoms known as halzoun or the marrara syndrome. The parasites do not mature in man and the illness is self-limiting within one or two weeks.

PSEUDOPARASITISM AND DELUSIONS OF PARASITISM

Patients often seek medical help when they find what they believe to be parasites upon their person or in faeces, urine and other bodily secretions. Frequently the specimens are found to be free-living creatures that have contaminated the specimen, such as urine or faeces after it has been passed, or were present in the receptacle into which the specimen was placed. Sometimes the objects are neither metazoan parasites nor free-living animals but are simply inanimate objects or dried tissue debris. In some patients it is almost impossible to reassure the patient that he is not parasitised. In its more extreme form parasitophobia, entomophobia or delusions of parasitism may indicate serious psychiatric disease. Thus it may be a manifestation of obsessional neurosis, depressive illness or even schizophrenia. Clinicians must be aware of this possibility when they encounter this problem, especially when it is recurrent.

FURTHER READING

Gordon, R.M. and Lavoipierre, M.M.J. (1962) *Entomology for Students of Medicine*. Oxford: Blackwell Scientific Publications.

Mattingly, P.F. (1969) *The Biology of Mosquito-borne Disease*. London: George Allen and Unwin Ltd.

Prathap, K., Lau, K.S. and Bolton, J.M. (1969) Pentastomiasis: A common finding at autopsy among Malayan aborigines. *Am. J. trop. Med. Hyg.*, **18**, 20–27.

Smith, K.G.V. (ed.) (1973) *Insects and Other Arthropods of Medical Importance*. London: British Museum (Natural History).

Zumpt, F. (1965) *Myiasis in Man and Animals of the Old World*. London: Butterworth and Co. Ltd.

5

The Epidemiology of Parasitism

The epidemiologist is concerned with the distribution of parasites in time and space, and the circumstances under which infection causes disease.

LEVELS OF TRANSMISSION

The critical parameter that determines the pattern of an infection in a community is the level of transmission as this limits the rate at which new infections are acquired (for discussion see pp. 213–218). Two terms are used to describe quantitatively the pattern of an infection within a community; they must be clearly distinguished. The **prevalence** is the proportion of the population infected at one point in time, while **incidence** is the number of new infections generated during a known period of time. Since they are both rates, prevalence and incidence must always be expressed with a denominator, for example 100, 1000 or 10 000 persons, as well as a numerator. In the case of incidence the period of time must be specified, frequently it is one year. There is a simple relationship between these two terms:

Prevalence = Incidence × mean duration of infection.

Two features shared by many parasitic infections, their long duration and the relatively low levels of protective immunity, have important consequences upon the patterns of infection they produce.

Transmission levels frequently vary in both space and time. Variation in space accounts for the focal nature of many parasitic infections, and is produced by the various local factors that are favourable or unfavourable to transmission; on a larger scale these same factors determine the geographic distribution of a parasite. Variations in transmission level with time are often seasonal, but there is a wide spectrum in the amount of change both for different infections and for the same infection in different places; the spectrum ranges from an almost constant or stable level to a wildly fluctuating one. The long duration of many parasitic infections implies that prevalence rates can remain moderately high despite low levels of incidence. For example if the duration of an infection is six months and the annual incidence is three per hundred then the prevalence rate under stable conditions will be 1.5 per cent; if the duration of infection is two or six years the respective prevalence rates would be six and eighteen per cent. Prolonged infections also reduce the effect, upon prevalence, of seasonal and other changes in incidence; long infections can bridge the gap between successive peaks in transmission.

As prevalence rates rise it is obvious that infected persons will themselves be exposed to further infection; in the absence of protective immunity this will produce multiple infections or **superinfection**; when this happens the simple relationship between prevalence and incidence, given above, no longer holds. Amongst the protozoan infections superinfection is common in malaria and probably also with the lumen dwelling species such as *Entamoeba histolytica*; because of much lower incidence rates and also, in some cases, protective immunity, superinfection is probably a rare event in infections caused by *Leishmania*, *Trypanosoma* and *Toxoplasma*. Amongst the metazoan parasites, superinfection is the normal means by which parasite loads are built up; the number of parasites carried by a host being referred to as the **intensity** of infection. In metazoan species whose parasitic adult stages have separate sexes, the levels of intensity must be sufficient to allow pairs to form, otherwise the life cycle cannot continue. Studies of the distribution of metazoan parasites among their hosts, in other words the frequency distribution of the intensity of infection, show almost without exception a non-random pattern. Nearly always one finds parasite aggregation within a small number of hosts, together with a larger number of hosts, than expected by chance, with either no infection or low levels of intensity. Mathematically the type of distribution observed can be fitted quite closely to a negative binomial curve. It is not entirely clear how this type of distribution is generated, but it probably results from the summation of several non-random factors that determine infection rates. The observed aggregation of parasites has two important practical consequences. Firstly a relatively large proportion of the total infective potential of a population is derived from a small number of hosts; if these can be identified and treated the level of transmission will fall significantly. Secondly it is amongst this same group of persons, with unexpectedly high parasite loads, that morbidity is most likely to be seen. This reasoning forms the basis of targeted chemotherapy, that is treatment of the most heavily infected persons in a community.

In general terms and under fairly stable conditions the mean levels of intensity in metazoan infections are more or less proportional to the level of transmission.

Endemic, sporadic and epidemic infections

Infections can be grouped under these three general headings; they are not mutually exclusive and one parasite, for example *Plasmodium vivax*, can be endemic in one situation and epidemic in others.

Endemic infections

An endemic infection is constantly present within a population and persists at a more or less stable level of prevalence. For the reasons already given endemicity is the commonest epidemiological situation in parasitic infections. Prevalence rates may change quite rapidly over short distances producing a focal pattern within a basically endemic situation. In malaria special terms have been introduced to describe the levels of endemicity; thus in holoendemic malaria, the highest level of endemicity, more than 75 per cent of children aged two to nine years have palpably enlarged spleens. Changes in the level of endemicity can occur naturally or as a result of control measures. When levels in transmission fall the decline in prevalence is usually gradual because of the long duration of most parasitic infections; this applies also to all control measures that do not include chemotherapy.

Sporadic infections

When levels of endemicity are very low, or very focal in their distribution, they may be described as sporadic. Most of the rarer zoonoses fall into this catagory; persons with particular occupations or recreational activities are at special risk when they inadvertently enter the natural ecosystem of the species. In contrast infections that are not zoonoses usually die out when transmission falls below a critical level.

The facultative parasitism by soil amoebae (*Naegleria*) is also sporadic. In the occasional unfortunate subject who bathes or dives in fresh water these ubiquitous amoebae may enter the nose and cross the olfactory epithelium to reach the meninges.

Opportunistic parasites also appear in a sporadic manner within the context of symptomless endemicity. These infections become clinically apparent more commonly, or even exclusively, in persons whose immune defences are impaired by disease or medical treatment. As therapeutic measures that depress immunity such as steroids, cytotoxic drugs and radiotherapy become more widely used throughout the world these infections will assume increasing importance.

Epidemic infections

Sudden increases in the level of transmission will produce an epidemic in the absence of protective immunity. While epidemics are comparatively rare in parasitic infections, several examples should be mentioned.

1. Malaria. Where levels of malaria transmission are normally so low that protective immunity within the community is low or absent, a sudden increase in transmission produces an epidemic. This occurs when the transmission season, each year, is either very short or there are periods of one or more consecutive years with no transmission. When an epidemic does occur all age groups are affected and morbidity may be high; this situation is often termed **unstable malaria**. In **stable malaria**, in contrast, at the other end of the malaria transmission spectrum, new infections continue more or less throughout the year and adults acquire considerable protective immunity while nearly all serious disease occurs in young children. Stable malaria reaches its most extreme form in equatorial Africa but also occurs elsewhere in the wet tropics. Unstable malaria is typically found in drier and more temperate conditions, or at high altitudes in the tropics.

2. Visceral leishmaniasis. In the Indian form of kala-azar, where there is no animal reservoir, epidemics sweep through the population at intervals of five to twenty or more years. The epidemic lasts for many months in each area it passes through. The only other part of the world where kala-azar is ever epidemic is East Africa, particularly Kenya; here human-to-human transmission arises secondarily from a zoonotic source.

3. Gambian sleeping sickness. While *T.b. gambiense* is basically a focal endemic infection with inter-human transmission, the situation is often unstable with unpredictable epidemics that may result in spread to new areas. The most notorious epidemics occurred in Uganda between 1901 and 1911, originating in Zaire and resulting from human population movements; in some areas up to 25 per cent of the population died. A lasting result was the establishment of new endemic foci.

4. Taenia solium. Recently an epidemic of epilepsy due to cysticercosis began in the highlands of Irian Jaya (western New Guinea) where people live in close association with pigs. The infection was introduced by the importation of infected pigs from neighbouring parts of Indonesia. This is an example of a parasite entering a new focus that particularly favours its transmission.

5. Trichinosis. Typically outbreaks of *T. spiralis* follow communal feasting upon infected and undercooked pork. This can happen at barbecues when meat is often incompletely cooked; in a less dramatic form outbreaks may derive from home-made sausages.

6. Other examples. Small outbreaks of toxoplasmosis have followed the ingestion of infected hamburgers. *Pneumocystis* may spread rapidly among malnourished or debilitated infants. Consumption of infected watercress, especially when collected in the wild, has led to outbreaks of fascioliasis in Europe. Exposure to water containing many schistosome carcariae may lead to epidemics of cercarial dermatitis. If a human *Schistosoma* species is involved an outbreak of the acute early systemic form of the disease can occur, especially when non-immunes are exposed. Contamination of piped water supplies by sewage has caused outbreaks of giardiasis.

GEOGRAPHICAL DISTRIBUTION OF PARASITES

The distribution of human parasites depends ultimately upon man's behaviour, and the physical and biological environment. These factors usually interact with one another, but it is often man himself who plays the dominant role. The distribution of vectors, intermediate and reservoir hosts are also controlled by factors falling under these three headings.

Knowledge of parasite distribution is of great importance to the clinician who must know where his patients come from, and where they have been. The public health worker must be aware of the effects of changing human ecology upon the frequency and distribution of parasites and should be able to predict future trends. The situation is always a dynamic one.

A few human parasites are cosmopolitan, for example *Toxoplasma*; a greater number have a limited distribution of variable extent. Some occur widely throughout the tropics and may be described as pantropical.

1. Physical environment

A. Temperature and humidity

These two variables frequently interact with one another.

(1) The viability of parasites in the external environment.

High temperatures with low humidity are usually the least favourable to the parasite. Examples where these factors may be critical to parasite survival include: the cysts of protozoa with direct life cycles (*Entamoeba histolytica, Giardia, Balantidium* and the various gut commensal species); the oocysts of *Isospora, Toxoplasma*, and *Sarcocystis*; the eggs and larvae of soil-transmitted nematodes; the eggs of trematodes and pseudophyllidean cestodes prior to their entry into the aquatic environment; cyclophyllidean cestode eggs prior to their ingestion by the intermediate hosts; and the transmissive form of *Pneumocystis carinii* when dispersed by aerosol.

(2) Rates of parasite development in the external environment, and in arthropod vectors.

The sporulation of oocysts and the rates of embryonation of nematode, pseudophyllidean cestode and trematode eggs, and also the development times for hookworm and *Strongyloides* larvae, are all temperature-dependent.

The development and maturation of filarial larvae within their vectors is affected by ambient temperature. When development is too slow, at low temperatures the vector will not survive long enough to effect transmission of the infective stage. Similarly in malaria the duration of the extrinsic cycle in the mosquito, that is the time between gametocyte ingestion and sporozoite formation, is directly controlled by temperature and this is often the major reason why malaria cannot persist in cooler climes.

B. The soil

For most parasites passing through a stage in the external environment it is the soil upon which the parasite is initially deposited. Temperature and humidity obviously affect the soil, but its own physical properties are also of great importance, particularly the particle size and texture as these affect the water-holding capacity and liability to dessication. Physical factors including rainfall and also biological ones, such as dung beetles, affect the rate at which human faeces deposited on the ground are broken up and their parasitic forms dispersed into the soil. Susceptibility to anaerobiosis is also relevant, and this may affect the risks of transmitting certain parasites when human faeces ('night soil'), in the raw state or after composting, are used as fertiliser.

C. The aquatic environment

Surface water in the form of pools, ponds, wells, lakes and rivers and also the capillary water films in the soil are essential habitats in many parasite life cycles. Parasite survival will depend upon various chemical qualities of the water, its pH and redox potential and also its temperature and flow rate.

(1) Trematodes — Miracidia after hatching from the egg must survive long enough to reach their snail intermediate host. Similarly cercariae emerging from infected snails must survive long enough to encyst as metacercariae if they are hermaphroditic flukes, or to penetrate the skin of their hosts if they are schistosomes.

(2) Pseudophyllidean tapeworms — The ciliated free swimming coracidium, hatching from the egg, must survive until ingested by *Cyclops* or other microcrustaceans.

(3) Guinea worm (*Dracunculus*) — The free swimming larvae, liberated by the female worm at the site of an open sore, must survive until ingested by *Cyclops*.

(4) Free-living amoebae (*Naegleria* and *Acanthamoeba*) normally live in organically-rich aquatic or wet environments, although they can withstand drying by forming cysts.

(5) Some larval nematodes, particularly those of hookworm and *Strongyloides*, live in the capillary water films in soil and on low vegetation. They can survive immersion in surface rain water for quite long periods but are extremely susceptible to dessication. Shaded sandy soils are the most favourable for these parasites.

2. Biological factors

The distributions in nature of appropriate vectors, intermediate hosts and reservoir hosts are some of the most obvious factors limiting the occurrence of parasites. This will apply to all parasite species having indirect life cycles and to those that are zoonoses; for the latter must have a reservoir host.

However while the presence of, for example, a particular vector species will be a necessary condition for the transmission of a parasite, the distribution of the parasite is always more restricted, because of the many other factors affecting the life cycle. A good example is anophelism without malaria, that is the presence of *Anopheles* vectors without the transmission of malaria; this can sometimes happen even when infected persons enter the area. It can occur when, for example, mosquito longevity is too short to allow completion of the extrinsic *Plasmodium* cycle, or when the human population protects itself against the biting mosquitoes.

3. Human ecology

A. *Population density and urbanisation*

In the past when man was exclusively a mobile hunter gathering species without permanent residence, most of his parasitic infections were zoonoses; faecal contamination of his own environment was minimal and directly transmitted intestinal protozoans and soil-transmitted helminths, were probably uncommon. The agricultural revolution produced large resident human populations with greater potential for direct person-to-person spread of infection, and greater environmental contamination by faeces; in addition the domestication of animals created new cycles of parasite transmission.

It might be thought that urbanisation would inevitably lead to a decline in human parasitism but this is not necessarily the case and it is only the feral zoonoses that disappear. Rapid urbanisation, especially in the tropics, is often associated with increased poverty, poorer housing and poor sanitation. The result is that people may be living in a more faecally polluted environment than in rural areas; for this reason infection rates and often disease rates with *E. histolytica* and *Giardia*

may be high, and epidemics of the latter species can occur when public water supplies become faecally contaminated. Food handlers and street vendors become a problem in urban areas, and amoebiasis is probably frequently transmitted in this way. Two soil-transmitted nematodes with simple life cycles, *Ascaris lumbricoides* and *Trichuris trichiura*, are often commoner in towns and cities. Social mores and domestic overcrowding favour the direct transmission of scabies, lice, *Trichomonas vaginalis*, *Hymenolepis nana* and *Enterobius*. In some towns, shared water supplies in the form of unprotected wells may favour guinea worm infection.

Open drainage ditches, septic tanks and other faecally contaminated water provide perfect breeding sites for the ubiquitous mosquito *Culex fatigans* and the current dramatic increase in bancroftian filariasis in many Asian towns and cities can be attributed to poor sanitation favouring this vector. The sandfly vector of urban oriental sore (*Leishmania tropica*) finds the moist interstices of poorly maintained and broken down houses, and piles of rubble, ideal breeding sites for its larvae. The extensive shanty towns of many South American cities favour *Trypanosoma cruzi* transmission since triatomine bugs live in the fabric of the mud and wattle houses where they feed freely on man and also upon the chickens, cats and dogs in the peridomestic environment; as a result the incidence of *T. cruzi* infection is increasing. Eating habits also change in cities, for example less well cooked meat may be served in special dishes at certain restaurants and this may produce more cases of taeniasis, toxoplasmosis and infections by *Sarcocystis*.

B. *Population movement*

The setting up of mining, agricultural or industrial centres in new areas sometimes favours parasitism. A zoonotic focus may be entered, as has happened recently with *Leishmania donovani* in Eastern Sudan producing many cases of kala-azar. Migrant workers are frequently poorly housed without adequate screening against mosquitoes; in consequence there may be outbreaks of malaria in relatively non-immune populations. Military operations carry similar risks; thus in recent years

Israeli soldiers have acquired cutaneous leishmaniasis (*L. major*) after sleeping in caves during war service; whilst British soldiers on jungle training in Belize have developed sores due to *Leishmania mexicana*. During the second world war Australian troops became heavily infected with hookworm while fighting in the Papua New Guinea forests. War conditions can also favour parasitism in more subtle ways; thus during recent disharmony in Eastern Nigeria people lived in the forest and ate freshwater crabs, the number of *Paragonimus* infections increased greatly in an area where it was previously little recognised.

Foreign travellers obviously put themselves at risk and may also introduce infection when their later destinations favour transmission. Immigrants to temperate countries from the tropics often bring infection with them but only rarely does this result in transmission. Where the recipient country can support transmission the risks may be considerable as when malaria-infected persons enter Northern Australia, Southern Europe or the Southern United States.

A full geographic history is essential in all persons with suspected parasitic disease.

C. Dams and irrigation

Many development programmes in the tropics involve irrigation systems, and the construction of dams to feed them, and to produce hydroelectricity. Certain health problems are inevitable but most can be foreseen. The migrant labour force is often poorly housed and sanitated, resulting in outbreaks of malaria and gastrointestinal infections. The flooding behind the dam and also the irrigation channels create new breeding sites for mosquitoes; as a result malaria and filariasis transmission may increase. Of great concern, especially in Africa, is that the snail intermediate hosts of schistosomiasis will increase their populations enormously and that the immigrant human population will bring *Schistosoma* infections with them. There are now several examples of greatly increased schistosomiasis incidence in these circumstances. The spillways and highly oxygenated water flow below a dam can create breeding sites for *Simulium* and hence the risk of onchocerciasis; however this should be preventable by

periodic insecticide application to the limited breeding area.

D. Agriculture

(1) *Animal husbandry*. Cattle raising produces only one real parasitic problem — the beef tapeworm (*Taenia saginata*); bovine cysticercosis is very important economically as it often renders carcases unsalable. Although in Africa *Trypanosoma b. rhodesiense* has been isolated from cattle it is unlikely that domestic herds are important reservoirs, the usual source of infection being wild game animals. *Sarcocystis hominis* infections in man derive from beef but are apparently benign.

Pigs can create several parasitic disease problems; the two most important being the pork tapeworm (*Taenia solium*) and trichinosis (*Trichinella spiralis*). In the Far East pigs are important reservoirs for two intestinal flukes, *Fasciolopsis buski* and *Gastrodiscoides hominis*. Most human infections with *Balantidium* are derived from pigs, or from the rats that are so often associated with them. *Sarcocystis suihominis* is a pig parasite, but is probably harmless in man.

Sheep farming produces several problems, the most important being hydatid disease (*Echinococcus granulosus*) which is common in most sheep-raising areas, unless carefully controlled. The related larval tapeworm *Multiceps* is also a sheep parasite, as are the two fluke infections *Fasciola* and the much less important *Dicrocoelium*. The relatively benign gut nematodes of the genus *Trichostrongylus* are normally acquired from sheep or goats. Sheep flesh is probably the commonest source of meat-acquired toxoplasmosis for man.

In certain countries, such as Libya, camels are important reservoirs of hydatid infection; however the strain of *E. granulosus* infecting horses is apparently non-pathogenic in man.

(2) *Fish farming*. This useful source of protein food carries certain health risks; whilst these are most evident in the Far East where the practice is most ancient, some will arise elsewhere when the practice is introduced. Fish ponds can be important breeding sites for mosquitoes transmitting malaria and filariasis. *Mansonia* mosquitoes, particularly, thrive where there is surface vegetation to which the larvae attach by means of their brea-

thing siphons; in some parts of Southeast Asia this is an important source of Brugian filariasis. The life cycles of the oriental liver flukes (*Clonorchis sinensis* and *Opisthorchis viverrini*) are maintained in fish ponds especially when human faeces are used as fertiliser. Where the water calthrop plant is grown in the ponds, transmission of the two intestinal flukes *Fasciolopsis buski* and *Gastrodiscoides hominis* can become established; the aquatic cycle being initiated by human or pig faeces added as fertiliser.

(3) *Human faeces used to fertilise agricultural land*. The use of fresh faeces, composted faeces or sewage sludge creates obvious problems in disease transmission. Protozoan cysts and helminth eggs vary greatly in their resistance to adverse conditions, *Taenia* eggs being the most resistant. Properly composted 'night soil' is relatively safe, the main risk being *Ascaris* infection. A related problem is the high rate of hookworm infection amongst agricultural labourers and workers on tea or rubber estates; here the source may be 'night soil' but more commonly it is promiscuous defaecation by the workers themselves; the common result is that in rural areas adult males have the highest hookworm loads.

E. Domestic environment

Many variables are important in this context. They include sanitation, water supplies, breeding places for rodents and for insect vectors such as triatomine bugs and mosquitoes. Home structure, window screening and bed nets will determine the access of winged vector mosquitoes and sandflies to a house and its occupants. Many indoor feeding mosquitoes rest on walls after their nocturnal blood meal but can only do so when conditions are suitable.

Pets are also significant. Thus dogs are the usual source of *Toxocara* infections in man, and also of hydatid disease and coenurus infection; the latter two conditions occuring particularly when dogs working with sheep are also treated as domestic pets. In many parts of the world dogs are the major reservoir of *Leishmania donovani* and an important one for urban oriental sore (*L. tropica*), and also for the liver fluke *Clonorchis sinensis*. Some dog hookworm species (*A. braziliense*) commonly cause cutaneous larva migrans in man, and a common dog tapeworm (*Dipylidium*) sometimes infects man. The dog heart worm, a filarial parasite *Dirofilaria immitis*, can also be transmitted to man. Dogs are suspected of being an important source of *Pneumocystis* infection.

Cats are perhaps of less significance, although oocysts of *Toxoplasma* in cat faeces are a common source of this infection in man. Cats are also important reservoirs of the liver fluke *Opisthorchis felineus* and of zoonotic Brugian filariasis.

F. Dietary customs

Local dietary behaviour is often critical for parasite transmission. This applies particularly to the hermaphroditic flukes whose metacercariae encyst upon certain fish, crustacea, molluscs or aquatic vegetation; and the tapeworms whose larval stages must be ingested in undercooked meat (*Taenia*) or fish (*Diphyllobothrium*). Other infections acquired from undercooked meat are trichinosis, *Toxoplasma* and *Sarcocystis*. Pickled or undercooked herrings are the source of *Anisakis* infections and the localised infection *Capillaria philippinensis* results from eating certain estuarine fish. *Angiostrongylus* infections can follow ingestion of certain molluscs or mollusc-contaminated salads. Raw sheep liver containing larval pentastomes can cause halzoun.

G. Occupational behaviour

Besides the problems associated with agriculture and animal husbandry certain other examples should be mentioned. Fishermen are at special risk from onchocerciasis and *Trypanosoma b. gambiense*, because of their frequent contact with the respective vectors, *Simulium* and riverine tsetse (*Glossina palpalis*). Irrigation workers and bathers are exposed particularly to schistosomiasis and cercarial dermatitis; persons diving in contaminated water carry the very small risk of contracting *Naegleria* meningoencephalitis.

Hunters and zoologists are at risk when they enter feral zoonoses, for example rural oriental sore (*L. major* and *L. aethiopica*) and Rhodesian trypanosomiasis, the latter being also a special hazard to the game park safari tourist. Persons entering the rain forests of Central and South America are exposed to *Leishmania mexicana* and *L. braziliensis* infections; those at special risk include collectors of wild rubber, timbermen and workers on road building programmes through virgin forest.

INFECTION AND DISEASE

In many microbial diseases it is possible to discuss the likely outcome of an infection simply in terms of the pathogenicity of the microbe and the susceptibility of the host at the time of initial infection. In parasitic disease the situation tends to be more complicated. Three important reasons for this are the long duration of many parasitic infections, and the frequency of reinfection and superinfection. In addition parasitic metazoa are fundamentally different from microbes since very few multiply within their host.

1. Pathogenicity of the parasite

Genetically distinct populations of parasites are known as **strains** and frequently these affect their hosts differently. In microbiology and also in protozoology a distinction is often made between **pathogenicity** and **virulence**; the former being an attribute of a species, while the latter is applied to strains within a species. Hence *Entamoeba histolytica* can be described as a pathogenic species that contains strains of different virulence. Often strains with differing disease potential are geographically separate, as is the case with *Trypanosoma cruzi*, where cardiomyopathy and megasyndromes show very different frequencies within the parasite's total distribution, or *Schistosoma mansoni* which produces much greater morbidity in Egypt than in West Africa. In other species, for example *Entamoeba histolytica*, it appears that several strains of differing virulence can circulate in the same ecosystem.

2. Host susceptibility

While the pathogenicity of a parasite is fixed genetic attribute, the susceptibility of a host is usually mainly non-genetic and may change during the course of an infection, particularly when it is a long one. Important variable host factors are nutritional status, intercurrent disease and pregnancy (p. 106). Previously mild or clinically inapparent infections can produce dangerous disease when host immunity falls; examples of such opportunistic infections are toxoplasmosis and strongyloidiasis, the latter being one of the few examples of a metazoan parasite multiplying, by autoinfection, within its host.

The lumen-dwelling protozoa (*E. histolytica*, *Giardia*, *T. vaginalis* and *Balantidium*) are unique in that they can switch from commensalism to a pathogenic form of parasitism. This interchange is often unpredictable, although it is likely that most primary infections with *Giardia* and *T. vaginalis* are initially symptomatic, even if only mildly so, and this is usually followed by commensalism. With *E. histolytica* an initial illness, even a mild one, is much less common, but tissue invasion and serious disease can occur later, sometimes after several years; host factors are presumably responsible but these can rarely be recognised.

3. Reinfection and superinfection

(a) Protozoa

As previously explained these phenomena are only common with the lumen–dwelling species and the malaria parasites. In both groups some protective immunity is usually acquired eventually but its effectiveness is variable. The absence of symptomatic giardiasis in adults, in places where the infection is common, is good evidence for acquired immunity; similarly tolerance to new *T. vaginalis* infections is gradually acquired. In contrast there is no definite evidence for acquired immunity in amoebiasis, and it is not clear what happens when superinfection occurs; possibly a resident commensal strain prevents the establishment of a second strain that is more pathogenic than the first.

In malaria the situation appears at first sight to be paradoxical, for immunity is acquired at an earlier age, and is more complete, when transmission levels are high, and hence reinfection and superinfection more common. However the better immunity at high transmission levels is gained at the cost of more deaths among infants and young children. Partial malaria control reduces the number of deaths by delaying the age of first infection and by spacing subsequent infections more widely. Complete immunity may never be gained in this context, which means that older children and adults may still suffer from mild clinical malaria. Only when transmission levels are very low will adults be liable to life-threatening infections. In most persons splenomegaly regresses as immunity is gained, hence when transmission is very high, palpable splenic enlargement is rare in adults; it becomes commoner as control measures are applied and immunity becomes less complete. Some individuals living in malarious areas show an atypical pattern of immunity, which controls parasitaemia but allows the spleen to enlarge progressively, so producing the tropical splenomegaly syndrome.

(b) Metazoa

These parasites are normally acquired by gradual accumulation rather than by a single exposure to many infective forms; although there are obvious exceptions such as trichinosis. Superinfection is essential for the survival of the species when the adult parasites are unisexual. In contrast superinfection is not necessary for those hermaphroditic species which practice self-fertilisation, such as some tapeworms, or in those parasites whose adults are free-living, as is the case with myiasis-producing flies.

In most metazoan infections the intensity of infection, or the number of parasites present, is the main determinant of morbidity. In schistosomiasis and in several of the commoner helminthic infections of the gut, it is possible to estimate the worm load by means of egg counts (p. 185). Hence the persons at greatest risk of developing disease can be identified and treated. When damage to the host is cumulative the duration of the infection becomes important, in addition to its intensity; examples are the progressive tissue damage by egg granulomas in schistosomiasis, and the continued blood loss in hookworm infection. In some helminthic infections it appears that adult worms must be present for protective immunity to be effective; this is known as **concomitant immunity**. The most thoroughly studied example of this phenomenon is schistosomiasis; in this infection adult worms initiate immunological mechanisms that destroy superinfecting schistosomulae in the skin or lungs. Thus at least in some species, it is possible that where transmission continues, persons with light worm loads are better off than those who have been successfully dewormed by chemotherapy.

Sometimes individual metazoan parasites damage vital body structures and in this context intensity of infection may not be relevant; examples are cysticerci in the myocardium or brain, *Toxocara* granulomas in the retina, or *Gnathostoma* larvae accidentally invading the nervous system.

FURTHER READING

Bradley, D.J. (1972) Regulation of parasite populations. A general theory of the epidemiology and control of parasitic infections. *Trans. R. Soc. Trop. Med. Hyg.*, **66**, 697–708.

Nelson, G.S. (1972) Human behaviour in the transmission of parasitic diseases. *Zool. J. Linn. Soc.*, **50** (Suppl. 1), 109–122.

Warren, K.S. (1973) Regulation of the prevalence and intensity of schistosomiasis in man; immunology or ecology? *J. infect. Dis.*, **127**, 595–609.

6

Host responses to parasites

IMMUNOLOGICAL RESPONSES EVOKED BY PARASITES

Parasites evoke a wide spectrum of immunological responses in their hosts. Their nature and the mechanisms involved are in no way unique to parasitic disease although they often differ quantitatively from those seen in other infections. Because of their biochemical and structural complexity, parasites can present a large number of antigens to their hosts.

Endogenous parasitic antigens are primarily structural, and apart from those on the parasite surface, most are only presented to the host's immune system when the parasite dies in the tissues. The multiplicity of structural antigens creates difficulties when relatively crude parasite extracts are used as antigen in serological tests. Some antigens will be sufficiently similar to those of related parasites, or even unrelated ones, that cross reactions are common. **Exogenous parasite antigens** are those substances released during the normal growth and development of the living organism. No parasite toxins have yet been identified, at least among those species living internally in man. An important group of exogenous antigens are enzymes released during the feeding process, for example from the buccopharyngeal glands of nematodes, and the salivary glands of ectoparasites. Other secretory products facilitate the movement of worms or schistosome eggs through tissue. Some are released from the anus and excretory pores, being derived from the living epithelial cells of these systems. The genital pores also release antigenic material, especially during oviposition or larviposition. Nematode moulting is another potent source of antigen; enzyme-rich moulting fluid is released when the old cuticle is shed.

The dosage, route and mode of antigen presentation will determine the type of immunological response, but little is known as to why certain parasites evoke a particular response.

The principal pathways by which parasite antigens activate the different cellular and humoral immune systems are shown in Figure 6.1. Most parasite antigens must be initially processed by macrophages, the exception being membrane-bound antigens which can directly activate the bursa-derived (B cell) lymphoid system. Interactions between the thymus-derived (T cell) lymphoid system and the B cell system are complex and include both suppression and facilitation.

Activation of B cell system

The result of activation of this system is a series of proliferating plasma cell clones secreting immunoglobulin. In many parasite infections specific antibodies have been detected in at least three immunoglobulin classes and sometimes four; the relative abundance of the immunoglobulin classes varies greatly in different infections and at different stages of an infection.

As might be expected, IgM antibodies are common in early primary infections; later they are often partly replaced by IgG antibodies. Use is made of this phenomenon in serodiagnosis; for example IgM antibodies in toxoplasmosis indicate active infection as opposed to a latent one, similarly current tissue invasion by *E. histolytica* provokes IgM antibody while past infections may be

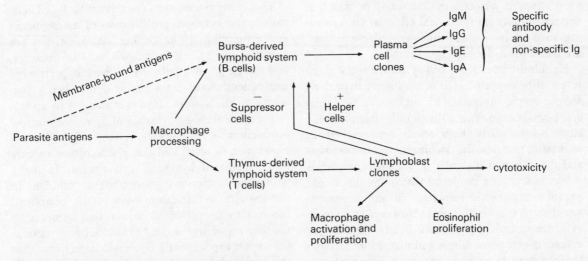

Fig. 6.1 Immunological pathways activated by parasite antigens
Abbreviations: B cells — bursa-derived lymphoid cells; Ig — immunoglobulin; T cells — thymus-derived lymphoid cells

evident serologically as IgG antibody. IgM responses are also prominent when parasites produce frequent antigenic changes of their surface coat, as in African trypanosomiasis; levels are also high in tissue nematode infections.

IgG antibodies are usually the most numerous and the ones reaching the highest titres. Most routine serological tests mainly detect IgG antibody. Their protective value is often considerable as evidenced by the absence of malaria in infants, up to the age of about 4 months, born to immune mothers; only IgG malarial antibody is transferred across the placenta. Very little is known about IgA antibodies to parasites; serum titres are usually low, but there is evidence that they are secreted into the gut, bronchial tree and vagina; their functional effects are uncertain.

Both helminths and ectoparasites provoke remarkably high titres of IgE antibody. The reason for this could be that antigen is presented mainly to immunological receptors in the skin and gut. IgE antibodies probably have important functional effects upon parasites.

Besides provoking specific antibody, parasites are notable for their stimulation of non-specific immunoglobulins. In several infections, the proportion of the increased immunoglobulin level that can be ascribed to specific antibody is less than 20

per cent. This has given rise to the hypothesis that some parasite antigens are B cell mitogens. However part of the high level, at least in the case of IgM, can be attributed to frequent antigenic change, as in African trypanosomiasis and perhaps malaria. Very high levels of non-specific IgM occur in the tropical splenomegaly syndrome (T.S.S.) and to a lesser extent in all persons repeatedly infected with malaria; they also occur in toxocariasis and several other tissue nematode infections. Autoantibody to various human tissues, including heart muscle, thyroid and gastric parietal cells can be demonstrated in serum from T.S.S. patients but there is no evidence so far that autologous tissue is damaged by this mechanism in any parasitic disease. Isohaemagglutinin titres are raised in toxocariasis. Heterophile antibodies to sheep red cells, and also anti-red cell agglutinins are produced in all the conditions mentioned. Other observed consequences of high levels of non-specific IgM are positive tests for rheumatoid factor, cryoglobulins and false positive Wasserman reactions; but these apparently have no functional effects. Detection of raised total serum levels of IgM by radial immunodiffusion are useful as screening tests for African trypanosomiasis, T.S.S. and toxocariasis. Non-specific IgG is common in several infections but reaches extreme proportions in visceral leishmaniasis in which it appears to have no functional effect at all; screening tests such as the formol-gel (aldehyde test) are based upon the high IgG levels.

Helminth infections can produce very high levels of non-specific IgE, much higher than those seen in atopic subjects. This appears to be a general phenomenon with all helminths having tissue stages; particularly high levels are reached in ascariasis, toxocariasis, trichinosis, schistosomiasis and filariasis. On the basis of animal experiments it was at one time proposed that helminths might provoke anamnestic responses in atopic persons sensitive to various allergens. However there is no evidence in man that asthma or any other atopic disease is exacerbated by helminths. More recently the converse hypothesis has been proposed that the high levels of IgE in worm infections might block most of the binding sites on tissue mast cells and thereby prevent a cell degranulation in the presence of atopic allergens, which must bind to two adjacent IgE molecules. Asthma and hay fever do appear to be fairly uncommon in the rural tropics, at least among young children, and *in vitro* the serum of patients with heavy helminth infections blocks mast cell degranulation in lung tissue. *Ascaris* and hookworm are the main candidates for this possible protective effect, but the evidence is still rather tenuous. From a diagnostic viewpoint a high level of total IgE in the absence of atopy is quite strongly suggestive of an helminthic infection.

Activation of T cell system

In a manner analogous to B cell activation, parasites promote lymphocyte transformation in a series of T cell lymphocyte clones. The activated lymphocytes (lymphoblasts) perform several immunological functions. Of great importance is specific cell-mediated cytotoxicity, which is responsible for the delayed cellular immune reactions seen in many parasitic infections. In addition to direct cytotoxicity, the local release of lymphokines causes non-specific cell damage, induces blast transformation of normal lymphocytes, activates macrophages and by inhibiting macrophage migration, facilitates their accumulation at the site of the lesion.

Two other phenomena are related to T cell activation: the systemic proliferation of macrophages and eosinophils. The former occurs within for example the spleen in malaria or leishmaniasis, and can be partly attributed to 'work hypertrophy' consequent upon extra tissue debris being presented to the system. However there is in several protozoan infections evidence of increased marrow production of monocytes, often reflected in a blood monocytosis, and this phenomenon appears to be mediated by the T cell system. In many helminthic infections eosinophils accumulate in the tissues, and are numerous in the peripheral blood; they are produced in increased numbers by the marrow. There is good evidence based particularly upon experimental *Trichinella* infections, that this eosinophil response is immunologically mediated by the T cell system. It is antigen specific, shows an accelerated anamnestic response on secondary challenge, and can be passively transferred by lymphocyte suspensions but not serum.

EFFECT OF IMMUNE RESPONSE UPON PARASITES

A. Protozoa

Destructive mechanisms are similar to those occurring in bacterial infections. In the case of extracellular parasites coating with antibody may lead to complement mediated cytolysis, or opsonisation and ingestion by phagocytes. Parasite immobilisation is common and may be especially important in flagellates. Even if the protozoan is not killed, it is more likely to be taken up by macrophages; trophozoites of *Entamoeba histolytica*, however, can apparently remobilise after temporary inactivation by antibody. Agglutination may be less common although it can be demonstrated *in vitro* with *Trypanosoma brucei* in the presence of antibody. Some antibodies have specific activity against certain parasite functions, thus multiplication of trypanosomes is inhibited by an antibody called ablastin. Antibody coating may also facilitate attack by 'killer' (K) cells. Sensitised T cells sometimes damage parasites specifically by direct contact or by the release of non-specific toxic mediators. Secretory IgA possibly damages intraluminal gut parasites such as *Giardia*, which may also be injured directly by T cells crossing the gut epithelium.

Intracellular parasites within macrophages, such as *Leishmania* and *Toxoplasma*, are destroyed *in situ* by macrophage activation, mediated by the T cell system. Although this mechanism is generated by exposure to a specific antigen, the macrophage-dwelling parasites are destroyed non-specific in its effects, hence any other macrophage-dwelling parasites are destroyed simultaneously.

B. Metazoa

Many effector mechanisms that destroy microbes are not much use against large parasites such as worms. Indeed with some of the larger species it is difficult to visualise how any immune mechanism can kill its target. Another consideration is that mechanisms demonstrated *in vitro* may have little effect within the host. Thus when small nematode larvae are incubated in immune serum, precipitates form around the mouth, anus and vulva, and sometimes the worm is killed. Similarly schistosome eggs *in vitro* are killed by precipitates of antibody — the so-called circumoval precipitation test, and schistosome cercariae become coated in a thick immune precipitate that kills the larvae — the 'cercarienhüllen reaction'. Whether such reactions occur *in vivo* is unknown. One thing that is clear is that antibody does not normally attach to the undamaged surface of the adult worm.

One manifestation of partial immunity in nematode infections is the delayed or arrested development of migrating tissue stages; the parasite survives but maturation is prevented. Whether this happens in man is uncertain; the hookworm *Ancylostoma duodenale* does have a period of arrested development lasting several months, but whether this is an intrinsic biological characteristic or an immunological phenomenon is not known. An example from veterinary medicine is *Toxocara canis* in the dog; migrating larvae are arrested in adult immune hosts, but in pregnant bitches immunity declines and the larvae reactivate so that many are transferred to the puppies by the transmammary and transplacental routes.

Cellular coating of larval helminths is now believed to be very important. In the presence of antibody several kinds of cells will attach to larval schistosomes, microfilariae, and also larval hookworms and *Strongyloides*. The principal cells involved are eosinophils, but macrophages and lymphocytes will also attach under certain conditions; the attached lymphocytes could include non-specific K cells. The worm surface is damaged by lysosomal enzymes released by the attached cells; this damage may be lethal. This is one mechanism by which schistosomulae are killed in the dermis or lungs following cercarial penetration. It is also likely that some hookworm larvae are killed by this mechanism as they pass through lymph nodes *en route* to the lungs from the feet. Microfilariae are usually only killed by this mechanism when their cuticle has been damaged; the microfilaricidal drug diethylcarbamazine has no direct lethal action, but it damages the cuticle in a subtle way that allows attachment of antibody and cells.

Another quite distinct mechanism is immune expulsion of worms from the gut. Worms attached to the gut wall may be directly attacked by cellular immune mechanisms in the mucosa. They may also provoke sudden increases in capillary permeability due to IgE-mediated mast cell degranulation. The latter mechanism allows high concentrations of serum antibody to come in contact with the worm; in addition release of pharmacological mediators could increase gut motility and expel the worms. IgE-mediated mast cell degranulation can also operate in local reactions in any tissue by causing oedema and assisting the local penetration of antibody and immunologically competent cells.

Immunity in arthropod infections also particularly involves IgE. The duration of ixodid tick feeding is shortened in sensitised animals, but it is doubtful whether comparatively rapidly feeding insects, such as mosquitoes, are affected by immune reactions. It can be argued, however, that the pruritic nature of reactions to bites alters host behaviour to minimise further exposure. In human scabies there is clear evidence that acquired immunity normally limits and finally eliminates the mite population; IgE mechanisms are almost certainly involved.

With many helminths a state of compromise is achieved between the host and its parasites. The host tolerates low or even moderate loads of adult worms but the presence of the latter maintains an immune mechanism which limits the survival of further incoming larvae; this is called **concomitant immunity**. Elegant transplantation experiments with schistosomes have shown that immunity against new infections is maintained only in the presence of adult worms which, although unharmed, provide the necessary antigenic stimulus. Death of worms in tissues can do considerable damage and it is sometimes in the host's interest not to kill the parasite. Examples are the severe reactions around dead filarial worms in lymph nodes, the eye damage occuring when onchocerciasis patients are given chemotherapy, and reactions around cerebral cysticerci which often remain clinically silent until the cysts die.

EVASION OF IMMUNE ATTACK BY PARASITES

Successful parasites have evolved mechanisms for limiting the damage done to them by the host's immune response. Prolonged infections and superinfection are only possible when some form of evasion is achieved.

1. Intracellular location

Many protozoa multiply intracellularly. *Plasmodium* and *Babesia* do so within erythrocytes, and *Toxoplasma*, *Trypanosoma cruzi*, *Isospora* and *Sarcocystis* do so within a variety of tissue cells. *Leishmania* and *Toxoplasma* multiply within macrophages. Antibody cannot harm intracellular parasites but they must all run the gauntlet of immunological attack, by cells and antibody, when their host cell ruptures and new ones must be entered. All protective immunity in malaria operates in the brief interval between a mature schizont rupturing an erythrocyte and the released merozoites gaining entry into a new red cell. Macrophage parasites have the advantage that their host cells may divide and disperse the parasites without them having to pass through an extracellular medium. However, in immune hosts, macrophages can be activated, by T cell systems, to destroy their parasites *in situ*. Even an interstitial location may be advantageous; titres of antibody to *Trypanosoma brucei* in tissue fluid are only 20 per cent of those in serum.

2. Lumen-dwelling

A great many parasites live within the body cavities that communicate with the outside world, particularly the gut. This not only facilitates dispersal of infective forms but it also limits immunological attack. Immune expulsion mechanisms do operate but in man, at least, they are apparently not very efficient. The role of secretory IgA in parasitic infections remains doubtful. *Entamoeba histolytica* has adopted an ideal lifestyle for, in its normal commensal form within the colonic lumen, it is unaffected by serum antibody or cellular immunity. Some resistance may develop to tissue invasion but the longevity of intraluminal infection is unaffected.

3. Antigenic variation

Trypanosoma brucei can adopt a series of over 20 different surface antigens. New antigenic forms appear when antibody responses have nearly eliminated the previous form. A genetic switch mechanism is involved and the sequence may vary although it always reverts to the same type in the vector. The prolonged persistance of *T.b. gambiense* is explained by this mechanism. A similar phenomenon occurs in many mammalian malarial infections and it could explain the recrudescences of human malaria.

4. Antigenic disguise

Some parasites appear to have evolved surface antigens that are so similar to certain host components that they are not recognised as foreign by immunological surveillance. Another strategy, adopted by adult schistosomes, is to take up host antigens, including blood group substances, to achieve the same result.

5. Inert cuticular surface

Most adult nematodes are covered by a thick cuticle which, when undamaged, is so poorly antigenic that very little immune response is mounted against it.

6. Location within cysts

Larval tapeworms are enclosed within capsules, comprising host and parasite components; when undamaged these are almost impermeable to loss of antigen or entry of antibody. Damage to the cyst wall allows antigen to escape, and parasite death usually has the same effect.

Toxoplasma forms tissue cysts in the brain and retina that are impervious, they persist through their host's life span. Occasionally they rupture and initiate new disease activity, especially when the host's immunity is compromised. The cysts of *Sarcocystis* within muscle are also impermeable to antibody.

7. Immunological tolerance

(a) Prenatal transfer

Parasite antigen is sometimes present in peripheral blood and it is likely that some is transferred transplacentally to the foetus, which may thereafter be partially tolerant to that antigen. Experimentally, this form of tolerance can be produced in schistosomal infections and there is suggestive evidence that this happens in man also. Filarial infections may also produce this form of tolerance. Tissue reactions to both of these parasites are often much less in indigenous subjects than in immigrants.

(b) Low-zone tolerance

In some parasitic infections the number of organisms is small, their growth is slow and the release of antigen into the circulation is at a very low level. Low-zone tolerance can be established by persis-

tent sub-immunogenic doses of antigen. Once established the tolerance could operate over a wide range of antigenic doses.

(c) High-zone tolerance

At the other extreme some parasites release huge amounts of antigen and immune complexes into the circulation. In this circumstance high-zone tolerance may be established in both B and T cell lines.

PERSISTENCE OF PARASITES WITHIN THEIR HOSTS

Protozoa

Only in cutaneous leishmaniasis can complete sterile immunity and resistance to reinfection be regarded as the normal outcome of infection. But even in this group of infections the parasites sometimes persist; thus *L.braziliense* can metastasise to the nasopharynx many years after the primary infection; *L. tropica* can cause chronic recidivans lesions; and certain predisposed persons infected with *L. mexicana* or *L. aethiopica* can develop the anergic form of disease known as diffuse cutaneous leishmaniasis (p. 143).

Lifelong persistence of the parasites with immunity to reinfection occurs in *Trypanosoma cruzi*, *Toxoplasma* and *Sarcocystis* infections; in the latter two, the parasites remain dormant and non-dividing within tissue cysts. In *T. cruzi* low-grade proliferation continues throughout life in certain tissue cells. Immunity to reinfection in the presence of current infection is known as **premunition**, a term that is applied mainly to protozoan infections. Premunition is virtually synonymous with concomitant immunity (p. 95), a term applied mainly to helminth infections.

In all other protozoan infections, reinfections are possible despite a variable degree of acquired resistance. Individual infections can persist for a long time; *E. histolytica* for at least 20 years as a colonic commensal, and *Plasmodium malariae* as a very low grade erythrocytic infection, liable to recrudescences, for up to 40 years.

Helminths

No examples of complete acquired immunity to helminths are known in man, and the persistence of an individual worm is determined mainly by its own longevity, for once having gained maturity they are usually unaffected by host immune mechanisms. *Clonorchis sinensis*, *Onchocerca volvulus* and *Echinococcus granulosus* can all survive, as individuals, for about 20 years. At the other end of the scale, the adults of *Enterobius vermicularis* and *Trichinella spiralis* live only a few weeks.

While reinfections can, to some extent, occur in all helminthic infections there are a few in which autoinfection accounts for their persistence. This occurs externally by transfer of eggs in *E. vermicularis* and *Hymenolepis nana* infections. In *Taenia solium*, external or internal autoinfection produces cysticercosis. In *Strongyloides stercoralis* infection, internal and perianal autoinfection account for its persistence for as long as 35 years; while each adult female worm lives only a few months. Internal autoinfection is also believed to occur in *Capillaria philippinensis* infections, so allowing very high loads to build up.

MECHANISMS OF HOST DAMAGE BY PARASITES

1. Direct physical and chemical damage to tissues

Intracellular protozoa usually kill the host cell within which they multiply; an exception being parasites within dividing macrophages. The anaemia in malaria and babesiosis is mainly due to direct red cell destruction. Protozoa living in other cells cause most of their damage from the local inflammatory reactions that follow cell rupture.

Some protozoa release cytolytic enzymes on contact with host cells. Thus invasive *Entamoeba histolytica* and *Balantidium coli* facilitate their passage by killing cells they meet; *E. histolytica* can also destroy host leucocytes. In all these examples the resulting cellular debris forms a rich papulum upon which the protozoan population feeds.

Vascular blockage is an important feature in falciparum malaria; capillaries, particularly those in the brain, become occluded by sticky parasitised red cells that adhere to the endothelium. Vascular narrowing of the pulmonary arterioles and of the hepatic radicles of the portal vein in schistosomiasis is secondary to granuloma formation. Other worms cause occlusions directly; thus *Dirofilaria immitis* can block small pulmonary arteries, and *Morerastronglylus costaricensis* the small mesenteric arteries. Small bowel obstruction can result from an impacted mass of *Ascaris* worms, and wandering individuals of this large species can block other hollow viscera that they may enter. Several bile duct parasites can cause intraluminal blockage and hydatid cysts can compress the biliary tract by external pressure.

The feeding activity of several adult worms may directly damage mucosal surfaces; examples are hookworm in the jejunum and *Fasciola* in the bile ducts. The irritant effect of large worms in the gut promotes peristalsis.

Larval cestodes damage local tissues as they expand; there is very little inflammatory response until the parasite leaks antigenic materials or dies. Migrating larval worms and other metazoa cause direct mechanical damage to tissues as they pass through them.

Many parasites damage tissues by provoking inflammatory changes that are not mediated immunologically. Although human parasites liberate no tissue toxins some of their metabolic products, for example the saliva of ectoparasites and the secretions of helminths relating to their tissue penetrating behaviour, do set up direct inflammatory changes. Capillary permeability is increased and inflammatory cells enter the area. In addition, inflammation is generated by the products of host cell death caused physically by the parasites, or by immunological mechanisms.

2. Tissue damage by immunological mechanisms

Immunopathological responses are of great importance in parasitic disease. This is now an area of intensive study and recent findings have greatly increased our understanding of the disease mechanisms. Examples of all four types of hypersensitivity response, as defined by Coombs and Gell, have been delineated. Mixed responses are common. Reactions are often precipitated by the death of parasites in tissue, and this can be an unwanted effect of chemotherapy.

Type 1 — IgE-mediated immediate hypersensitivity

Tissue mast cells, primed with IgE, degranulate when antigen molecules form bridging links between adjacent IgE molecules. The granules release histamine, heparin, and serotonin; and plasma kinins are activated. The best examples of this type of reaction are immediate sensitivity reactions to insect bites, and local or generalised anaphylaxis in response to leakage of hydatid cyst fluid. Diagnostic skin tests giving immediate reactions to intradermal injection of parasite antigen are mediated in this way; they can be elicited in most helminthic infections, as these nearly always induce a strong IgE response. By contrast protozoa induce very little, if any, IgE in their hosts and immediate skin test responses are very unusual, although they have been reported in active invasive amoebiasis.

There are numerous examples of this type of immunopathology in helminthic disease; they include the acute phase of schistosomal infections that appears soon after egg laying begins, the acute lymphadenitis and acute lymphangitis produced by lymphatic-dwelling filarial worms, the acute myositis of trichinosis and the acute lung pathology caused by the larvae of *Ascaris* and other nematodes as they migrate through lung tissue into the alveoli. In many examples, however, the reaction is a mixed one and Type 3 (immune complex mediated) reactions are occurring more or less simultaneously.

IgE antibodies initiate the immune expulsion mechanism that eliminates some helminths from the gut.

Type 2 — Complement mediated cytolytic reactions

When antibody combines with antigens on the surface of host cells, the complement system may be activated and the cell destroyed. This is the least common form of immunopathology in parasitic disease. Although non-specific immunoglobulin responses are common in some parasitic infections and reactivity to host tissues can be some-

times demonstrated by immunoflourescence, no damage is done, except to red blood cells. Immunologically-mediated haemolysis occurs in malaria and trypanosomiasis, and perhaps also in schistosomiasis, babesiosis and other infections. Complement can sometimes be demonstrated on the red cell surface, and less commonly immunoglobulin. However it is not clear whether the parasitic infection induces antibody with true red cell specificity, or whether parasite antigen or immune complexes attach non-specifically to the red cell. The result is the same; complement-mediated lysis, or opsonisation and removal by the reticuloendothelial system. The process is arrested when the parasitic infection is eliminated.

Type 3 — Immune complex reactions

Combination of antibody with parasite antigen may initiate a sequence of changes that lead to inflammation, oedema, infiltration by neutrophil polymorphs and damage to tissue cells. The outcome is greatly influenced by whether the complexes are formed in the tissues, to produce a typical **Arthus response**, or are formed in the circulation.

Complexes of antigen and antibody initiate the release of vasoactive amines by three mechanisms; the activation of complement, platelet aggregation, and activation of the kinin system via Hageman factor. The activation of complement also releases compounds chemotactic to polymorphs which infiltrate the area, degenerate and release their lysosomal enzymes. It is the combined effect of lysosomal enzymes and vasoactive amines that produces the Arthus reaction. Damage to small blood vessels is often prominent and endogenous pyrogen is liberated so that fever is a common accompaniment. When tissue immune complex reactions occur in helminthic infections local infiltration by eosinophils is common. The complexes are themselves chemotactic to eosinophils, and these cells are believed to modulate the severity of the reaction by destroying some of the complexes before severe tissue injury is done.

An Arthus reaction can occur in the dermis when skin tests for helminths are performed or it can follow an insect bite. The inflammatory response appears between two and 24 hours later, being intermediate between the immediate sensitivity component and the delayed cellular response (Type 4 reaction).

This type of tissue reaction is common in many helminth infections, especially when worms die in the tissues. Thus it is partly responsible for the acute lymph node and lymph vessel reactions of lymphatic filariasis, the myositis of trichinosis and the lung pathology produced by migrating nematodes, such as *Ascaris*. Tropical pulmonary eosinophilia, an abnormal sensitivity reaction to filarial infection, is a typical reaction of this kind. In the acute phase of schistosomiasis an illness much resembling serum sickness is produced with fever, severe malaise, urticaria and generalised lymphadenopathy. The chemotherapy of filariasis is particularly liable to precipitate reactions of this type; in the lymphatic-dwelling species a lymphatic reaction is produced; in onchocerciasis the reaction is in the dermis and eye, following local destruction of microfilariae. The skin reaction in onchocerciasis is very vigorous and relatively few microfilariae in the dermis can provoke severe itching, hence the use of this reaction in the **Mazzotti diagnostic test**; the ocular reactions during the treatment of onchocerciasis may be very severe and iridocyclitis can precipitate blindness. Treatment of sleeping sickness patients can precipitate an immune complex mediated encephalitis.

Circulating immune complexes in parasitic diseases can produce glomerulonephritis; the most well studied examples being those caused by quartan malaria (*P. malariae*) and by *Schistosoma mansoni*. Transient glomerular damage by this mechanism, probably also occurs in acute falciparum malaria and during the treatment of *Trypanosoma b. rhodesiense* and *Loa loa* infections. It is likely that other examples of immune complex mediated renal damage will soon become apparent.

Type 4 — Delayed cell-mediated immune reactions (CMI)

This type of reaction is mediated by specifically sensitised T lymphocytes and these cells accumulate in the local lesion. Lymphokines liberated by these cells cause the accumulation and activation of macrophages. The result is a local granuloma.

CMI reactions in parasitic disease rarely lead to giant cell formation. While specifically sensitised T lymphocyte populations can be demonstrated in many parasitic infections, using the *in vitro* test for lymphoblast transformation to antigen; in relatively few infections are CMI reactions of great importance pathologically. The two notable exceptions are leishmaniasis and schistosomiasis.

The CMI response underlies the 'delayed' skin test responses seen after intradermal injection of parasite antigen; like the tuberculin test, they are maximal between 48 and 72 hours after testing. Delayed skin test reactions occur in toxoplasmosis, amoebiasis and many helminth infections, but in these they are of little diagnostic use. In contrast the leishmanin test in cutaneous leishmaniasis is a valuable diagnostic tool.

The lesions of cutaneous leishmaniasis evolve in parallel with the CMI response. Initially the lesion is papular and heavily infiltrated with lymphocytes, and also with macrophages, many of them parasitised. The vigorous CMI response in the dermis eventually causes ischaemic necrosis of the overlying epidermis to produce an ulcer. Later activated macrophages destroy all the parasites and the lesion heals. Persons unable to mount a specific CMI response develop the diffuse or anergic form of disease; in this condition there is little lymphocytic infiltrate, the epidermis remains intact and the *Leishmania* amastigotes continue to proliferate.

The egg granuloma, the basic lesion of schistosomiasis, is mainly a CMI response. The egg lies at the centre, slowly degenerates and later disappears; eventually the lesion is replaced by fibrosis. Experimentally the egg granuloma can be simulated in mice by the intravenous injection of latex particles coated with schistosomal antigen; typical granulomas are produced in the lung where the particles are arrested. Granulomatous reactions leading to fibrosis produce the typical schistosomal pathology in the walls of the urinary tract, gut, hepatic radicles of the portal vein and the pulmonary arteries.

CMI contributes to the inflammatory changes seen in trichinosis, lymphatic filariasis and trypanosomiasis. In toxoplasmosis rupture of infected cells, particularly in the retina, causes local CMI reactions.

3. Induction of Neoplastic changes

Only two human parasites are known to cause cancer.

Clonorchis and *Opisthorchis* flukes can cause cholangiocarcinomas originating in the bile ducts.

Schistosoma haematobium can initiate squamous cell bladder cancers. There is some evidence that *S. japonicum* can initiate colonic cancers, but this has been disputed.

HOST SUSCEPTIBILITY

A. Genetic factors

Studies with inbred strains of laboratory animals have shown that the susceptibility to many parasitic infections, and also the host immune response to them is under genetic control. In man it is likely that genetic factors explain some of the varied disease patterns seen in different individuals and populations. This is an area where more work needs to be done, the HLA system is potentially important but no definite associations are yet reported.

Among the blood group genes, persons without Duffy group substance are much less susceptible to *P. vivax* malaria and this probably explains the virtual absence of this malarial species in West Africa where the indigenous population is mainly Duffy negative. Blood group A persons appear to be more susceptible to giardiasis. Persons heterozygous for haemoglobin S, who have sickle cell trait AS, show a reduced prevalence of *P. falciparum*, much lower levels of parasitaemia and a virtual absence of cerebral malaria. This is an example of balanced polymorphism, the geographical distribution of the sickle cell gene corresponds quite closely with intensity of malaria transmission. At equilibrium a stable gene frequency is maintained when excess deaths from malaria in AA persons are exactly balanced by deaths from sickle cell anaemia in SS persons. There is now good evidence that deficiency in the red cell enzyme glucose 6 phosphate dehydrogenase is related to malaria in a similar way; and possibly also haemoglobins C and E. The interactions between red cell characteristics and malaria parasites can now be studied using *in vitro* cultures. *P. fal-*

ciparum grows less well in the respective red cells; in AS cells the parasites also induce premature sickling and this hastens the removal of the parasites from the circulation.

B. Immunodeficiency

Several types of abnormal immune response can predispose to parasitic infection. The effects of pregnancy and protein energy malnutrition are included here because they probably operate through impairment of CMI responses. The known relationships are listed here; others will doubtless be found.

1. *Pneumocystis* — Overt infections are almost entirely confined to (a) severely debilitated or malnourished infants; (b) patients on steroid and immunosuppressive drugs; (c) persons with hypogammaglobulinaemia (IgG or IgM), or specific defects in CMI response.

2. *Babesia* — The very rare infections derived from cattle (*B. bovis*) have nearly all been in splenectomised persons. Rodent babesiosis (*B. microti*) however, can occur in normal persons.

3. *Toxoplasma* — Latent infections are reactivated in persons with lymphatic tumours or those taking immunosuppressive drugs.

4. Malaria — splenectomy predisposes to increased levels of parasitaemia and sometimes fulminating infections with *P. falciparum*. Pregnancy also increases parasitaemia and morbidity.

5. *Entamoeba histolytica* — Tissue invasion is more common in the following situations: (a) patients taking steroid enemas, systemic corticosteroids, or immunosuppressive drugs; (b) debilitating disease; (c) late pregnancy and the puerperium; (d) protein energy malnutrition.

6. Giardiasis — Severe in (a) primary hypogammaglobulinaemia, especially the variable non-selective form and patients with nodular lymphoid hyperplasia; (b) selective IgA deficiency.

7. *Isopora belli* — Prolonged infections are more likely in persons with lymphoid tumours.

8. *Acanthamoeba* — This soil amoeba is opportunistic in persons with debilitating disease and lymphoid tumours.

9. *Strongyloides* — Hyperinfection is common in the following situations: (a) during steroid and

immunosuppressive therapy; (b) lymphoid tumours; (c) other malignancies and debilitating diseases; (d) protein energy malnutrition.

10. Scabies — Hyperinfection ('Norwegian scabies') can occur in persons taking steroids and immunosuppressive drugs, in mongolism and in gross debility.

C. Age, sex and pregnancy

Most age and sex relationships with parasitism derive from differing levels of exposure and acquired immunity. One of the factors restraining malarial parasitaemias in young infants is the presence of haemoglobin F in erythrocytes; *in vitro* studies show that this haemoglobin supports the growth of *P. falciparum* less readily than does haemoglobin A. Above the age of puberty amoebic liver abscesses are at least five times commoner in males than females; before puberty the sex incidence is equal. Amoebic dysentery does not show this sex difference. Pregnancy predisposes to malaria, invasive amoebiasis and symptomatic trichomoniasis (p. 173).

D. Nutritional status

The three parasitic infections most likely to be exacerbated by protein energy malnutrition in children are invasive amoebiasis, strongyloidiasis and pneumocystosis; their importance in this context has been underestimated, and depressed CMI may be the underlying mechanism. Although repeated malarial infections can severely impair nutritional status, a paradoxical situation occurs in the severly malnourished child who rarely gets very high *P. falciparum* parasitaemias, and almost never dies of cerebral malaria. It appears that the grossly malnourished host cannot support the parasite's own nutritional requirements. Similarly patients with terminal cancer cannot easily be experimentally infected with *Leishmania donovani*.

Experimentally a milk diet has a prominent protective effect against malaria in several mammalian species. Such a diet is deficient in para-amino benzoic acid, an essential nutrient for *Plasmodium*, and when this is added to the milk diet the protection disappears. Whether breast-fed infants are protected against malaria in this way is not known. Some reports suggest that severe iron deficiency is protective against malaria in man, and that iron therapy, or an iron rich diet, may precipitate severe malaria; however this relationship has been disputed.

E. Local diseases predisposing to parasitism

Several examples are known:

1. *Entamoeba histolytica* — Invasive amoebiasis may be superimposed upon colonic and rectal malignancies.

2. *Strongyloides* — Small bowel stasis predisposes to autoinfection and the dangerous hyperinfection state can result, especially when the helminthic infection itself causes paralytic ileus. Other relevant forms of stasis are mechanical obstruction, chagasic megacolon, the abuse of antidiarrhoeal drugs, or even simple constipation with or without diverticulosis.

3. *Trichomonas vaginalis* — Cervical cancers predispose to heavy infections with this parasite.

4. *Acanthamoeba* — This facultative parasite can be a secondary invader of corneal ulcers, gastric mucosal lesions or even cerebral infarcts.

5. 'Norwegian scabies' — Persons with peripheral neuropathy, including that due to leprosy, may develop this state of hyperinfection.

6. Hypochlorhydria — This predisposes to giardiasis and, possibly, also to guinea worm infection.

FURTHER READING

Beeson, P.B. and Bass, D.A. (1977) *The Eosinophil*. Philadelphia: W.B. Saunders Co.

CIBA Foundation Symposium (1974) No. 25 Parasites in the Immunised Host: Mechanisms of Survival. Amsterdam: Associated Scientific Publishers.

Cohen, S. and Sadun, E.H. (eds) (1976) *Immunology of Parasitic Infections*. Oxford: Blackwell.

Edington, G.M. and Gilles, H.M. (1976) *Pathology in the Tropics*, 2nd edition. London: E. Arnold (Publishers) Ltd.

Marcial-Rojas, R.A. (ed.) (1971) *Pathology of Protozoal and Helminthic Diseases*. Baltimore: Williams and Wilkins

Mims, C.A. (1977) *The Pathogenesis of Infectious Disease*. London: Academic Press.

Taylor, A.E.R. (ed.) (1968) Immunity to parasites: Sixth Symposium of the British Society for Parasitology. Oxford: Blackwell Scientific Publications.

Warren, K.S. (1972) The immunopathogenesis of schistosomiasis. A multidisciplinary approach. *Trans. R. Soc. trop. Med. Hyg.*, **66**, 417–432.

Weir, D.M. (1977) *Immunology. An Outline for Students of Medicine and Biology*, 4th edition. Edinburgh: Churchill Livingstone.

World Health Organization (1977) Immune complexes in disease. *Tech.Rep.Series* no. 606. Geneva: WHO.

7

Local effects of parasitism 1

A. GASTROINTESTINAL DISEASE

The clinical presentations of the numerous parasites affecting the gut are diverse; some parasites can present in several different ways. The anatomical location of the different parasites is shown in Table 7.1. While there are several fairly clearly defined modes of presentation, some infections simply produce poorly localised abdominal pains, or less commonly a non-specific diarrhoea. An important consideration is that the identification of an infection by stool microscopy does not necessarily imply that it is the cause of a patient's symptoms; this applies particularly to many light

Table 7.1 Anatomical location of gastrointestinal parasites

Lumen only	Small bowel (normally)	*Ascaris*
	Colon and rectum	*Entamoeba histolytica* } commensal *Balantidium* } forms *Enterobius*
Mucosal attachment	Small bowel	*Giardia* Tapeworms (adult) Hookworm, *Trichostrongylus* *Fasciolopsis, Echinostoma* *Heterophyes, Metagonimus*
	Ileo-caecal region	*Ternidens* (+ transient mucosal invasion)
	Large bowel	*Trichuris, Gastrodiscoides*
Epithelial cell invasion	Small bowel	*Isospora belli* *Sarcocystis hominis, S. suihominis*
Mucosal invasion	Stomach or small bowel	*Anisakis*★
	Small bowel	*Trichinella*★, *Strongyloides* *Capillaria philippinensis*
	Large bowel	*Entamoeba histolytica, Balantidium* *Oesophagostomium*★
Smooth muscle cells, autonomic nerve plexuses	Oesophagus and large bowel (mainly)	*Trypanosoma cruzi*★
Mesenteric veins (adults), gut wall and mucosa (eggs)	Ileum and colon Colon (mainly)	*Schistosoma japonicum* *S. mansoni, S. intercalatum*
Mesenteric arteries (adults), gut wall (eggs)	Ileo-caecal region (mainly)	*Morerastrongylus*★
Peritoneal lesions	–	*Paragonimus*★ (ectopic) *Armillifer armillatus*★ (pentastome) Hydatid cyst★ (secondary)

Parasites not normally diagnosed by stool examination are marked with an asterisk★

helminthic infections which are often completely symptomless. Exclusion of other pathologies is often necessary before attributing a patient's symptoms to a gut parasite. Some of these infections often present with non-gut manifestations, for example hookworm presenting as iron deficiency anaemia, and intestinal schistosomiasis presenting as hepatosplenomegaly. Another common presentation is as wasting and growth retardation (p. 168).

The majority of the commoner infections are normally recognised by stool microscopy (Table 7.1). Egg counts per gramme of faeces are of value when morbidity is being assessed in hookworm, *Ascaris, Trichuris, Trichostrongylus* and schistosomal infections. In other instances the finding of even scanty parasites in stool concentrates may be highly significant (*Strongyloides, Capillaria philippinensis, Entamoeba, Balantidium* and *Isospora*). Microscopy of duodenal aspirates or 'string tests' can be of value in infections of the upper jejunum and duodenum (*Giardia, Strongyloides*). Proctoscopy and sigmoidoscopy are very useful procedures in amoebiasis and balantidiasis, and gastroscopy has found useful in *Anisakis* infections; but otherwise endoscopy is of limited value. Radiological studies of the gut are of relatively little value except to demonstrate certain local lesions, the chagasic megasyndromes, or in the acute abdominal situations of gut obstruction or perforation: however radiology is often necessary to exclude other conditions. Serology is of some value in intestinal amoebiasis and is useful in the chagasic syndromes; otherwise it is currently of little value. Blood eosinophilia can occur in any of the helminthic infections but very high levels are suggestive of strongyloidiasis, fasciolopsiasis or trichinosis. When secondary complications have appeared, and in those infections where man is an abnormal host (*Oesophagostomium, Anisakis, Morerastrongylus* etc.) diagnosis is sometimes only made at laparotomy in an emergency context.

Visible parasites and pruritus ani

Only the most fastidious observers are likely to notice any but three kinds of parasite in their stool. *Ascaris* is immediately recognisable by its large size and superficial resemblance to a large and rather pale earthworm. Tapeworm proglottids (*Taenia and Diphyllobothrium*) may be passed singly or in short ribbons; some patients will make drawings of their parasites showing remarkable detail. *Taenia saginata* proglottids have the disconcerting habit of migrating spontaneously through the anus, an event preceded by its subjectively recognisable passage down the anal canal; the proglottids of this worm continue to move actively for some time after they are passed, *T. solium* is far less active.

Threadworms (*Enterobius*) will usually be recognised on the stool surface or in undergarments or night attire. Mothers frequently notice them on the perianal skin of their children. The size, colour and wriggling movements of *Enterobius* are unmistakable.

Pruritus ani due to *Enterobius* results not only from the nocturnal migrations of the female worm upon the perianal skin, but is also due to sensitisation especially when worms are ruptured by scratching. Most of the other manifestations of this parasite, lethargy, nervousness etc. are due to sleep loss together with anxiety — mainly parental. *Taenia saginata* also produces pruritus ani and both infections can be recognised by finding eggs on cellophane anal swabs. External autoinfection by *Strongyloides* larvae produces perianal lesions but these usually extend to the buttocks; the linear urticarial tracks, produced by each larva, will normally be visible.

Acute gastroenteritis — Trichinosis (Trichinella spiralis)

For up to two weeks after eating undercooked infected meat, usually pork, patients may complain of nausea, vomiting, abdominal pains and watery diarrhoea. During 'common source' outbreaks, this infection may be mistaken for other types of food poisoning; fever is common and may suggest typhoid fever, eosinophilia appears after about 10 days followed soon after by myositis and other manifestations. The gut phase of the infection coincides with the invasion of the small gut mucosa by the adult worms and the viviparous larviposition into the tissues by the female worm. It is very rare indeed for adult *T. spiralis* or their larvae to be found in stool specimens. Recognition of the early illness is important, and often possible during outbreaks, since prompt chemotherapy will arrest the infective process and prevent larval dissemination to the tissues.

Dysentery

The dysenteric syndrome comprises the passage of frequent liquid or semiformed stools containing blood, and commonly mucus. It is caused by several parasites that produce ulceration of the colon. The differential diagnosis in acute illness will be mainly shigellosis and in more chronic ones nonspecific ulcerative colitis and neoplasm.

1. Amoebiasis

Invasion of the colonic mucosa by *Entamoeba histolytica* is most common in the rectosigmoid and caecum, but the whole colon may be affected or any part of it. Superficial erosions extend into the submucosa where they expand to form flask-shaped ulcers, later there may be extensive undermining of the submucosa and patchy mucosal loss. The inflammatory exudate is predominently lymphocytes and macrophages, secondary bacterial infection is variable and neutrophils are sometimes plentiful. Amoebae are seen at the periphery of the lesions extending into healthy tissue. Very extensive involvement produces toxic megacolon, the bowel wall becomes extremely friable and multiple perforations can occur. Less commonly deep localised lesions perforate acutely. Erosion of large blood vessels is relatively uncommon, but blood transfusion is sometimes necessary.

Symptoms vary greatly in severity from mild relapsing bowel upsets with blood-stained stools to fulminant dysentery. High fever and tenesmus are less common than in bacillary dysentery. Moderate tenderness over the affected colon is common. Stools are often foul-smelling, and usually haematophagous amoebae will be found together with red cells amd macrophages. When amoebae are not found in the stool, proctoscopy or sigmoidoscopy should be performed and scrapings taken from any lesions that are seen. Fresh wet preparations must be searched for living amoebae; their recognition in histological sections is

difficult. Amoebic ulcers often have pouting raised edges; the intervening mucosa is usually normal in appearance. Serology is positive in about 70 per cent of patients.

The chemotherapy of uncomplicated amoebic dysentery is relatively straightforward (p. 198). Parasitological cure is essential otherwise relapses are common. Acute perforation can be dealt with surgically. But the more common multiple perforations of a dilated colon cannot be repaired; conservative management with gastric suction, intravenous fluids and emetine injections will often succeed but mortality rates of 30 per cent are common in this situation.

More chronic local lesions known as **amoebomas** may develop in isolation or in the context of relapsing dysentery; they are proliferative granulomatous reactions and can be detected by endoscopy or barium enema. Response to chemotherapy is rapid. Amoebic strictures are more fibrotic reactions usually situated in the rectosigmoid. A few patients who are successfully treated parasitologically continue to have dysenteric symptoms. This **post-dysenteric colitis** may be helped by salazopyrin, it is usually self-limited and further chemotherapy is unnecessary.

2. Balantidiasis

This relatively rare infection gives rise to pathological and clinical findings very similar to those of amoebic dysentery. Ulcers tend to be deep and early perforation is not uncommon. The ciliated trophozoites will be found in stools or rectal scrapings.

3. Trichuriasis

Heavy infections with *T. trichiura* will produce dysentery, especially in children. The worms are attached to the colonic mucosa by their anterior ends which lie embedded in the mucosa. Acute inflammatory reactions surround the sites of attachment from which blood oozes; the worm is not a blood feeder. Eggs will easily be detectable in the stool. Care must be taken to exclude concurrent infection with amoebiasis; *E. histolytica* trophozoites can invade the mucosa at the sites of worm attachment. Heavy *Trichuris* infections can produce rectal prolapse and the worms may then be seen on the everted oedematous mucosa.

4. Intestinal schistosomiasis — S. mansoni, S. japonicum and S. intercalatum

The passage of eggs from the radicles of the mesenteric veins across the gut wall to the lumen causes inflammatory responses to antigens released by the eggs. Many eggs are killed and become surrounded by eosinophilic micro-abscesses and granulomas; when these are numerous the mucosa becomes locally ulcerated, or hyperplastic reactions produce sessile or pedunculated polyps. Extensive focal granulomatous reactions with fibrosis produce rigidity of the gut wall or stenosis; serosal lesions can cause intestinal adhesions. At the lower end of the bowel anorectal and ischiorectal abscesses and fistulae may develop together with polyps in the anal region. Lesions are generally more severe in *S. japonicum* infections because of its higher egg output, and in this species the ileum is commonly affected.

The symptoms are usually colicky pains and bloody diarrhoea, they may continue intermittently for several years. In heavy infections eggs are easily found in the stools but in lighter infections stool concentration methods must be used or rectal snips taken through a proctoscope and examined as fresh squash preparations between two glass slides. Sigmoidoscopy may show a reddened granular mucosa with elevated yellowish pin-point granulomas, and sometimes ulceration or polyps; biopsy may be necessary to exclude malignancy. Polyps are readily demonstrable by barium enema. Response to chemotherapy is good but fibrotic scarring may persist.

5. Other helminths

Heavy infections with the fluke *Gastrodiscoides hominis* and the nematode *Oesophagostomium* can cause dysentery, but more commonly colicky pains and diarrhoea without blood are produced. *Gastrodiscoides* lives attached to the colonic mucosa by means of its suckers; *Oesophagostomium* lies embedded in the caecal mucosa and can lead to

surgical problems. Hyperinfection in strongyloidiasis can produce bloody stools especially when the colon is involved.

Malabsorption syndromes

Only four human parasites have been convincingly shown to produce malabsorption.

1. Giardiasis

Giardia trophozoites live attached to the epithelial cells of duodenal and jejunal villi and crypts by means of their ventral suckers. In symptomatic infections there is moderate shortening and blunting of the villi and the crypts are deepened. A moderate infiltrate of lymphocytes and plasma cells occurs in the submucosa and there are increased numbers of intra-epithelial lymphocytes. Malabsorption of fat and xylose probably results from functional immaturity of the villus cells which have a high turnover rate. Primary infections are usually symptomatic, especially in children but in areas where transmission rates are high many infections, at least in adults, are asymptomatic. In epidemics symptoms begin five to 10 days after infection. Common presenting features are nausea, abdominal bloating, borborygmi and frequent loose, offensive and rather pale stools. Meals often precipitate nausea and dyspepsia, and these symptoms may be followed by a loose stool. Symptoms may last a few days or continue for up to three months; in children and certain predisposed subjects the illness can be very prolonged and resemble coeliac disease.

Giardia cysts or trophozoites can usually be found in the stools but repeated examinations may be necessary, duodenal samples can also be examined.

2. Strongyloidiasis

Female worms living in the submucosa of the jejunum set up local inflammatory responses with oedema, infiltration by macrophages and eosinophils and secondary epithelial changes. The eggs laid locally in the submucosa hatch near to the epithelial surface and set up further local damage.

Several clinical presentations are possible with this parasite but a malabsorption syndrome resembling tropical sprue is one of the more important and often occurs in the absence of these other features. Stools are bulky and pale and there is malabsorption of fat and xylose; hypoproteinaemia is common and may result from a protein-losing enteropathy. There is a rapid exfoliation of epithelial cells from the mucosa. Rhabditiform or filariform larvae can be found in stools or duodenal samples and eosinophilia is common.

3. Capillariasis — Capillaria philippinensis

This infection was recognised in man in 1963 in the northern Philippines, and is now known to occur also in Thailand. The adult worms live, like *Strongyloides*, embedded in the jejunal mucosa and similar inflammatory changes are set up. The eggs superficially resemble *Trichuris*, but sometimes they hatch in the gut and establish internal autoinfection. While outbreaks derive initially from eating infected fish, human-to-human transmission does occur. Patients present with steatorrhoea and the effects of a severe protein-losing enteropathy, namely severe muscle wasting, hypoproteinaemia, weakness and weight loss. Eggs are not continuously demonstrable in the stool and their periodic occurrences may coincide with successive generations of egg-producing females. Serological tests may be of some value but cross reactions with other helminths have so far proved troublesome.

Supportive management is important in these patients as they are frequently fluid and electrolyte depleted. Chemotherapy is difficult because complete elimination of the parasite is essential.

4. Isosporiasis — Isospora belli

This under-recognised coccidian parasite undergoes its asexual and sexual cycles within the epithelial cells of the jejunum and duodenum. The lamina propria is infiltrated with lymphocytes, plasma cells and eosinophils; the epithelium shows broadening of the villi or a clubbing of their tips, or even a completely flat mucosa. The symptoms resemble those of giardiasis and are usually self-limited although some infections are prolonged or even fatal. The characteristic oocysts are found in the stool but these are easily missed or confused with those of non-pathogenic *Sarcocystis hominis*.

Megasyndromes — Trypanosoma cruzi

Megaoesophagus and megacolon are the two principal gut manifestations of chronic Chagas' disease. They appear many years after the initial acute infection; about half of these patients have evidence of cardiac involvement. Parasite multiplication within smooth muscle cells sets up focal areas of inflammatory myositis and these are believed to destroy adjacent parasympathetic nerve ganglia and their post-ganglionic fibres. The result is partial denervation with dilation and altered motility of the oesophagus and colon, and rarely the stomach or small bowel. Serology is positive and xenodiagnosis is the only way of demonstrating parasites in the blood.

Oesophageal involvement produces chronic dysphagia, initially for solids and then for soft foods. Swallowing becomes painful and there may be regurgitation. Hypersalivation is common and the parotid glands enlarge. Patients become emaciated and are liable to aspiration pneumonia. Treatment may be successful with balloon dilation or cardiotomy to relieve the block at the lower end of the oesophagus. Excision of part of the oesophagus and replacement by colonic or small bowel segments may be necessary.

Megacolon produces retention of faeces and gas; faecal impaction is common. Volvulus and intestinal obstruction are also frequent complications. Faecal impaction can be cleared by enemas but these may be complicated by septicaemia. Resection of affected segments of bowel eventually becomes necessary.

Acute abdomen

Acute abdominal presentations can occur with several gut parasites. In some instances diagnosis is only possible at laparotomy and by biopsy and subsequent histology; in others recognition before surgery may be possible and this may prevent unnecessary intervention.

1. Localised pain with or without a mass

Pain in the right iliac fossa, sometimes with a palpable mass, has several causes and appendicitis may be closely simulated. Ectopic *Ascaris* worms may migrate into the appendix or into a Meckel's diverticulum. True amoebic appendicitis is rare but caecal amoebomas can block the appendix or present as a tender mass. Amoebomas may also initiate an intussusception; surgery can sometimes be avoided if *E. histolytica* infection is confirmed. *Enterobius* worms are quite often found in surgically removed appendices, but this parasite is responsible for very few cases of appendicitis; tapeworm proglottids, especially *Taenia saginata*, may also enter the appendix but only exceptionally do they cause appendicitis. Schistosomal polyps and granulomas may also block the appendix and present as tender masses.

Oesophagostomium, a monkey nematode, lives in encapsulated granulomas in the walls of the caecum and colon and may present as tender caecal masses; in man the worms eventually die producing fibrosis and sometimes calcification. Another monkey parasite, *Ternidens deminutus*, produces similar lesions but they are much smaller and most infections are asymptomatic. Eggs of *Ternidens* are quite commonly found in the stool, in *Oesophagostomium* infections they are rarely found; the eggs of both these parasites closely resemble hookworm eggs. Lesions due to ectopic *Paragonimus* or the pentastome *Armillifer armillatus* can present as acute abdominal pain.

Morerastrongylus costaricensis lives in the smaller mesenteric arteries particularly those supplying the ileocaecal region. Eosinophilic granulomas, which may contain eggs and fragments of worm, are set up in the bowel wall and these present as masses in the right iliac fossa, with fever and eosinophilia; mesenteric arteritis can lead to thrombosis and gut infarction. Human infections with this rat parasite have been described from Costa Rica, Panama and Honduras. Diagnosis and treatment is surgical.

'Herring worm' infections in man due to *Anisakis* set up eosinophilic granulomas in the wall of the stomach and small intestine. Infections follow ingestion of raw herring and other fish containing infective larvae. Patients present with acute upper abdominal or epigastric pain with vomiting and sometimes signs of obstruction or peritoneal irritation. In Japan lesions are commonest in the stomach and they can sometimes be recognised at gastroscopy; occasionally removal of the worm may be possible by this route. Serology has been of some value but usually surgery is necessary. The excised lesions are up to 1.5 cm in diameter and are very oedematous with superficial ulceration and petechial haemorrhage.

Parasites entering the pancreatic duct produce severe upper abdominal pain and sometimes acute pancreatitis. This complication has been reported in *Ascaris* and *Clonorchis* infections.

2. Intestinal obstruction

Ascariasis is an important cause of small bowel obstruction, and in many tropical countries it is the commonest cause of this phenomenon in children aged one to five years; it cannot occur in light infections. A bolus of worms becomes impacted in the gut, often in the terminal ileum, and sets up reflex spasmodic contractions of the intestinal smooth muscle. Patients usually have a history of episodic colicky pains that have previously subsided spontaneously. Obstruction may be precipitated by intercurrent illness or anthelminthic treatment, particularly tetrachlorethylene used for hookworm infection.

Symptoms begin abruptly with colicky periumbilical or right lower quadrant pain, vomiting, abdominal distension, constipation and sometimes a palpable mass. About 40 per cent of patients vomit *Ascaris* worms or pass them *per rectum*. Most patients have radiological signs of obstruction and sometimes the worms can be seen contrasted by the gas-filled loops of intestine. High egg counts will be present in the stool. Management should usually be conservative initially and at least two-thirds of all patients can normally be treated without surgery. The first priorities are nasogastric suction and intravenous fluids; piperazine can then be administered via the nasogastric tube. In this way many obstructions will resolve within 12 to 36 hours. If laparotomy is necessary the preferred technique is to massage the worms through the ileocaecal valve; enterotomy and worm extraction through a short incision on the antimesenteric border of the bowel should be avoided when possible as any residual worms can easily penetrate the suture line. Local resection and end-to-end anastomosis is required when the gut wall is in poor condition or there is infarction of the gut, intussusception or volvulus.

Other parasitic conditions causing obstruction are amoebomas of the colon, schistosomal granulomas and polyps of the colon and ileum, *Oesophagostomium* granulomas of the caecal region, and very rarely in infections with the large tapeworms *Diphyllobothrium* and *Taenia*. In the later stages of hyperinfection with *Strongyloides* severe diarrhoea progresses to a paralytic ileus, in which the oedematous wall of the small bowel becomes atonic with consequent obstruction and sometimes septicaemia or peritonitis; vomiting may be profuse. Lastly chagasic megacolon should be mentioned as a cause of obstruction.

3. Intestinal perforation and peritonitis

Deep amoebic ulcers of the colon can perforate suddenly to cause acute peritonitis, but more commonly multiple slow leaks occur in a diffusely dilated colon; surgery is recommended in the former situation, but not the latter (p. 110). Similar phenomena occur in the much rarer balantidial infections. Peritonitis can also result from a ruptured amoebic liver abscess, and sometimes occurs in hyperinfections with *Strongyloides*.

Ascaris worms may penetrate a weakened bowel wall for example in typhoid or tuberculosis of the gut, or they can escape from suture lines. To avoid post-surgical complications patients with known or suspected *Ascaris* infections should be dewormed before elective gastrointestinal surgery is performed.

Non-acute abdominal pain

All parasites that damage the bowel wall by invasion, attachment or production of local lesions can produce gut pains whose character will depend upon their location. Parasites causing malabsorption can cause pain by altering gut motility. Large parasites in the small bowel can produce pain by stimulating reflex peristalsis and this is the prob-

able explanation of the recurrent and often severe colicky pains in ascariasis. The giant intestinal fluke (*Fasciolopsis*) has the same effect. The relatively mild pains noted by patients with the large tapeworms (*Taenia* and *Diphyllobothrium*) are also due to reflex gut spasm: this is almost always the only symptom these worms produce.

Several parasites of the duodenum and jejunum can produce epigastric pains and dyspepsia that closely simulate a duodenal ulcer; unnecessary radiology can be avoided by finding them. This presentation is typical of primary hookworm infections but also occurs in *Strongyloides*, *Trichostrongylus* and *Fasciolopsis* infections.

Simple diarrhoea

Diarrhoea with stools that are not blood-stained and do not show features of malabsorption is not commonly due to parasitic infection. It can be produced however by the organisms causing dysentery when infections are light or the lesions confined to the proximal bowel. Thus in amoebiasis, when ulcers are located only in the caecum and ascending colon the patient may complain of episodic stool looseness. Similarly with those infections causing malabsorption, a low grade infection can present clinically as simple diarrhoea; only biochemical tests will reveal the true defect. The acute gastroenteritis of trichinosis has already been mentioned.

One important parasite to consider is *Strongyloides*. Hyperinfection occurs particularly in debilitated and immunosuppressed persons, including malnourished children. Because of internal autoinfection, inflammation and oedema of the gut wall can extend down from the jejunum to the ileum and sometimes the colon. A profuse and often watery diarrhoea results and leads to dehydration and electrolyte loss; the stools may contain mucus and sometimes blood. The illness may be a fulminating one and can progress to paralytic ileus and leakage into the peritoneum or septicaemia. *Strongyloides* larvae must be looked for repeatedly and are usually numerous. Patients with lymphoproliferative disorders and those receiving steroids, cytotoxics or radiotherapy must be carefully watched for this complication. Preferably they should be screened for *Strongyloides* before this situation arises. Paradoxically patients with the hyperinfection syndrome often do not show blood eosinophilia. Supportive care is critical in these patients and thiabendazole is the only effective anthelminthic; antibiotics and perhaps metronidazole may be required if gut perforation is suspected.

B. LIVER DISEASE

Parasites damage the liver by several mechanisms; Table 7.2 shows how the parasites responsible relate to hepatic pathology.

Table 7.2 Anatomical location of liver parasites, and the types of secondary pathology

1. Biliary tract lumen
   — *Clonorchis*, *Fasciola*, *Opisthorchis*, *Ascaris*
2. Space occupying lesions in liver parenchyma
   — *Entamoeba histolytica* (amoebic abscess)
   Echinococcus (hydatid cyst)
3. Larva migrans
   — Nematodes: *Ascaris*, *Toxocara*, *Strongyloides*, *Capillaria hepatica*, *Gnathostoma*
   Trematodes: *Fasciola*
4. Egg granulomas and fibrosis — *Schistosoma mansoni*, *S. intercalatum*, and *S. japonicum*
   (eggs carried to liver via portal vein)
5. Intracellular:
   a. Hepatocytes — *Toxoplasma*, *Plasmodium* (not pathological)
   b. Kupffer cells — *Leishmania donovani*

   Liver damage by secondary mechanisms:
   1. Acute hepatocellular damage
      — *Plasmodium falciparum*, *Trypanosoma b. rhodesiense*
   2. Sinusoidal infiltration
   — *Plasmodium* (repeated infection)

Biliary tract syndromes

1. Clonorchiasis and opisthorchiasis

These flukes migrate from the duodenum up the common bile duct to the distal biliary passages where they mature. They feed upon cellular debris and epithelial secretions. The presence of the flukes initially provokes some desquamation of the biliary epithelium which later shows hyperplasia and sometimes adenomatous changes, goblet cells proliferate and much mucus is secreted. Cystic dilatations of the smaller bile ducts appear and these are surrounded by proliferating fibrous tis-

sue. Flukes become impacted in the bile ducts producing obstruction and sometimes secondary bacterial cholangitis. Chronic infections may lead to calculus formation, the stones are of a soft sandy consistency and often associated with biliary mud. Asymptomatic biliary carriers of *Salmonella typhi* are common in clonorchiasis. In heavy chronic infections extensive peribiliary fibrosis may lead to a form of biliary cirrhosis and even portal hypertension. Another late complication is cholangiocarcinoma.

Early infections present with epigastric pain, tender hepatomegaly, malaise and fever; eosinophilia is common. Later the illness is characterised by recurrent episodes of hepatic pain, biliary colic, fever and jaundice and the liver becomes chronically enlarged. Pyogenic cholangitis may lead to septicaemia. Many light infections are asymptomatic. Eggs will usually be found in the stools or duodenal juice, except in early infections. Levels of serum alkaline phosphatase are often raised. Cholangiography may show cystic biliary dilatation and filling defects due to the flukes. Chemotherapy is unsatisfactory and parasitological cure can rarely be obtained. Surgical drainage of the biliary tract may be necessary and allows evacuation of many of the flukes.

Dicrocoelium infections are usually symptomless but otherwise resemble mild clonorchiasis.

2. Fascioliasis

The pathogenesis of this infection differs from clonorchiasis in three ways. Firstly the flukes are larger and cause more mechanical damage. Secondly their passage to the biliary tract occurs through liver tissue; after penetrating the gut wall the young flukes traverse the peritoneum and then enter the liver through its capsule; some lose their way and end up in the lung or anterior abdominal wall. Thirdly man is an abnormal host and tissue reactions are vigorous; some flukes die in the liver parenchyma before reaching their destination.

The usual presentation in early infections is tender hepatomegaly, fever and eosinophilia; eggs are often absent from the stool at this stage and they may indeed never appear. Serological tests are often helpful. In established infections the manifestations are similar to those of clonorchiasis. Adult flukes can damage the biliary epithelium severely and blood loss can produce anaemia.

3. Ascariasis

Biliary obstruction, often by a solitary worm, is the second commonest surgical complication of *Ascaris* infections. Most patients are children, worms are stimulated to migrate up the bile duct in several stress situations including the postoperative period. Patients present with severe colicky right upper quadrant pains, liver enlargement and tenderness. If the block is not relieved jaundice develops and biliary obstruction may be complicated by pyogenic cholangitis or pyogenic liver abscess. Many worms probably reverse their migration and re-enter the bowel; the eggs they leave behind are believed to act as potent nidi for calculus formation. Biliary strictures are a late sequel.

The diagnosis is suggested by a high faecal egg count or the appearance of worms in vomit or faeces. Early cases should be managed conservatively with nasogastric suction, intravenous fluids and piperazine via the gastric tube. When symptoms persist or cholangiograms repeatedly show the presence of biliary tract worms, then surgical intervention is necessary but unless obstruction is complete or there are septic complications this can be deferred for two weeks.

Space-occupying lesions

1. Amoebic liver abscess

Entamoeba histolytica trophozoites are carried passively from colonic ulcers to the liver via the portal vein. Very few succeed in establishing themselves, and lodgement in a pre-existing focus of liver damage is perhaps necessary. Amoebae cause a lytic necrosis with little inflammatory response apart from some lymphocytes. The lesion extends peripherally with amoebae at its advancing edge; the central part becomes filled with chocolate-brown, bacteriologically sterile, liquefied liver substance. Most lesions are solitary and many of these occur in the upper right lobe of the liver;

they can reach 12 cm or more in diameter. Most patients do not have clinically apparent intestinal amoebiasis; those that do often have multiple liver abscesses. Untreated, nearly all liver abscesses eventually rupture into adjacent structures; most commonly this is through the diaphragm into the lung, but they may penetrate the chest or abdominal wall, the pericardium or rupture into the peritoneal cavity. Jaundice occurs only when lesions are multiple or major segments of the biliary tract are compressed.

Symptoms usually evolve over a period of one to four weeks, but some lesions are relatively chronic and others only become apparent after rupture. The clinical features are tender liver enlargement and fever. Pleuritic pain is common and frequently referred to the right shoulder tip; most patients show a raised erythrocyte sedimentation rate and a polymorphonuclear leucocytosis. A normocytic anaemia slowly develops. Localised liver tenderness is a very helpful sign and should be specifically looked for, particularly by palpation of the intercostal spaces. Helpful radiological signs are a raised immobile right hemidiaphragm and changes in the right lung base. Isotope or ultrasound scans reveal filling defects in most patients but interpretation can be difficult. Amoebic serology is very helpful as over 95 per cent of cases give positive results. Stool microscopy is of no direct value in diagnosis: for reasons that are not understood over 50 per cent of patients with liver abscess show neither cysts or trophozoites in their stools. Liver function tests are often normal.

Diagnostic percutaneous needle aspiration is only necessary when other diagnostic methods are not available. Important differential diagnoses are primary and secondary neoplasms of the liver and pyogenic liver abscess. Clinical response to chemotherapy is usually rapid, any concurrent intestinal amoebic infection must be eradicated. Therapeutic needle aspiration is sometimes necessary, the indications are:

1. Very big abscesses and those in the left lobe
2. Rupture or imminent rupture
3. Failure to respond to chemotherapy after five days.

The principal complications of aspiration are bacterial secondary infection, and rarely haemorrhage. Laparotomy and surgical drainage may be necessary when the abscess continues to refill despite repeated percutaneous aspiration, or when the diagnosis is uncertain and attempts at needle aspiration have failed or are anatomically hazardous. An indwelling soft rubber drain is rarely required after surgical drainage, but if used it must be connected to a sterile underwater seal and removed early.

Follow-up liver scans show that lesions take up to four months to disappear completely; sometimes a bizarre hepatic calcification is seen many years afterwards. Scar tissue is minimal in the absence of secondary infection.

2. Hydatid cysts

a. Echinococcus granulosus. About 50 per cent of all primary hydatids occur in the liver, most in the right lobe; they often do not become clinically apparent until five to 20 years after infection. The high frequency of hepatic cysts results from the fact that hexacanth embryos must traverse the liver after leaving the gut in portal blood. Young hepatic cysts are unilocular but most mature ones are multivesicular and contain daughter cysts, the formation of daughter cysts may result from leakage of bile across a damaged laminated membrane; partial rupture into the biliary system is probably quite common. Rarely daughter cysts form on the external surface of the primary cyst, making total removal of the parasite very difficult; such external daughter cysts have a normal laminated membrane differentiating them from the multilocular cysts of E. multilocularis.

Uncomplicated cysts present as painless hepatic enlargement, sometimes if the cyst is on the liver surface it presents as a pedunculated mass separate from the liver. Later, pain is produced if neighbouring structures, are involved, and obstructive jaundice can occur if cysts are near the porta hepatis. Allergic symptoms and eosinophilia suggest partial rupture. Some lesions are silent and found incidentally at autopsy or as radiological shadows. Only about 40 per cent of hepatic cysts are radio-opaque and scanning methods are much more sensitive. Most hepatic cysts produce seropositivity. Uncomplicated cysts may be left without surgery unless they are either very big, or producing, allergic manifestations or threaten to rupture. Needle aspiration must never be attempted, as leakage can cause anaphylaxis. When surgery is performed complete excision should be the objective; a potential plane of cleavage lies between the laminated membrane and the adventitious fibrous wall. To prevent spillage and dissemination of protoscolices to form future secondary daughter cysts, the scolices must be killed with iodine; after packing off the site 20 ml of fluid is drawn off by syringe and replaced by the same volume of a 1 per cent aqueous solution of iodine — this will kill the scolices within one minute. Other scolicidal solutions that may be used are 2 per cent formalin or 0.5 per cent silver nitrate.

Several dangerous complications can occur in untreated hydatid cysts; in all of them allergic features may be prominent. In order of frequency they are:

1. Intrabiliary rupture producing biliary colic and jaundice.

2. Suppuration, usually secondary to partial biliary rupture, presenting as hepatic pain, fever, toxaemia and sometimes septicaemia.

3. Intraperitoneal rupture causing an acute abdominal situation and later daughter cyst formation throughout the peritoneum.

4. Rupture into the thorax or less commonly into the gut or major blood vessels.

Following intrabiliary rupture or direct extension into the gut, daughter cysts and brood capsules may be found in the stool after washing the whole specimen with a stream of water. All complicated hepatic cysts require surgery, the technical difficulty is often considerable.

b. Echinococcus multilocularis. Over 90 per cent of cysts due to this much rarer human parasite are in the liver. No thick fibrous wall encapsulates the lesion which extends by exogenous budding to produce the so-called alveolar or malignant hydatid. The liver becomes honeycombed by a mass of small interconnected cysts, in a loose fibrous stroma. Clinically it simulates hepatic malignancy; obstructive jaundice and portal hypertension are recognised sequels, and local hepatic necrosis is common. Secondary spread to lungs and brain can occur. Surgical excision may be impossible.

Larva migrans

Relatively acute tender hepatomegaly with eosinophilia and fever is a syndrome produced by the immature stages of several worms as they pass through liver tissue. All these larval worms reach the liver from the gut. Damage is partly mechanical and partly due to allergic sensitisation and local inflammatory responses. True biliary parasites can present a similar picture.

1. Nematodes

In ascariasis this is a transient phenomenon appearing one to five days after embryonated eggs are swallowed. Most larvae pass through the liver sinusoids to the lungs but some are immobilised and destroyed locally. In toxocariasis the liver phase is prominent and much more prolonged. Many larvae never escape from the liver, tissue reactions are vigorous and trails of inflammatory cells are left by the larvae. Neutrophils, eosinophils and macrophages adhere to the parasite but many remain alive surrounded by a cuff of these cells; dead larvae produce eosinophilic micro-abscesses. Overt hepatic involvement can persist for several months; other features include pneumonitis and splenomegaly and the blood eosinophil count is usually very high. Specific serology is useful and other non-specific serological changes are suggestive. Percutaneous liver biopsy is very rarely of any value. However, abnormal areas of the liver surface that may appear as white plaques five to 10 mm in diameter can be biopsied at laparoscopy or laparotomy to yield identifiable larvae histologically. In strongyloidiasis the liver pathology is usually overshadowed by gut or lung manifestations, however hepatic granulomata are formed and may be found in biopsies. In gnathostomiasis the hepatic stage may precede the more pathognomonic skin manifestations and larvae pass through the liver before they are disseminated throughout the body.

Capillaria hepatica is a unique member of this group of nematodes, for the liver is its final destination. Recognised infections are rare in man but could be common where rodents are eaten or food is contaminated by dirt or soil containing eggs derived from dead rodents. The worms live in the hepatic parenchyma and lay eggs into the tissues to produce granulomas. Eggs never appear in the stool. At laparoscopy lesions appear as large whitish spots on the liver surface; eggs which resemble those of *Trichuris* may be seen in biopsies.

Stool examination will be negative in all these conditions except in strongyloidiasis.

2. Trematodes

In fascioliasis liver migration forms part of the normal syndrome of early acute infections; eggs are usually absent from the stool.

Hepatic schistosomiasis — S. mansoni and S. japonicum

All hepatic pathology in intestinal schistosomiasis is caused by immunological and cellular reactions to eggs that reach the liver by embolisation in portal blood from adult worms ovipositing in the terminal radicles of the mesenteric veins of the gut wall. Schistosomulae reach the portal system after leaving the lungs via arterial blood; the worms mature and pair up in the intrahepatic part of the portal vein but no hepatic damage is caused until the worms migrate to their final destination and begin egg laying. The type of host response depends on the stage and intensity of infection and the extent of previous exposure. Because of its higher egg output damage is greater with *S. japonicum*.

The acute disease occurs mainly in heavy primary infections; liver pathology forms part of a systemic illness (**Katayama fever**) which may be fatal. Reactions around the eggs show infiltration of lymphocytes and eosinophils and are surrounded by foci of hepatocellular necrosis. Clinically the liver becomes enlarged, tender and painful; other features are fever, high blood eosinophilia, splenomegaly, diarrhoea, and allergic symptoms. The liver gradually regresses in size as the immunological response becomes less intense.

The chronic form of disease is the one normally encountered; many patients give no history of acute illness. Chronic hepatic schistosomiasis develops insidiously as eggs and their tissue reactions accumulate in the liver. The primary lesion is an egg granuloma which heals by fibrosis as the egg is destroyed and disappears. The liver initially becomes enlarged for a period of several years, it becomes hard and eventually shrinks to below normal size. Confluent fibrous scarring around the finer radicles of the portal vein produces a vascular block; extension of this perivascular fibrosis around the larger branches of the portal vein produces the typical macroscopic lesion known as **Symmers' fibrosis** or **pipestem fibrosis**. The cut liver surface shows white rings around branches of the portal vein that resemble the stem of a clay pipe. Lobular architecture is well preserved and most granulomas are near the portal spaces; schistosome pigment may be seen. The functional effect is portal hypertension due to a presinusoidal intrahepatic block; the wedged hepatic vein pressure is normal. Total liver blood flow is maintained by an increased arterial blood flow. Hepatocellular function is well maintained until the very late stages, and serum albumin and bilirubin levels remain normal for a long time. Progression to cirrhosis does not occur.

The only clinical feature in many patients with chronic disease is firm, non-tender hepatomegaly and usually some enlargement of the spleen. As the process progresses the spleen enlarges and the liver shrinks, eventually becoming impalpable. In the late disease portal hypertension leads to haematemesis and melaena, which are often well tolerated, or to features of hypersplenism. Ascites, peripheral oedema and jaundice are very late features. Many patients survive a series of gastrointestinal bleeds over a period of years and yet maintain good hepatocellular function, provided blood transfusions are given when necessary.

Diagnosis of hepatic schistosomiasis is based upon finding eggs in stool specimens or rectal biopsies; they will always be found unless previous chemotherapy has been given. Although liver biopsy may show fibrosis and granulomas, it normally has no place in diagnosis. Chemotherapy will usually arrest hepatic damage and portal pressure may be lowered except in very late cases. Although dead worms become impacted in the intrahepatic portal veins after chemotherapy, no permanent damage results. Surgical procedures to reduce portal pressure may be necessary after repeated bleeding episodes but they should never be performed prophylactically. Splenectomy with splenorenal anastomosis is the preferred procedure giving a much lower incidence of hepatic encephalopathy than portocaval shunts; full chemotherapy must be given prior to surgery. Simple splenectomy will eliminate hypersplenism and reduce portal pressure, but this procedure may be followed by portal vein thrombosis.

Simple hepatomegaly and hepatocellular damage

Several protozoan infections produce generalised liver enlargement. There may be associated parenchymal cell damage, although commonly liver function remains normal.

1. Visceral leishmaniasis — Leishmania donovani

Liver enlargement is an invariable feature of this disease, and proceeds in parallel with splenomegaly as the disease progresses. In chronic cases the enlarged liver extends below the level of the umbilicus. Microscopically the hepatic sinusoids are moderately dilated and there is gross hyperplasia of the Kupffer cells many of which contain proliferating amastigotes. In the portal tracts focal collections of lymphocytes and plasma cells accumulate. In chronic cases some parenchymal damage occurs and hepatocytes are occasionally seen to be parasitised. Jaundice and lowered serum albumin levels are rare late features. It is now evident that periportal fibrosis may be a sequel of long standing infections following therapy but it is disputed whether this ever leads to cirrhosis. Liver biopsy is not normally used to diagnose *L. donovani* infection; marrow or splenic aspiration being the preferred methods.

2. Malaria

Pre-erythrocytic schizogony in all plasmodial species, and secondary exo-erythrocytic schizogony in *P. vivax* and *P. ovale* infections, take place in hepatocytes which they destroy. Pathologically neither are of any consequence and in fact parasitised cells are so scanty that they have never been found in natural human infections.

In acute malaria mild or moderate hepatomegaly is common but regresses quickly after treatment. Only in severe falciparum malaria is hepatocellular function impaired. Microscopically there is vascular congestion, periportal infiltration, and Kupffer cell enlargement and hyperplasia, the latter containing parasitised and unparasitised red cells together with masses of haemozoin. In severe falciparum malaria degeneration and necrosis of centrilobular hepatocytes occurs. This may be due to anoxia secondary to anaemia, vascular stasis and arterial hypotension. The result is further liver enlargement, and sometimes the appearance of jaundice, a moderate rise in serum transaminase levels and depressed levels of certain clotting factors. Progression to hepatic coma never occurs, but the appearance of jaundice in a febrile patient sometimes leads to a mistaken diagnosis of viral hepatitis.

Where people are repeatedly infected with malaria a persistent mild or moderate hepatomegaly occurs, but this slowly regresses together with a reduction in spleen size, as immunity is built up. Microscopically the sinusoids are congested and Kupffer cells containing haemozoin are concentrated periportally where they are visible macroscopically as greyish-black dots. As immunity increases and parasitaemia becomes less frequent so the amounts of haemozoin decrease in the periportal areas which show an increasing lymphocytic infiltration. These chronic changes have no effect on liver function and no residual damage remains when regression is complete. A few older subjects living unprotected from malaria in endemic areas do not show a regression in liver size and nearly all these patients show progressive splenomegaly. This condition is believed to be an abnormal immunological response to repeated malaria challenge, and is variously called 'big spleen disease' or tropical splenomegaly syndrome (p. 132). The liver histology is specific for this condition and biopsy can be a useful way of confirming the diagnosis. The hepatic sinusoids are greatly dilated and heavily infiltrated with clusters of lymphocytes and some plasma cells; the Kupffer cells are enlarged and hyperplastic. Haemozoin is scanty and parasites are almost never seen; the sinusoidal reticulum is normal. The portal tracts are moderately infiltrated with lymphocytes and plasma cells. The sinusoid infiltrate may resemble lymphatic leukaemia. Liver size and pathological changes regress completely with prolonged malaria chemosuppresion.

3. Trypanosomiasis

Moderate hepatomegaly may occur in *T.b. rhodesiense* infection and the acute phase of *T. cruzi* infection. Histology is non-specific. In Rhodesian trypanosomiasis jaundice and other evidence of parenchymal damage is not uncommon, several factors including heart failure and hypotension may contribute, but damage may be partly due to disseminated intravascular coagulation.

4. Toxoplasmosis

In acquired toxoplasmosis hepatic enlargement is unusual. It is much commoner in congenital infections and in infections in immunocompromised hosts. *Toxoplasma* trophozoites proliferate within hepatocytes and set up focal inflammatory changes when they rupture. In heavy infections parenchymal damage may be sufficient to produce jaundice. Splenomegaly is invariably present when the liver is involved.

FURTHER READING

Knight, R. and Wright, S.G. (1978) Progress report. Intestinal protozoa. *Gut*, **19**, 940–953.

Knight, R., Schultz, M.G., Hoskins, D.W. and Marsden, P.D. (1973) Progress report. Intestinal parasites. *Gut*, **14**, 145–168.

Marsden, P.D. (1975) Parasitic diseases of the liver. In L. Schiff (ed) *Diseases of the liver*, pp. 1078–1088. Philadelphia, Toronto: J.B. Lippincott Co.

Marsden, P.D. (ed.) (1978) Intestinal parasites. Clinics in Gastroenterology, Vol. 7, Number 1. London: W.B. Saunders Co. Ltd.

World Health Organization (1969) Amoebiasis. *Tech. Rep. Series* no 421.

8

Local effects of parasitism 2

A. PULMONARY DISEASE

Pulmonary eosinophilia syndromes

Several helminths can cause a disease characterised by patchy pulmonary infiltration and a high blood eosinophilia. The duration and severity of these illnesses varies considerably. The shorter and more benign illnesses conform to the original descriptions of Löffler's syndrome. Pulmonary eosinophilia caused by helminths can be divided into two groups. One of these, diffuse filarial lung disease, is a well characterised disorder that is generally chronic and responds to specific chemotherapy; the other, multifocal helminthic pneumonitis, is produced by several different helminthic parasites and presents as an acute or sometimes recurrent disorder of variable severity.

The helminthic causes of pulmonary eosinophilia have to be differentiated from other illnesses with similar presentations, including extrinsic allergic alveolitis, drug reactions with pulmonary infiltration, chronic asthma with sensitivity to *Aspergillus*, periarteritis nodosa and certain unexplained pulmonary eosinophilia syndromes.

1. Multifocal helminthic pneumonitis

The pulmonary infiltration is produced by tissue reactions around migrating larval worms. Pathologically alveoli become filled with fluid, red blood cells and an acute inflammatory exudate in which eosinophils are prominent. The disorder presents clinically with cough, chest pains, dyspnoea and wheeze; sputum is scanty, mucoid and sometimes blood-stained; fever may be present and scattered rhonchi and râles may be heard; blood eosinophilia is usually prominent and the sputum may contain numerous eosinophils and Charcot-Leyden crystals.

Radiologically there is patchy shadowing in the lung fields, often more prominent in the perihilar region; the appearances often change rapidly over the course of a few days.

(a) *Larval nematodes* — *Ascaris*, hookworm, *Strongyloides*, *Toxocara*, *Trichinella* and *Gnathostoma*. Ascariasis is the commonest cause of this syndrome and will be seen especially in children. The condition is sometimes seasonal and coincides with the onset of transmission; the pig ascarid *A. suum* can produce the same type of illness. Only heavy or primary exposure to hookworm larvae is likely to produce significant lung symptoms. In both ascariasis and hookworm the condition is self-limiting and lasts for up to two weeks; no specific treatment is indicated. In strongyloidiasis symptoms may be persistent or recurrent because of autoinfection; in toxocariasis they can last for several months. Pneumonitis in trichinosis is part of the systemic illness produced by larval dissemination throughout the body from the gut; in this infection dyspnoea can be aggravated by respiratory muscle involvement. *Gnathostoma* larvae are about 4 mm long and may produce linear tracks in lung tissue.

Diagnosis will often be made on the epidemiological history and presence of other features. Stool microscopy will be negative except in long-standing strongyloidiasis but may become positive later when *A. lumbricoides* or hookworm have produced the syndrome. Larvae may be found in sputum or gastric washings of patients with *Ascaris* pneumonitis, and less commonly when hookworm or *Strongyloides* is responsible.

Serology is useful in toxocariasis and trichinosis; rather non-specific serological tests for nematodes, using for example crude *Ascaris* antigen, will be positive in many of these conditions. Serum IgM levels are often high, especially in toxocariasis, most of this immunoglobulin is non-specific (p. 97).

Specific chemotherapy is indicated only in strongyloidiasis and toxocariasis but supportive treatment and occasionally steroids may be required in all these conditions. It is suspected that pulmonary strongyloidiasis and probably also *Ascaris* pneumonitis predispose to bacterial pneumonia.

(*b*) *Larval trematodes — Schistosoma, Fasciola, Paragonimus* (early lesions). Schistosomulae traverse the lung soon after cercariae penetrate the skin. Pneumonitis is part of the systemic illness produced in the early stages of schistosomiasis. Immature *Fasciola* flukes may miss the liver during their migrations and enter the lungs after traversing the diaphragm; lesions are usually at the right lung base. In early paragonimiasis young flukes traverse the lungs, producing a patchy pneumonitis, on their migration to peribronchial tissues.

The epidemiological history will usually be helpful in these conditions and serology is sometimes of value.

2. Diffuse filarial lung disease — 'Tropical pulmonary eosinophilia'

This condition is caused by an exaggerated hypersensitivity response to *Wuchereria bancrofti*, *Brugia malayi* and probably also some zoonotic *Brugia* species. It occurs sporadically in most areas where these filarial infections are endemic, young adults are often affected and Indians show a racial susceptibility. The adult filarial worms are in the lymphatic system and the lung pathology results from local destruction of microfilariae in the pulmonary vascular system; the peripheral blood never shows microfilaraemia. Pathologically there is a perivascular inflammation with mixed acute and granulomatous features, eosinophils are prominent and some fibrosis occurs in chronic lesions; fragments of microfilarae may be found.

This condition presents clinically with paroxysmal nocturnal cough and bronchospasm, malaise, low fever and later more persistent dyspnoea; sputum is usually scanty but haemoptysis may occur. Radiologically there is miliary mottling, an increase in reticular markings and prominence of bronchovascular markings. A high blood eosinophilia is the hallmark of the disease and absolute counts may reach 20 000/mm^3 or more, and nearly always exceed 3000. Filarial serological tests are always strongly positive. The condition is often very debilitating and may last many months or even years. Sometimes other features of filarial disease, such as hydrocele or inguinal adenopathy, are present.

The differential diagnosis includes other helminths causing multifocal pneumonitis, but few of these produce such a chronic illness; if blood eosinophilia is overlooked pulmonary tuberculosis may be suspected. Lung biopsy is rarely necessary unless required for the exclusion of other disorders.

The clinical response to a full course of diethylcarbamazine is usually excellent and a therapeutic trial is frequently justified; symptoms may be exacerbated in a few patients when treatment is started. The prognosis is good but it is now evident that a few patients with long-standing disease develop pulmonary hypertension.

Peribronchial cysts and bronchiectasis — Paragonimus

After crossing the lungs, *Paragonimus* flukes come to lie in pairs within cystic spaces that communicate with the bronchial system. The cysts measure up to 1 cm in diameter and are surrounded by a fibrous capsule; they are commonest near the hilum or at the periphery of the lung. Inflammatory and granulomatous reactions around the worms and their eggs lead to progressive peribronchial damage and later bronchiectasis; other pulmonary complications include local atelectasis, secondary bacterial infections, pleural adhesions, pleural effusions and pneumothorax.

Clinically, patients present with gradual onset of cough, dyspnoea and haemoptysis; sputum is plentiful and often rusty-brown in colour. Moderate loss of weight is common but fever is unusual except in early cases or when complications occur. Finger-clubbing is quite common and persistent râles may be heard in the chest. Symptoms may continue for many years; when very few worms are present patients may be almost symptomless. Radiologically there may be patchy shadowing, prominent hilar markings, or more pathognomonic lesions comprising nodular opacities, ring shadows or small irregular calcific foci. Clinically and sometimes radiologically paragonimiasis can resemble pulmonary tuberculosis. The diagnosis is normally made by finding the characteristic operculated eggs in the sputum, or in the stools when expectorated sputum has been swallowed. Serological tests are of some value but skin tests remain positive for a very long time. Specific therapy is usually successful but some permanent lung damage may remain.

Focal lesions in lung parenchyma

1. Hydatid cysts

About 40 per cent of patients infected with *Echinococcus granulosus* have lesions in the lungs. Most cysts are solitary, they are commonest in the lower lobes, particularly on the right side; many are situated peripherally in the lung but others are near the hilum. Lung hydatids are especially common in children; they are unilocular and often nearly spherical in shape because of low tissue resistance and when uncomplicated there is little tissue reaction. Radiologically they appear as homogeneous rounded opacities surrounded by normal lung parenchyma; cyst wall calcification is very rare.

Small and even moderately sized cysts are often clinically silent and may be detected by routine chest X-rays. The symptoms of uncomplicated cysts are paroxysmal dry cough, haemoptysis and chest pains that may be poorly localised or pleuritic; later there is exertional dyspnoea. Physical signs may resemble those of pleural effusion if the cyst is situated inferiorly; radiological differentiation is easy, attempted aspiration may be disastrous. Diagnosis is normally based upon radiological findings together with serological and intradermal tests. Unless pulmonary hydatids are small and

clinically inactive they must be removed surgically otherwise serious complications are inevitable as the cyst continues to grow. A simple enucleation is usually possible; following incision of the adventitia extrusion of the complete cyst may be facilitated by increasing intrapulmonary pressure using a cuffed endotracheal tube.

Eventually most pulmonary hydatids leak or rupture suddenly into a bronchus. Slow leakage produces increasing cough and haemoptysis and protoscolices or isolated hooklets may be found in the sputum; secondary infection is common and daughter cysts may form. Massive rupture presents as a paroxysm of coughing with a rush of salty fluid into the mouth, haemoptysis may be profuse and aspiration of hydatid fluid into alveoli produces pulmonary oedema with cyanosis and often anaphylactic shock; pieces of hydatid membrane ('grape skins') may be found in the sputum. More rarely hydatids rupture into the pleural cavity or into major intrathoracic blood vessels. All complicated cysts must be treated surgically and lobectomy is usually necessary. Hepatic hydatids sometimes extend through the diaphragm and present as right lower lobe lesions. Rarely secondary cysts occur in the lung or pleural cavity, either in the neighbourhood of primary lesions, or after embolisation to the lungs following intravascular rupture of a primary cyst into the venous side of the circulation.

2. Amoebiasis of the lung

Pulmonary amoebiasis is always secondary to liver abscess. Most lesions are in the right lower and middle lobes, they nearly always result from direct extension of hepatic lesions through the diaphragm; rarely there is no direct connection and amoebae are blood-borne to the lung. Pleural adhesions usually form as the subdiaphragmatic lesion extends upwards. The necrotic cytolytic amoebic lesion progresses through lung tissue until a bronchus is invaded to form a hepato-bronchial fistula through which the liver abscess may be partly drained spontaneously. Less commonly an amoebic empyema is formed and this may be preceeded by a serous effusion.

Chest symptoms and signs may be the presenting features of an unsuspected liver abscess, but in most patients simultaneous liver pathology is clinically evident. The clinical features are fever, pleuritic chest pain, cough, haemoptysis and later when a hepato-bronchial fistula becomes established, expectoration of larger amounts of reddish brown sputum ('anchovy sauce'); rarely bile may appear in the sputum. Radiology is very helpful and changes include a raised, immobile and often deformed right hemidiaphragm, patchy consolidation in the right lower lung fields and later cavitation in this region; pleural fluid is sometimes present. *E. histolytica* trophozoites should be searched for in the sputum but care must be taken to distinguish them from the mouth commensal *E.gingivalis*. The haematological and serological changes will be similar to those of uncomplicated liver abscess. When the hepatic lesion is not clinically apparent pulmonary amoebiasis can be mistaken for various right lower zone lung pathologies especially bacterial pneumonias and bacterial lung abscess. Chemotherapy is the same as for liver abscess; surgical intervention is rarely necessary except to drain an empyema. Residual lung damage after chemotherapy is unusual but sometimes bronchiectasis or a persistent lung cavity may necessitate local lung resection.

3. Focal pulmonary filariasis — Dirofilaria immitis

In man the dog heart worm does not develop fully, and cannot establish itself in the human heart. However immature worms become embolised in the pulmonary arteries and here they die setting up necrotic inflammatory reactions. Several dozen cases have now been described from North and South America, Australia and Japan. Although most patients have few symptoms the lesions produce prominent radiological shadows that may resemble neoplasms. Cases may be detected on routine radiographs on which they appear as more or less rounded, well-defined, solid, non-calcified 'coin' lesions reaching a diameter of up to several centimeters. Excision biopsy is usually necessary to exclude cancer; the degenerated immature worm may be difficult to find but lies in an arteriole surrounded by necrotic granulation tissue.

Protozoan interstitial pneumonitis — Pneumocystis carinii and Toxoplasma gondii

1. Pneumocystosis

An acute or subacute lung infection with inflammation and oedema of interstitial tissues and a prominent exudation of foamy proteinaceous material into the alveoli. The lungs become firm and rubbery in consistency. Overt infections only occur in immunodeficient subjects and malnourished or premature infants; in the former the interstitial cellular reaction is mainly lymphocytes and macrophages, and in the latter it is predominantly plasma cells. In neither form are polymorphonuclear leucocytes seen.

The major clinical features are tachypnoea and an unproductive cough together with fever, dyspnoea and later cyanosis. Deterioration may be rapid or take place over a period of weeks. Physiologically there is an alveolar capillary block with hypoxia and often hypocarbia due to hyperventilation. Radiologically bilateral perihilar haziness progresses to denser shadowing in which air bronchograms may be seen; in addition segmental infiltrates and pleural effusions may be present. The parasite can sometimes be demonstrated, as a cystic structure 5–6 μm in diameter containing up to 8 sporozoites, in stained preparations of sputum or bronchial washings. More commonly transbronchial or open lung biopsy is necessary to find the organism and to exclude other pathogens found in such patients; percutaneous needle lung biopsy is now less favoured because of the risks involved. Now that co-trimoxazole is known to be effective in this condition it may sometimes be justifiable to do a therapeutic trial; however parenteral administration is necessary to achieve adequate blood levels of trimethoprim, and the search for other pathogens must continue. Serological diagnostic methods are not yet satisfactory, many false negatives occur and only a rising antibody titre is confirmatory. Full supportive management is critical in these patients.

2. Toxoplasmosis

Pneumonitis is one of the features of disseminated toxoplasmosis in the immunocompromised host and presents clinically in a manner resembling pneumocystosis with similar radiological and clinical findings. However other features of toxoplasmosis including myocarditis, encephalitis or hepatosplenomegaly may be present. Differentiation is important because co-trimoxazole is not effective in toxoplasmosis while the combination of pyrimethamine with sulphadiazine is.

Secondary bacterial and aspiration pneumonias

Patients with advanced kala-azar and late Gambian sleeping sickness often die of bacterial pneumonia. In both conditions the host is immunologically compromised; other factors are the presence of reticulo-endothelial infiltration within the interstitial lung tissue in kala-azar, and depressed levels of consciousness and malnutrition in trypanosomiasis. Pulmonary tuberculosis is more common than expected in both of these diseases, and also in paragonimiasis.

Aspiration pneumonia occurs in late mucocutaneous leishmaniasis especially in patients with gross destruction of the oropharynx or lesions of the larynx. Patients with megaoesophagus due to *Trypanosoma cruzi* infection frequently aspirate oesophageal contents into their lungs; initially this presents as nocturnal cough but later overt aspiration pneumonia may kill the patient.

Pulmonary oedema — Plasmodium falciparum

Pulmonary oedema is an uncommon but serious complication of severe falciparum malaria. In its advanced form it is often fatal. Several factors may be responsible, they include anoxic damage and increased permeability of pulmonary capillaries, over-enthusiastic administration of intravenous saline solutions, and inappropriate secretion of antidiuretic hormone. Pathologically capillary haemorrhages are seen and the capillaries are blocked by parasitised erythrocytes, alveolar septa are infiltrated with mononuclear cells, and the alveoli filled with fluid and lined by a hyaline membrane.

Patients may slowly become dyspnoeic with basal râles or develop an acute respiratory distress syndrome. Supportive management includes oxygen, fluid restriction especially parenterally, and if necessary intravenous frusemide or mannitol. Alternatively dialysis can be used to remove excess fluid from the body; in extreme situations mechanical ventilation with positive end-expiratory pressure has been successful.

Many clinicians believe that this dangerous complication can be largely prevented by avoidance of injudicious over-hydration with parenteral fluids.

B. CARDIAC DISEASE

Diffuse myocarditis

1. Chagas' disease — Trypanosoma cruzi

The primary acute form of the disease mainly affects children, it carries a mortality of about 10 per cent in clinically apparent infections. At autopsy the heart is enlarged, flabby and dilated. Microscopically the interstitium is oedematous and diffusely infiltrated with lymphocytes and plasma cells; muscle fibres show hyaline necrosis and degeneration and amastigotes may be seen with them. Clinically the acute myocarditis reveals itself as tachycardia, arrhythmias and electrocardiographic changes; in relatively few patients is it the direct cause of death. Parasites can usually be found in the blood and prolonged courses of chemotherapy can probably eliminate the parasite and improve the long-term prognosis.

The heart in cases of chronic chagasic cardiomyopathy is dilated and hypertrophied. Characteristically the cardiac apex is dilated and thinned to form an aneurismal dilatation that may affect both ventricles; the pulmonary conus may also be dilated. Mural thrombi are common at the ventricular apex and in the atria and can be the source of emboli. The atrioventricular valve rings are dilated but the valves themselves are not directly affected. Microscopically some muscle fibres are seen to be hypertrophied while others show focal necrosis and granular degeneration. Cellular infiltrates are focal and comprise monocytes, lymphocytes and plasma cells; patchy fibrosis may be seen. Conducting tissue appears to be selectively damaged by the inflammatory foci, injury being most marked in the sino-atrial and atrio-ventricular nodes, the right bundle branch and the anterior ramification of the left bundle branch. Parasites are very rarely found in sections from chronic heart cases.

Many milder cases are clinically silent or detectable only on the electrocardiogram. Symptoms and signs appear progressively after the age of 20 years; they include palpitations, dizziness, precordial pains, cardiac enlargement, mitral and tricuspid incompetence, thromboembolism and right-sided cardiac failure; dyspnoea is uncommon. The annual mortality in those with known cardiac involvement is 0.7 per cent; death is sudden in 38 per cent of patients and most of the remainder die in congestive cardiac failure. Chest X-rays show generalised cardiomegaly. The most frequent electrocardiographic changes are right bundle branch block, ventricular extrasystoles, first degree atrio-ventricular block and changes in the T wave and ST segment; in severe cases complete A–V block, atrial fibrillation or left bundle branch block may occur. Serological tests for *T. cruzi* are positive and xenodiagnosis may be positive in 50 per cent. Chemotherapy is of no value and supportive management is difficult. Procainamide is useful for extrasystoles, digoxin should be used cautiously and can easily induce unwanted cardiac effects, especially when concurrent use of diuretics has caused hypokalaemia. Propranolol and other β-blockers may produce bradycardia, shock and even death. Isoprenaline is useful for Stokes-Adams attacks but cardiac pacemakers are the favoured treatment for heart block, although sometimes they are poorly tolerated and they can precipitate the release of emboli.

2. African trypanosomiasis — Trypanosoma brucei

Acute myocarditis is common in Rhodesian trypanosomiasis and may contribute to a fatal outcome, while in Gambian sleeping sickness milder and more chronic changes are found at autopsy but these are rarely evident clinically. In *T.b. rhodesiense* infections, the cardiac pathology is similar to that seen in acute *T. cruzi* infections. The heart is dilated and shows degeneration of cardiac fibres with cellular infiltration and oedema in the interstitium; in addition quite extensive lymphocytic perivascular infiltrates may be present in the myocardium and pericardium. A small pericardial effusion is common and may be associated with pleural effusions.

Clinically *T.b. rhodesiense* myocarditis manifests as cardiac enlargement, congestive cardiac failure and arrhythmias such as atrial fibrillation. Extrasystoles and first degree atrio-ventricular heart block are common electrocardiographic changes. Parasites can always be demonstrated in thick blood films. Digoxin is fairly well tolerated and this together with diuretics will usually tide the patient through until specific chemotherapy exerts its favourable effect. Significant long term after effects are unknown.

3. Toxoplasmosis — Toxoplasma gondii

Toxoplasmal myocarditis is clinically very significant in the disseminated form of the disease occurring in immunocompromised hosts, and in such patients it may be accompanied by hepatosplenomegaly, encephalitis or pneumonitis. In the ordinary acquired toxoplasmosis a very mild myocarditis is probably common but not clinically apparent, however in a few patients it is significant. In either situation toxoplasmal organisms proliferate intracellularly within cardiac muscle cells and when these rupture intense inflammatory foci cause damage to neighbouring cardiac cells.

The clinical features are those of acute myocarditis and supportive management will be important. Chemotherapy should always be given if there is evidence of cardiac involvement.

4. Trichinosis — Trichinella spiralis

In heavy infections with *T. spiralis*, myocardial involvement is common and is an important cause of death in fatal cases. The larvae that disseminate to the myocardium set up multifocal interstitial inflammatory lesions; other features of the disease are invariably present. No true cysts are formed in cardiac muscle. This complication may present with cardiac enlargement, arrhythmias or cardiac failure. Corticosteroids should be given to suppress the cellular reaction, together with specific chemotherapy. There is no residual cardiac damage in trichinosis once the acute phase has passed.

5. Sarcocystosis

Species of *Sarcocystis* cause myocardial damage in a number of herbivorous mammals, the intermediate hosts; they proliferate within cardiac muscle fibres. *Sarcocystis* parasites have sometimes been found in the myocardium of man, but they are probably often overlooked. Possibly some cases of unexplained myocarditis in man are due to this parasite; sarcocysts in man are attributed to the species *S. lindemanni* (p. 30).

Pulmonary hypertension

1. Schistosomiasis

Schistosoma haematobium eggs may be swept directly to the lungs from the vesical venous plexus via the inferior vena cava, right side of the heart, and the pulmonary artery. In intestinal schistosomiasis due to *S. mansoni* and *S. japonicum* eggs can only reach the lungs when portal hypertension has created collaterals through which eggs pass from the portal vein to the systemic venous circulation. In practice damage to pulmonary vessels is usually less with *S. haematobium* than with either *S. mansoni* or *S. japonicum*, despite the fact that it is a late feature of the latter infections.

Egg granulomas in the pulmonary arteries set up necrotising lesions with destruction of the intima and vascular occlusion; some vessels recanalize producing angiomatoid lesions. Multiple lesions increase pulmonary arterial pressure producing medial hypertrophy, hyaline thrombosis and further arteritis. Later the pulmonary artery shows aneurismal dilatation, arteriosclerosis and the right ventricle becomes hypertrophied. Patients complain of exertional dyspnoea and faintness, and later develop right-sided heart failure. Some show mild or moderate cyanosis due to arteriovenous pulmonary anastomoses or bronchopulmonary shunts. Patients with severe portal hypertension may have, in addition, porto-pulmonary shunting and some develop finger-clubbing. Clinically a left parasternal heave is prominent and the second heart sound widely split with its pulmonary component accentuated; right ventricular hypertrophy and failure may be present. Radiologically the pulmonary conus is prominent, as are hilar shadows due to dilated branches of the pulmonary artery which show abnormal branching and truncation peripherally. The electrocardiogram shows right ventricular hypertrophy and strain; arrhythmias are rare. Differentiation from other causes of cor pulmonale and even congenital heart disease is not always easy. Chemotherapy arrests the disease process but otherwise management is supportive.

When patients with uncomplicated *S. haematobium* infection are given chemotherapy adult worms embolise to the lung, no permanent damage is done but some patients develop dyspnoea and cough. Radiologically, transient pulmonary shadows appear and presumably these represent tissue reactions around dead worms.

2. Filariasis

Some patients with diffuse filarial lung disease ('tropical pulmonary eosinophilia') have developed pulmonary hypertension after chemotherapy. Many cases are probably clinically silent but others develop the usual symptoms and signs of a primary pulmonary hypertension. It is presumed that vasculitis, resulting from microfilarial destruction in periarteriolar tissue, is responsible. Possibly some cases of unexplained cor pulmonale in endemic areas are due to chronic filarial lung disease that has never been recognised or treated.

In dogs the heart worm *Dirofilaria immitis* causes severe pulmonary hypertension. This infection is being increasingly recognised in man as a cause of 'coin' lung opacities. Although the worm cannot mature fully in man, it is possible that heavy infections might sufficiently damage the pulmonary vessels to produce significant haemodynamic effects.

Anaemic heart disease

Severe hookworm anaemia is a common cause of heart failure in many tropical countries. Its recognition is of great importance and its management not always easy. Cardiac output at rest begins to increase at haemoglobin levels below 7 g/dl and heart failure normally appears at levels below 3 to 5 g. Peripheral vascular resistance falls because of hypoxia and the cardiac output is increased by an elevated stroke volume and tachycardia, the latter especially in children; the total blood volume is not increased. Salt and water retention occurs because of reduced renal blood flow and possibly also secondary aldosteronism. Hookworm-induced hypoproteinaemia contributes to the oedema.

Patients normally present in a high cardiac output state. Their complaints are exertional dyspnoea, palpitations, dizziness, precordial pains and ischaemic leg pains. A puffy oedema of the face, hands, and arms is common, especially in children. In compensated patients the hands are warm and cardiac output high, systolic murmurs can be heard over the enlarged heart and also a venous hum in the neck. When compensation fails the cardiac output falls, the extremities become cold and there may be evidence of cerebral hypoxia. Orthopnoea and pulmonary oedema are unusual unless induced by injudicious intravenous fluids; a raised jugular venous pressure in present in all patients but does not necessarily imply cardiac failure. Both bed rest and diuretics can cause decompensation in previously ambulant patients; bed rest promotes a diuresis by increasing renal blood flow.

Blood transfusion is necessary in most severely anaemic hookworm patients; usually no more than two units are necessary to tide the patient through until iron therapy produces its effect. The risk of circulatory overload is high and packed or sedimented red cells must be used. Exchange transfusion is the ideal method, but slow intravenous infusion with an appropriate dose of frusemide is usually successful. The intraperitoneal route may be used but absorption of red cells is relatively slow. Digoxin is of little value in management for it cannot exert an inotropic effect upon a severely anoxic myocardium. Anthelminthics should be withheld until the haemodynamic status has improved.

Pericarditis and pericardial effusions

1. Amoebiasis

Amoebic abscesses in the left lobe may extend upwards to involve the pericardium; less commonly involvement comes from the right lobe of the liver or a lung abscess. Initially there is a serous effusion but this is a prelude to suppurative amoebic pericarditis. Patients may present in shock due to cardiac tamponnade, or with a more gradual onset of pericardial signs; retrosternal pain is common and also a friction rub. The diagnosis is most difficult when the underlying liver abscess is not previously apparent; in this circumstance tuberculous pericarditis might be suspected. Pericardial aspiration is essential in all patients with this complication, it may have to be done as an emergency measure and repeated aspirations are often necessary; the liver abscess must also be aspirated. Chemotherapy is the same as for liver abscess. Constrictive pericarditis is an uncommon late sequel and sometimes requires pericardiectomy.

2. Trypanosomiasis

Serous pericardial effusions are quite common in acute myocarditis due to *Trypanosoma cruzi* and *T.b. rhodesiense*. Cardiac failure in these conditions may be a contributory factor. No special treatment is necessary.

Focal myocardial lesions

1. Hydatid cysts

About 1 per cent of all hydatids occur in the myocardium and are usually solitary. Some cysts die and form an inspissated mass of caseous material, but the remainder continue to grow and within one to five years rupture into a cardiac chamber or less commonly into the pericardium; such rupture can cause fatal anaphylaxis. Pericardial rupture may lead to daughter cyst formation that later affects cardiac function. Intracardiac rupture is commoner on the right side of the heart and leads to multiple secondary pulmonary cysts. Rupture into the left side of the heart causes disastrous dissemination throughout the arterial circulation and multiple brain cysts are a frequent sequel.

Because of their poor prognosis there is a strong case for considering surgical resection of myocardial hydatids; however the majority are clinically silent until they rupture.

2. Cysticercosis — Taenia solium

The myocardium is quite a common site for cysticerci in man but they are usually clinically silent; cysts will always be present elsewhere. Multiple cysts may cause myocardial failure by mechanical means but the most common manifestation is a conduction defect or arrhythmia resulting from critically sited cysts. Supportive care may be required.

3. Heterophyiasis

Focal cardiac granulomas around the ectopic eggs of the small intestinal fluke *Heterophyes heterophyes* (p. 56), and certain related species have been reported several times, especially from the Philippines. Most lesions are in the myocardium but some are in the cardiac valves. In some patients these lesions cause cardiac failure.

FURTHER READING

Danaraj, T.J., Pacheco, G., Shanmugaratnam, K. and Beaver, P.C. (1966) The etiology and pathology of eosinophilic lung (tropical eosinophilia). *Am. J. trop. Med. Hyg.*, **15**, 183–189.

Islam, N. (1964) *Tropical Eosinophilia*. East Pakistan: Islam A. Chittagong.

Shaper, A.G., Hutt, M.S.R. and Fejfar, Z. (eds) (1974) *Cardiovascular Disease in the Tropics*. London: British Medical Association.

9

Local effects of parasitism 3

A. SPLENIC PATHOLOGY

Introduction

Splenomegaly is an important clinical sign in parasitic disease. However, it is a common finding in only three: malaria, the hepatosplenic stage of intestinal schistosomiasis and visceral leishmaniasis. A spleen that is palpable is usually at least two or three times its normal size.

Four mechanisms contribute to splenic enlargement; more than one may operate simultaneously.

1. Pooling of red cells in splenic cords and sinuses

Red cells passing from the terminal splenic arterioles enter the sponge-like splenic cords of Billroth that contain loose reticular tissue packed with many macrophages and monocytes. They leave the cords by crossing a fenestrated basement membrane, to enter the splenic sinuses and so pass to the splenic vein. In many infections red cells are damaged physically or become coated with antibody, immune complexes or complement. Such cells may be culled by macrophages in the splenic cords. As a consequence macrophages proliferate, the cords thicken, and an increasing proportion of normal red cells are temporarily trapped during their passage through the spleen. The result is splenic enlargement and sequestration of many red cells. White cells and platelets may be culled and sequestered in a similar way.

2. Proliferation of lymphatic tissue, plasma cells and reticuloendothelial cells

Antigenic material reaches the spleen from two sources. Some parasites are destroyed within the spleen (*Plasmodium*, *Trypanosoma*, *Leishmania donovani* and *Toxoplasma*); alternatively antigens or immune complexes may be blood-borne. The type of cellular response depends upon the infecting agent, the mode of antigen presentation, the stage of the infection and previous exposure. The presence of foreign material promotes macrophage proliferation directly. Specific responses of T and B lymphocytes may be primary or secondary. T lymphocytes proliferate in the periarteriolar lymphatic sheaths surrounding the central arteries; they secondarily activate and promote proliferation of cord macrophages. B lymphocytes proliferate in the germinal centres of the white pulp and produce plasma cells.

These cellular proliferations cause the spleen to enlarge. Macrophage proliferation enlarges the splenic cords and increases red cell sequestration.

3. Portal hypertension

Raised portal venous pressure dilates the splenic sinuses and delays the transit of red cells through the splenic cords. Red cells, white cells and platelets accumulate in the cords where some are destroyed, causing macrophages to proliferate. Lymphocytes also proliferate, mainly (perhaps) due to the disease process producing the portal vein block.

4. Space-occupying lesions

These include cysts, abscesses, infarcts and subcapsular haematomas.

There are three possible consequences of splenic enlargement.

Splenic pain and discomfort

Usually enlarged spleens are painless and non-tender, but pain may be produced by acute inflammation, sudden enlargement, or local infarction. Very big spleens, as seen in some parasitic diseases, cause considerable discomfort and a dragging sensation in the left upper abdomen.

Splenic rupture

Fortunately this is rare, but it may occur after minor trauma, especially in *P. vivax* malaria; the tear is nearly always near the hilum.

Hypersplenism

A haematological syndrome that can occur in any splenic disease; in a mild form it is common. The term denotes a pancytopenia, or at least a depression of one or more of the formed elements in the blood, in the presence of splenic enlargement. Three mechanisms are involved:

a) Sequestration of blood cells in the spleen; in huge spleens this may amount to half the total red cell mass.

b) Haemolysis of normal or abnormal cells by a hypertrophied macrophage system within the splenic cords.

c) Expansion of plasma volume due to raised splenic blood flow and pooling; in consequence blood cells are diluted.

Theoretically hypersplenism is cured by splenectomy, but this is sometimes undesirable, particularly in the tropics. Where malaria is endemic, continuous chemosuppression must be given to all patients undergoing splenectomy.

Acute proliferative splenomegaly

1. Acute malaria

The spleen is always enlarged in acute malaria, but it may not be palpably enlarged, particularly in early falciparum malaria in non-immunes. Absence of a palpable spleen should never suggest that malaria is not the cause of fever. In fatal cases the cut surface is greyish red in colour and germinal centres are prominent. Parasitised and unparasitised red cells, and haemozoin fill the splenic cords and splenic sinuses, and are also seen within macrophages. Areas of vascular thrombosis, infarction and haemorrhage are common.

2. Trypanosomiasis

Mild or moderate splenomegaly accompanies liver enlargement in *T.b. rhodesiense* infection, and in acute forms of *T. cruzi* infection. *T. cruzi* amastigotes proliferate within splenic macrophages.

3. Toxoplasmosis

In some acquired infections, and in most congenital infections and those in immunocompromised hosts, splenomegaly accompanies hepatomegaly. Organisms proliferate in the cells of the spleen.

4. Toxocariasis

In visceral larva migrans due to this dog parasite some spleen enlargement is common. Immunologically-based proliferative changes predominate, but larval granulomas may also be present.

5. Acute schistosomiasis — 'Katayama syndrome'

Hepatosplenomegaly is common in this systemic illness that appears soon after *S. japonicum* or *S. mansoni* worms begin oviposition. The spleen shows sinusoidal dilatation and thickening of the splenic cords, which are infiltrated with proliferating macrophages, and eosinophils. Circulating immune complexes may underlie these changes; spleen size will regress even without chemotherapy. Occasionally mild splenomegaly occurs in early acute *S. haematobium* infections. Immune mechanisms must be responsible as the eggs of this species never reach the spleen.

Chronic proliferative splenomegaly

1. Malaria

Persistent splenomegaly is a very common finding in persons repeatedly exposed to malaria, especially in children. The prevalence of splenic enlargement is used by malariologists to estimate levels of transmission. The spleen is firm and non-tender; its size gradually diminishes as immunity increases. In young children, abundant haemozoin makes the sectioned spleen jet black in colour, but as levels of parasitaemia diminish and the child becomes older, pigment slowly disappears, first from the sinusoids and later from the splenic cords. The capsule becomes wrinkled and may show evidence of previous perisplenitis; patchy fibrosis sometimes persists within the splenic substance.

2. Tropical splenomegaly syndrome

Some adults and adolescents, living unprotected in malarious areas, develop progressive splenic enlargement instead of the normal regression in size. The spleen can reach an enormous size and extend to the right lower abdomen; moderate liver enlargement is invariable. Repeated episodes of infarction cause pain and later adhesions between the spleen and the parietal peritoneum, especially beneath the diaphragm. The spleen is firm and the cut surface red, haemozoin is absent. The splenic sinuses are congested, and the cords are packed with red cells; erythrophagocytosis and haemosiderin deposits are prominent. Lymphocytes and plasma cells are plentiful. Infarcts and patchy fibrosis are common.

Patients have no fever or parasitaemia, except during pregnancy. Their main complaints are weakness, symptoms of anaemia, and splenic pain or discomfort. Many patients are wasted, after an infarct a splenic friction rub may be heard. Anaemia is moderate, 6–10 g/dl, and normocytic normochromic; there is leucopenia with a relative or absolute lymphocytosis, and often thrombocytopenia. Malarial antibody titres are very high, as is the total IgM level. Liver biopsy changes are diagnostic (p. 120). Untreated the long-term morbidity and mortality is considerable.

Long term malaria chemosuppression results in regression in spleen size, weight gain and reversal of hypersplenism. Improvement should begin within three months, antimalarial drugs must be continued for one year at least, and ideally for life. Splenectomy has sometimes been performed in these patients, it is technically very difficult because of adhesions, and is unnecessary. Some of the patients who fail to respond eventually develop chronic lymphatic leukaemia or lymphosarcoma, but the relationship is uncertain. A normal lymphoblastic transformation to phytohaemagglutinin is a useful test to distinguish tropical splenomegaly syndrome from malignant disorders.

3. Visceral leishmaniasis

Progressive splenomegaly is invariable as the disease progresses. There is gross hyperplasia of the cord macrophages and sinus endothelial cells, and these are heavily parasitised with dividing amastigotes. Red cell sequestration is considerable. There is little lymphocytic response and the germinal centres are normal; plasma cells are sometimes plentiful. Some infarcts may be seen, and also areas of extramedullary erythropoesis.

The enlarged spleen is non-tender. Hypersplenism results in pancytopenia. Transfusion of fresh blood is particularly useful when thrombocytopenia produces mucosal bleeding. Needle splenic puncture to demonstrate parasites is the classic diagnostic method. Amastigotes are more plentiful than in the bone marrow, and the procedure is very simple and painless, but it can cause bleeding. It should not be used unless the spleen is easily palpable and platelet count, bleeding time and coagulation studies are considered satisfactory.

Portal hypertension

1. Hepatosplenic schistosomiasis (see also p. 118)

In S. mansoni and S. japonicum infections a progressive presinusoidal intrahepatic portal block results from fibrosis around egg granulomas.

Besides sinusoidal congestion the splenic cords show considerable reticuloendothelial hyperplasia. Germinal centres are difficult to find. Egg granulomas may be seen and some schistosome pigment. Areas of infarction and haemorrhage are common, and also venous thrombosis. The spleen may be very big and cause discomfort.

The degree of hypersplenism is variable but rarely severe, red cell life span is reduced. Most patients tolerate bleeds from oesophageal varices well and defects of blood coagulation are not common. Liver function is well maintained. A chronic Salmonella septicaemia can complicate schistosomal splenomegaly. The surgical treatment of portal hypertension due to schistosomiasis is discussed on page 119.

2. Other infections

In heavy infections with *Clonorchis* and *Opisthorchis* biliary cirrhosis may produce moderate portal hypertension. Large hydatid cysts near the porta hepatis, particularly those due to *Echinococcus multilocularis*, can compress the portal vein; rarely amoebic liver abscesses in this location do likewise.

Although portal hypertension is rarely of much importance in these infections, it can account for the spleen being palpable.

Space-occupying lesions

1. Hydatid cysts

About 2 per cent of hydatids occur in the spleen. Most are unilocular; as they enlarge, splenic tissue is pushed to one side. They may extend downwards as an abdominal mass compressing adjacent structures, or upwards, elevating the left diaphragm and compressing the lung, to present as left chest pain and dyspnoea. They are not radio-opaque. Many diseases can be simulated. Rupture is into the peritoneum. Splenectomy may be difficult because of adhesions.

2. Amoebic abscesses

These are very rare and usually occur in association with liver abscess. Early rupture occurs into the peritoneum.

B. ANAEMIA

Introduction

Several mechanisms can contribute to a lowering of haemoglobin level in parasitic disease.

1. Splenic sequestration and destruction of normal red cells

Any form of splenic enlargement will produce this effect, more or less in proportion to splenic size.

This mechanism is important in malaria and is a major factor in the tropical splenomegaly syndrome. It is also important in visceral leishmaniasis and to a lesser degree in hepatosplenic schistosomiasis. In these conditions leucocytes and platelets are sometimes similarly affected and a pancytopenia results.

2. Haemolysis

(a) Direct by intra-erythrocytic parasites (*Plasmodium* and *Babesia*).

(b) Indirectly through immunological mechanisms.

Reticuloendothelial cells remove red cells coated by immune complexes, antibody or complement. This mechanism is probably important in malaria, the more acute forms of trypanosomiasis, visceral leishmaniasis, babesiosis and perhaps in hepatosplenic schistosomiasis and toxocariasis.

Overwhelming intravascular haemolysis can occur in falciparum malaria to produce haemoglobinaemia and haemoglobinuria ('blackwater fever'). A similar phenomenon may occur in babesiosis.

3. Blood loss and consequent iron deficiency anaemia

Hookworm infection is the prime example. Heavy *Trichuris* infection and urinary and intestinal schistosomiasis also cause appreciable blood loss. Acute bleeding occurs from varices in hepatosplenic schistosomiasis, and also from amoebic and balantidial ulcers of the colon.

4. Secondary folate deficiency

Continued haemolysis in repeated malarial infections increases the folate requirements for erythropoiesis, and these may exceed supply. Chronic blood loss can have the same effect.

5. Vitamin B_{12} deficiency

The fish tapeworm (*Diphyllobothrium latum*) can reach 8 or 10 metres in length. It splits the intrinsic factor-B_{12} complex and incorporates the vitamin into its own body. Free B_{12} not taken up by the worm cannot be absorbed. Levels of serum B_{12}

decline over a period of several years and a few patients develop megaloblastic anaemia and even neurological changes. The location of the worm affects the outcome, since those higher in the small bowel deprive the host of more vitamin. Other factors contributing to fish tapeworm anaemia are reduced folate absorption and release of the haemolytic substance lysolecithin by the worm. In addition to anthelminthic treatment, patients with B_{12} deficiency must be given an adequate course of this vitamin by injection.

6. Bone marrow replacement

In late visceral leishmaniasis the marrow space is heavily infiltrated with macrophages, many of them parasitised. Normal marrow components are crowded out with depression of erythropoesis, leucopoesis and megakaryocyte formation. Bone marrow aspiration to demonstrate amastigotes is usually the diagnostic method of choice.

In three conditions anaemia is a major disease component. These will be considered in more detail.

Malaria

In acute falciparum malaria direct destruction of parasitised red cells is of prime importance and the rate of fall in haemoglobin level is usually proportional to the intensity of parasitaemia; when this exceeds 5 per cent the fall may be very rapid. In *P. vivax*, *P. ovale* and *P. malariae* malaria, intensity of parasitaemia very rarely exceeds 1 per cent and direct parasitisation can play little part in anaemia production. Patients with these three infections can, however, develop a progressive anaemia of moderate degree; immunological mechanisms and splenic sequestration must predominate.

The anaemia in malaria is primarily normochromic, normocytic. Between paroxysms and very soon after chemotherapy there is a brisk reticulocytosis reaching levels of 10 per cent; the large polychromatic cells may suggest a macrocytic anaemia. In acute paroxysms leucopenia is common and affects particularly polymorphonuclear cells; lymphocyte counts probably remain normal but monocytosis is common: Thrombocytopenia of moderate degree is common even in *P. vivax* malaria, while in *P. falciparum* levels may be depressed sufficiently to produce purpura. Splenic sequestration may be the major cause of leucopenia and thrombocytopenia in acute paroxysms, and the polymorphs show a shift to the left. Temporary marrow suppression could also be relevant in acutely ill patients and would explain the absence of reticulocytes in paroxysms. Malaria pigment is commonly seen in polymorphs and monocytes in heavy falciparum malaria and may persist for a few days after parasitaemia has cleared; occasionally this is a useful retrospective diagnostic clue in recently treated patients whose parasitaemia has cleared.

The evidence for immunological mechanisms in malarial anaemia includes lowered levels of serum complement in acute paroxysms and sometimes its presence on the red cell surface. Direct Coombs tests are sometimes positive and antibodies to tanned red cells are often detectable. In animals injection of malarial antigen alone can produce anaemia; in human malaria, antigen and immune complexes can be detected in serum. Splenic sequestration and non-immunological damage is also important when there is considerable splenic enlargement and this is persistent. Osmotic fragility of non-parasitised cells is increased.

Concurrent iron deficiency is common and this may give mixed blood film appearances. Malaria causes no iron loss from the body except in sweat, but gut absorption is halted during acute paroxysms. Malaria pigment (haemozoin) contains about 12 per cent elemental iron and although eventually this is all made reavailable it is temporarily sequestered from the available iron pool.

Continuing haemolysis in those with repeated or persistent parasitaemia leads to extension of hyperplastic marrow in the long bones. Secondary folate deficiency is common where dietary folate is inadequate, the marrow becomes megaloblastic and the blood film macrocytic; children and pregnant women are specially susceptible. Serum haptoglobin levels fall, because of haemoglobin release, and may become undetectable. Levels of unconjugated bilirubin are raised but only in the presence of parenchymal liver damage does significant jaundice occur. *Salmonella* septicaemia appears to be unusually common following malarial haemolysis, as it is in other haemolytic disorders. Very severe intravascular haemolysis can occur in non-immunes with falciparum malaria; the binding capacity of haptoglobin is exceeded, free haemoglobin is present in the serum and is lost in the urine, producing the syndrome of blackwater fever. In the past many cases were precipitated by quinine therapy; but a few cases occur without quinine and some kind of sensitisation must be involved. This condition must not be confused with drug-induced haemolysis in glucose-6-phosphate dehydrogenase deficient persons.

In the tropical splenomegaly syndrome parasitaemia is exceptional except during late pregnancy, and anaemia is due to splenic red cell sequestration, an expanded plasma volume and the culling of normal red cells by a hyperplastic reticuloendothelial system. The Coombs test is negative, haemoglobin levels range between 6–10 g/dl and response to prolonged antimalarial therapy is good.

The treatment of malarial anaemia normally requires only the elimination of the malaria parasite and where appropriate long-term chemosuppression. Short courses of folic acid may be required but not iron unless body iron stores are depleted. Blood transfusion is occasionally necessary in acute falciparum malaria. Blackwater fever is predominantly a renal problem (p. 162).

Visceral leishmaniasis

A pancytopenia is the usual finding in this infection. Haemoglobin levels fall progressively and may reach 3 g/dl; red cells are normochromic, normocytic. For most of the illness the marrow is hyperplastic and blood reticulocyte counts are raised. Normal red cells are sequestered and destroyed in the progressively enlarging spleen; there is some evidence that immunological mechanisms also play a part. Leucocytes and platelets are also removed by the spleen, white cell counts may fall below 2000/mm³ and neutrophils are particularly affected leading to secondary septic complications. Monocytosis is common and also a relative lymphocytosis. In India amastigotes may be found in circulating monocytes and less often in neutrophils; buffy coat films can be used diagnostically but organisms are scanty. Thrombocytopenia may contribute to bleeding.

In the very late stages of the infection the marrow may be replaced by macrophages accentuating the pancytopenia. Foci of extramedullary haematopoiesis are sometimes found in the spleen and liver.

Hookworm

Hookworm infection produces a simple blood loss iron deficiency anaemia, giving a microcytic hypochromic blood film. There is no good evidence that the worms release toxins that damage circulating red cells or suppress the marrow. The rate at which anaemia appears in hookworm infection depends upon the intensity and duration of infection, body iron stores and the availability of dietary iron. Even moderately heavy infections will not produce anaemia if plenty of dietary iron is available.

Feeding hookworms in the gut produce local traumatic bleeding, a process that is enhanced by the release of anticoagulant substances. Red cells ingested by the worms pass mainly straight through the gut and anus, the worms gaining their nutrients from plasma components. A variable proportion of the haemoglobin iron is reabsorbed by the human host, estimates vary up to 50 per cent, the remainder is permanently lost. Less iron is reabsorbed when worms are located lower down the small bowel.

With continued iron loss, body iron stores are progressively depleted, marrow iron becomes scanty or absent on microscopy, and serum ferritin levels fall. Later there is a fall in serum iron and a rise in iron binding capacity. Red cells become microcytic and hypochromic with some anisocytosis and poikilocytosis. In a previously healthy adult male it may take two or three years before a heavy hookworm infection produces anaemia, in children and pregnant women the period is very much less. Stool egg counts are useful in the assessment of the role of hookworm in an iron deficient patient; a count of 1000 eggs per gram, for either *Ancylostoma* or *Necator*, is equivalent to a daily blood loss of about 2.2 ml. Blood loss is directly proportional to the egg count.

The effects of hookworm anaemia are firstly upon physical and mental work capacity and secondly upon haemodynamic status; very low haemoglobin levels may lead to heart failure (p. 127). In addition iron deficiency may itself predispose to certain bacterial and other infections; although this relationship has been disputed it is the subject of considerable current research.

Oral iron medications are absorbed normally and this is the ideal form of iron replacement. The rate of rise in haemoglobin level is the same with oral and parenteral iron, about 1.5 g/dl per week. Unfortunately many patients will not persist with oral iron especially when this must be continued for up to three months to replace iron stores. Thus parenteral iron is preferred when replacement is urgent or there is doubt whether tablets will be taken; a single total dose intravenous infusion of Imferon will often be the preferred method.

C. LYMPHATIC PATHOLOGY

Tender lymphadenitis and lymphangitis

1. Lymphatic filariasis

The adult lymphatic-dwelling filarial worms (*Wuchereria bancrofti* and *Brugia malayi*) normally live in the afferent lymphatics, particularly those draining into the inguino-femoral, axillary and epitrochlear nodes (Fig. 9.1). If there is no tissue reaction the worms live unharmed, and their microfilariae pass through the glands and then, through the efferent lymphatics, to reach the blood. Sometimes this state of harmony persists throughout the infection, accompanied perhaps only by a mild reactive hyperplasia of the adjacent node. More frequently, there are repeated episodes of painful tender lymph node enlargement, **acute lymphadenitis**, lasting for several days and accompanied by fever, systemic upset and eosinophilia. Tender cords become palpable below the affected gland and these are acutely inflamed afferent lymphatics; this **acute lymphangitis** may become visible as red lines extending peripherally from the node. These acute episodes can be precipitated by death of the worms, local trauma, the moulting fluids of developing worms, or by chemotherapy.

Sometimes when intra-abdominal nodes are affected, acute inflammation presents as abdominal pain and fever, or sometimes fever alone ('filarial fever'); an important diagnostic clue is high blood eosinophilia.

The more severe acute episodes can be very vigorous and septic adenitis or cellulitis may be simulated; ulceration of overlying skin is by no means unusual.

The acute reactions in lymphatic filariasis probably result from both IgE-mediated hypersensitiv-

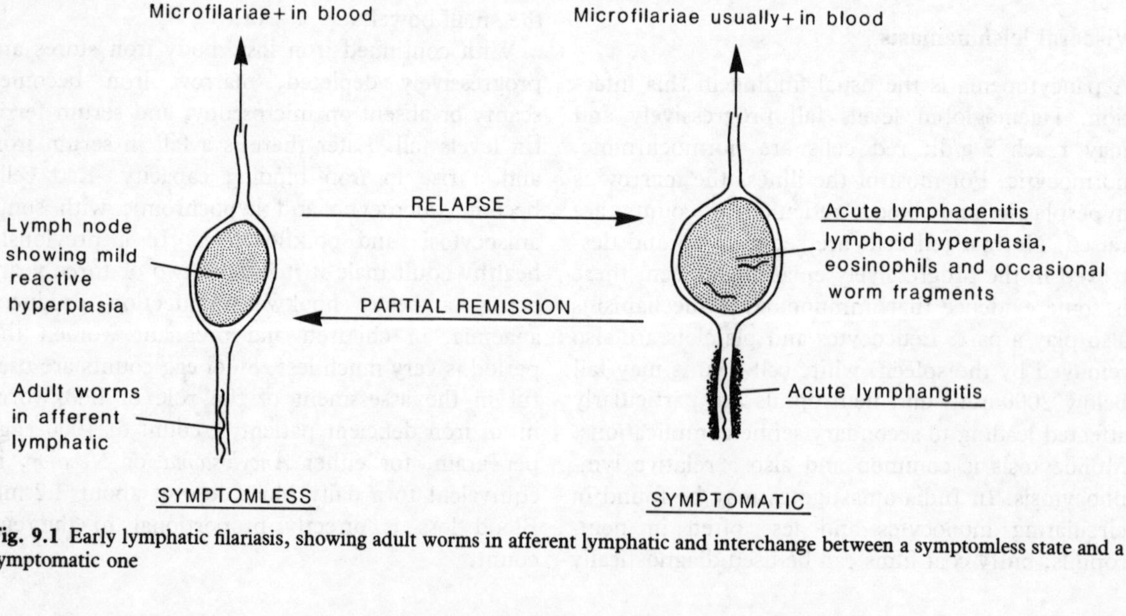

Microfilariae+ in blood　　　　　　Microfilariae usually+ in blood

Lymph node showing mild reactive hyperplasia

Adult worms in afferent lymphatic

RELAPSE

PARTIAL REMISSION

SYMPTOMLESS

Acute lymphadenitis lymphoid hyperplasia, eosinophils and occasional worm fragments

Acute lymphangitis

SYMPTOMATIC

Fig. 9.1 Early lymphatic filariasis, showing adult worms in afferent lymphatic and interchange between a symptomless state and a symptomatic one

ity and immune-complex Arthus reactions. In addition T and B lymphocytes proliferate in the nodes and, together with the repeated acute inflammatory episodes, this leads to chronically enlarged nodes in which degenerating worm fragments may be found. In some patients hypersensitivity to filarial antigens continues to build up and the blood becomes amicrofilaraemic, either because all the microfilaria are killed in lymph nodes or elsewhere; or because the adult worms themselves are destroyed immunologically. The majority of patients however, continue to show microfilaraemia and suffer repeated acute inflammatory episodes that lead, over a period of years, to more chronic changes.

2. Secondary septic adenitis and lymphangitis

Infected scabies and infected insect bites often lead to an ascending lymphangitis and adenitis; usually Streptococcus pyogenes is responsible. Patients with lymphoedema due to lymphatic filariasis also suffer repeated septic episodes, again caused by S. pyogenes; these often originate between the toes or in moist folds of elephantoid tissue. Unlike the filarial sensitivity reactions, septic lymphangitis moves up the limb and there is no eosinophilia. Penicillin must be given to prevent further damage to the lymphatic system. Patients with lymphoedema due to filariasis usually have raised antistreptolysin titres.

Children with head lice often have palpable posterior occipital nodes. In onchoceriasis, lymphadenitis is common, due either to secondary impetigo, or to hypersensitivity reactions against microfilariae and immune complexes carried to the nodes by dermal lymphatics.

Simple lymphadenopathy

Several protozoan infections may cause painless lymphadenopathy by promoting proliferation of lymphoid cells, plasma cells and macrophages. Sometimes the inflammatory changes are suggestive of a particular infection but they are by no means specific. Organisms can be very difficult or impossible to find in histological sections, and if nodes are removed for the exclusion of other conditions, such as lymphoma, then impression smears must be made of the sectioned gland immediately after it is removed. Impression smears should be examined as wet, and as stained preparations. Animal inoculations may be helpful, and also culture in suspected visceral leishmaniasis. Lymphatic filariasis can also present as simply lymphadenopathy but other features of the disease are nearly always present, and cervical gland enlargement is most unusual.

1. American trypanosomiasis — T. cruzi

A generalised lymphadenopathy forms part of the initial acute illness. The regional nodes draining the chagoma and inoculation site are affected first but the involvement soon becomes generalised. An enlarged pre-auricular node forms part of the Romana sign produced by conjunctival inoculation. Trypanosomes will be present in blood films except in the earliest stages. T. cruzi proliferate as amastigotes in lymph node macrophages, but all forms of the parasite might be seen in impression smears.

2. African trypanosomiasis — T.b. rhodesiense and T.b. gambiense

Here also an initial regional node may be related to the primary chancre, and this progresses to a generalised lymph node enlargement. Lymphadenopathy is by no means always present in T.b. rhodesiense infections but it is in T.b. gambiense. In the latter infection the long illness is characterised by episodes of fever and parasitaemia, and relapsing lymph node enlargement. Affected nodes are intially firm and rubbery but later they become smaller and fibrotic. As the infection progresses, nodes in the posterior triangle of the neck become the most noticably affected, and this sign (Winterbottom's) had been recognised as early as 1803 to be a precursor of sleeping sickness and death.

Needle aspiration of a cervical node is a classic diagnostic method in T.b. gambiense infections because parasitaemia may be intermittent and scanty. A rubbery node should be chosen, as fibrotic ones are often negative. Suction by syringe is usually unnecessary; the needle lumen will fill spontaneously if the gland is gently massaged for half a minute with the needle *in situ*. A finger is placed over the butt of the needle as it is withdrawn and the contents are expressed, by syringe, onto a slide.

3. *Visceral leishmaniasis — L. donovani*

In all forms of this infection, except those occuring in India, lymphadenopathy is a common feature, especially in the earlier stages of the disease. The glands are firm and rubbery but later become fibrotic. The cervical nodes are often prominently involved. Microscopically macrophage proliferation predominates over other cell types, and multinucleate giant cells may be seen. Amastigotes are usually numerous within the macrophages. Needle aspiration can be performed in the same manner as for *T.b. gambiense* infections.

4. *Toxoplasmosis*

In the acquired form of this infection generalised lymphadenopathy is very common; it is a less common feature of toxoplasmosis in the immunocompromised host, and is absent in congenital infections. Cervical nodes are particularly affected and this, together with systemic symptoms, creates a clinical picture similar to infectious mononucleosis. The glands are firm and nontender. Gland architecture is well preserved; necrosis and giant cells are absent. Cell proliferation is mainly histiocytic and groups of large eosinstaining reticulum cells are prominent. Organisms are very rarely seen in sections or smears, and animal inoculations are necessary to demonstrate them.

   Diagnosis is usually made serologically. Most acquired infections subside spontaneously and chemotherapy is only necessary when systemic symptoms or involvement of other body systems necessitates it.

Chronic filarial lymphatic lesions

Most patients heavily or repeatedly infected with *Wuchereria bancrofti* or *Brugia malayi* eventually develop one or more late disease manifestations (Fig. 9.2). Diagnosis is often difficult to establish with certainty because microfilaraemia may disappear, possibly for immunological reasons, in late infections, especially in lymphoedematous patients. The association of several late disease features, and a history of previous acute manifestations is highly suggestive. Skin tests and serology are currently of little value because many adults in endemic areas will give positive results. Features of chronic filariasis nearly always occur in adults. In order to frequency they are:

1. *Chronic lymphadenopathy*

Nodes in the inguino-femoral, axillary and epitrochlear region may reach a great size; especially those in the groin. Microscopy shows lymphoid hyperplasia, patchy fibrosis and fragments of dead worm surrounded by eosinophilic granulomas. The nodes are non-tender and enlargement is generally bilaterally symetrical.

2. *Genital lesions* (p. 160)

These include hydrocele, lesions of testis and spermatic cord, lymph scrotum and scrotal lymphoedema.

3. *Lymph varix — (lymphadenocele or varicose lymph node)*

Distension of the node capsule to form a lymphfilled sac results from lymphatic block higher up the lymphatic chain. These lesions are commonest in the groin, where a femoral hernia can be simulated, but they also occur in the axilla and epitrochlear regions. The enlarged node can be felt within the sac which empties by gravity when the part is elevated. Aspiration gives clear lymph, or sometimes chyle from groin varices; microfilariae are sometimes found in the fluid. Varicose lymph nodes are nearly always due to filariasis.

4. *Chronic lymphangitis*

This manifests as non-tender cords, up to half a centimeter in diameter, extending down the inner thigh from the groin, or medially in the upper arm between the axillary and epitrochlear nodes. These cords are fibrotic tissue reactions to previous episodes of acute lymphangitis; although fre-

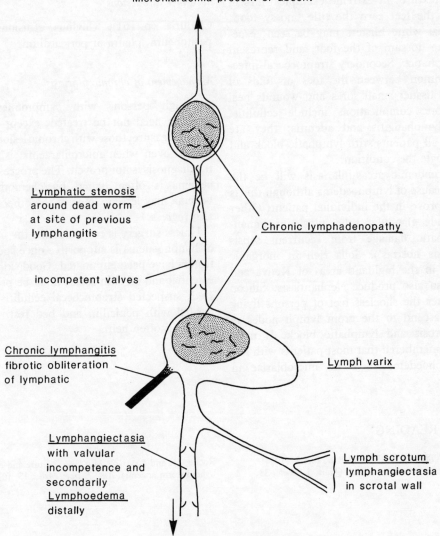

Microfilaraemia present or absent

Lymphatic stenosis
around dead worm
at site of previous
lymphangitis

Chronic lymphadenopathy

incompetent valves

Chronic lymphangitis
fibrotic obliteration
of lymphatic

Lymph varix

Lymphangiectasia
with valvular
incompetence and
secondarily
Lymphoedema
distally

Lymph scrotum
lymphangiectasia
in scrotal wall

Fig. 9.2 Late lymphatic filariasis

quently overlooked, they are useful signs because they are specific for filariasis.

5. *Lymphoedema*

This results from valvular incompetence of the lymphatic chain due to a more proximal block. Protein-rich fluid accumulates in the subcutaneous tissue and eventually sets up fibrous reactions. Initially the oedema is episodic, and often associated with fever, malaise and painful acute reactions in the draining lymph nodes. This early oedema may

be tender and it pits on pressure. After several episodes, the oedema becomes firm and non-pitting, but even at this stage it may still pit at its upper limit indicating that the process is still active. Most commonly lymphoedema is limited to the lower limb below the mid-calf, but it can extend upwards to the mid thigh. Involvement of the arms, scrotum, vulva and breasts are all much less common.

Chronic lymphoedema produces skin changes that give the condition its name, elephantiasis. Acanthosis and hyperkeratosis give the skin its dry, warty texture; in extreme examples filiform papillae on the feet earn the title 'mossy foot'. Subepidermal white blisters may be seen, especially on the dorsum of the foot, and represent dilated lymphatics. Secondary streptococcal infection is common between the toes or folds of elephantoid tissue; small sores and wounds heal poorly. Septic complications include cellulitis, ascending lymphangitis and adenitis; they are common in all patients with lymphatic block and they exacerbate the condition.

In most endemic areas filariasis will be the commonest cause of lymphoedema although this is difficult to prove in the individual patient. Other causes include glandular tuberculosis, malignancies, lymphatic damage from recurrent sepsis ('elephantiasis nostras'). Soils rich in inorganic silicates, as in the highland areas of Kenya and Ethiopia, can also produce elephantiasis. Silicon particles enter the shoeless feet of persons living there, and ascend to the groin lymph nodes to produce fibrosis and lymphatic block. It must always be remembered that most patients with late filarial lymphoedema show no microfilariae in their blood.

6. Other rare lesions

Chyluria (p. 161). Chylous effusions into the peritoneum, pleura or pericardium.

Management of chronic filariasis

Although persons with symptomless microfilaraemia need not be treated, except as a public health measure, those with chronic lesions should be treated even when microfilaraemia is absent and the diagnosis is not proven. The progress of lymphoedema is often halted by chemotherapy and oedema may lessen; some of the other lesions will also regress.

Unless surgery is contemplated the management of lymphoedema is supportive once specific causal factors have been eliminated. Good skin hygiene is essential and all skin sepsis must be promptly treated; suspected streptococcal cellulitis should be treated with penicillin and bed rest. Supportive bandages often help.

FURTHER READING

Gilles, H.M., Williams, E.J.W. and Ball, P.A.J. (1964) Hookworm infection and anaemia. *Quart. J. Med.*, 33, 1–24.

Roche, M. and Layrisse, M. (1966) Nature and causes of hookworm anaemia. *Am. J. trop. Med.*, 15, 1031–1100.

10

Local effects of parasitism 4

A. SKIN DISEASE

Parasites damage dermal tissues in several ways. The relationship of these organisms to the skin takes several forms and these are shown in Table 10.1. Three groups of parasitic disease, cutaneous leishmaniasis, cutaneous filariasis and the parasitic arthropods are of special dermatological importance. These will be considered first before the differential diagnosis of parasitic skin disease is considered more generally.

Table 10.1 Relationship between the skin and the parasites causing skin pathology

A. True parasites of dermal tissues — skin natural site of parasite entry and exit
    1. Epidermis — scabies and other mites. *Tunga penetrans* (blood feeder)
    2. Dermal macrophages — cutaneous leishmaniasis
    3. Dermis and subcutaneous tissue — myiasis
    4. Subcutaneous, microfilariae in dermis — *Onchocerca*, *Dipetalonema streptocerca*
    5. Subcutaneous, microfilariae in blood — *Loa loa*
B. Lesions at sites of entry
    1. Vector-borne protozoa
       — *Trypanosoma* (transient lesions)
       Leishmania donovani (sometimes)
    2. Helminth larvae — hookworm, *Strongyloides*, *Schistosoma*
C. Lesions at site of exit — guineaworm (*Dracunculus*)
D. Dissemination from viscera
    — *Taenia solium*, *Gnathostoma*, *Entamoeba*, *Leishmania donovani* (late), *Dirofilaria repens* and *tenuis*, *Spirometra*. Ectopic flukes
E. Allergic reactions to blood–feeding anthropods — lice, mosquitoes, etc.
F. Sensitivity reactions to internal parasites
    — *Ascaris*, *Echinococcus*, etc. *Trypanosoma*
G. Secondary changes due to lymphatic block
    — *Wuchereria*, *Brugia*
H. Secondary bacterial infections
    — Superimposed on the lesions of many parasites causing ulceration and pruritus

Cutaneous leishmaniasis (due to the *L. tropica*, *L. mexicana* and *L. braziliensis* species complexes)

After inoculation into the dermis by the sandfly (*Phlebotomus* etc.) vector, the infective promastigotes enter dermal macrophages and transform into amastigotes. Thereafter parasite multiplication continues within dermal macrophages and histiocytes. The normal evolution of the uncomplicated dermal lesion is shown in Figure 10.1

The initial lesion is a non-itchy papule which appears two to six weeks after the infective bite; microscopy shows the lesion to be heavily infiltrated with macrophages and histiocytes which proliferate locally. Many of these cells contain parasites. Within three weeks lymphocytes infiltrate into the periphery of the lesion together with some plasma cells. The local immune response, which finally eliminates the parasites, is mediated by specifically sensitised T lymphocytes. As cell mediated immunity builds up infected macrophages and their parasites are destroyed and the vigorous cellular reaction causes local necrosis so that the overlying epidermis ulcerates. The lesion then extends peripherally with the strong inflammatory reaction continuing under the slightly raised edges of the lesion; satellite lesions are common; these begin as papules but may later fuse with the main lesion as it extends. The edges of the ulcer are well defined, and its base is often covered by a slough and evidence of bacterial infection. Parasites become progressively more scanty and eventually the lesion heals after a period of activity lasting between three months and two years. The scar is slightly depressed and shows a thin epidermis and some fibrosis in the upper dermis. The leishmanin skin test becomes

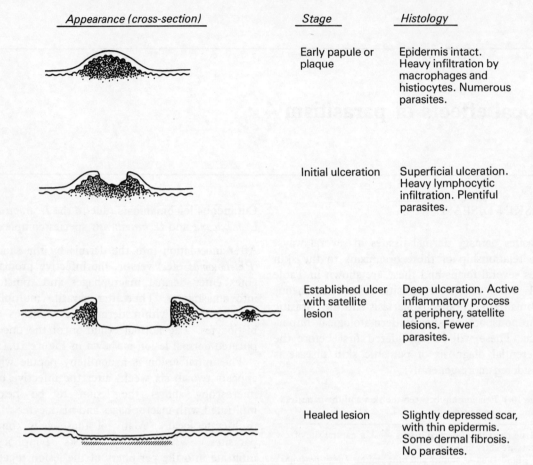

Appearance (cross-section)	Stage	Histology
	Early papule or plaque	Epidermis intact. Heavy infiltration by macrophages and histiocytes. Numerous parasites.
	Initial ulceration	Superficial ulceration. Heavy lymphocytic infiltration. Plentiful parasites.
	Established ulcer with satellite lesion	Deep ulceration. Active inflammatory process at periphery, satellite lesions. Fewer parasites.
	Healed lesion	Slightly depressed scar, with thin epidermis. Some dermal fibrosis. No parasites.

Fig. 10.1 Normal evolution of lesion in cutaneous leishmaniasis

positive soon after ulceration begins, it reflects the patient's cell mediated sensitivity to leishmanial antigen. Lesions are commonest on exposed parts of the body, especially the hands, lower arms and legs, face and ears.

The characteristics of the lesion depend to a considerable degree upon the species and subspecies of the infecting parasite (Table 2.2). In the Eastern hemisphere cutaneous lesions are caused by members of the *L. tropica* complex, the condition has many local names but is generally referred to as oriental sore. The most benign lesions, which rarely exceed 2 cms in diameter, are caused by *L. tropica* (= *L.t. minor*) which produces the so-called 'dry' or 'urban-type' lesions, and also by *L. aethiopica*. Larger, more rapidly spreading and sometimes multiple lesions are produced by *L. major*; this is sometimes known as the 'moist' or

'rural-type' of the disease. In the Western hemisphere, the *L. mexicana* complex usually produce mild disease; the commonest form is due to *L.m. mexicana;* which occurs particularly among wild rubber collectors and is known locally as chiclero's ulcer. The *L. braziliensis* complex produce mild to moderately severe disease and sometimes lesions are multiple; those due to *L. peruviana* of the high Andes are generally mild. In two of the subspecies, *L.b. guyanensis* and *L.b. panamensis*, local lymphatic spread can occur producing indurated lymphatic cords, often with multiple ulceration along the course of limb lymphatics, a condition known locally as 'pian bois'. In infections due to *L.b. braziliensis* there is the risk of spread to the nasopharynx to produce mucocutaneous leishmaniasis (p. 151).

Although the healing rate of all cutaneous

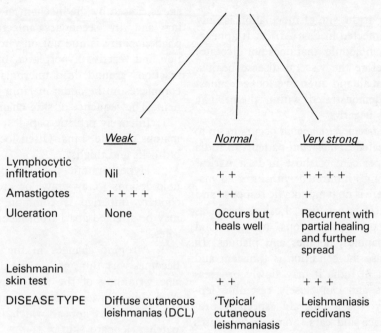

CELL MEDIATED IMMUNE RESPONSE

	Weak	Normal	Very strong
Lymphocytic infiltration	Nil	+ +	+ + + +
Amastigotes	+ + + +	+ +	+
Ulceration	None	Occurs but heals well	Recurrent with partial healing and further spread
Leishmanin skin test	—	+ +	+ + +
DISEASE TYPE	Diffuse cutaneous leishmanias (DCL)	'Typical' cutaneous leishmaniasis	Leishmaniasis recidivans

Fig. 10.2 Spectrum of cellular immune response in cutaneous leishmaniasis

lesions is determined, to some degree, by the strength of the patient's cellular immune response, there are two atypical forms of cutaneous leishmaniasis, both of them uncommon, which appear to be caused almost entirely by an abnormal host immune response. These atypical forms represent the two ends of the immunological spectrum; their main characteristics are shown in Figure 10.2, which contrasts them with the normal response which lies between these extremes.

a. *Leishmaniasis recidivans*. This is a relapsing form of oriental sore, that occurs with some strains of *L. tropica*, particularly those found in Iraq and Israel; its overall frequency is about one per cent of all *L. tropica* lesions. The host's immune response appears to be good, or even excessive, but the parasites are not completely eliminated. The lesion continues to spread over a period of many years, with partial healing and then new activity at the margins of the previous lesion. The clinical and histological appearances are very similar to those of cutaneous tuberculosis, the parasites are very scanty.

b. *Diffuse cutaneous leishmaniasis (DCL)*. This condition is associated with an antigen-specific immunological defect that allows parasites to multiply uncontrolled within the dermis. No ulceration occurs, and within the dermis lymphocytes are very scanty, but parasites and macrophages are very numerous; the leishmanin skin test remains negative. Papular, nodular and plaque-like lesions may extend all over the body. In the Eastern hemisphere this lesion only occurs with *L. aethiopica*, but it accounts for less than 0.01 per cent of all infections with this parasite. In the Western hemisphere it is considerably more common but is only produced by *L. mexicana amazonensis* and *L.m. pifanoi*; the latter is a rare subspecies that has only been isolated from patients with DCL.

The diagnosis of cutaneous leishmaniasis can only be confirmed by finding amastigotes (p. 184) or culturing *Leishmania* promastigotes (p. 186) in material obtained from the lesions. Needle aspiration is the simplest method but not always positive. Most parasites are found in the active non-ulcerated parts of the lesions. The leishmanin test (p. 189) is useful in later lesions, but does not distinguish between current and past infection.

Cutaneous lesions due to *Leishmania donovani*

A primary lesion at the site of inoculation is only seen in patients infected in East Africa. It appears as a papule or small nodule, that does not ulcerate, a few months before the visceral disease begins. The lesions are small and often overlooked; amastigotes can be demonstrated within them. The leishmanin test is negative.

Post-kala-azar dermal leishmanoid occurs in up to 20 per cent of treated *L. donovani* patients in India and in about 2 per cent of those in East Africa. The dermis becomes infiltrated with infected macrophages but there is no lymphocytic response and the leishmanin test is negative. Lesions begin as hypopigmented or erythematous macules and transform into papules, nodules and plaques. In the African disease the condition is transient and self-limiting, but in India it may slowly progress over many years and can closely resemble lepromatous leprosy; the lesions are especially prominent on the face and ears. Some Indian cases remit spontaneously but others require further chemotherapy; the parasites are not drug-resistant.

Cutaneous filariasis

A. Onchocerciasis

Adult worms. Fibrous nodules (**onchocercomata**) containing several adult worms become palpable in the subcutaneous tissues a year or more after exposure to infection begins. The nodules are smooth, rounded, non-tender and measure up to 3 cm in diameter. They are freely mobile and located particularly over bony prominences including the iliac crest, sacro-iliac region, greater trochanters, knees, shoulders and chest wall.

Nodulectomy is an effective way of reducing the worm load in onchocerciasis, the procedure is simple and safe as the nodules are superficial. Nodules on the skull are of special importance because of their proximity to the eyes.

Onchodermatitis. Microfilariae of *O. volvulus* live in the dermis but only cause damage when they die and set up sensitivity reactions that include infiltration by eosinophils, lymphocytes and plasma cells. Lesions progress and evolve over a period of many years and severity is generally proportional to worm load. Quite a lot of the damage is caused by the mechanical effects of scratching and by secondary infection. Local lymphadenopathy is due not only to secondary infection and reactive hyperplasia, but to Arthus-type reactions around dead microfilariae and immune complexes in the node; melanin pigment is prominent. The sequence of skin changes is:

1. Intensely pruritic papules, appearing erythematous on pale skins. Often located initially over buttocks and thighs.

2. Hyperkeratotic papules, plaques and lichenoid lesions ('craw-craw' or crocodile skin). Secondary impetigo is common. The whole skin may be affected apart from face, scalp, palms and soles.

3. Atrophic changes in the epidermis, which becomes very thin, and in the dermis; produces a fine wrinkling of the skin, noticeable especially over shins, lower abdomen and knees. Speckled achromic spots appear which fuse into irregular patches (leopard skin).

4. Late and secondary changes. Gross inguinal adenopathy. Pendulous folds of atrophic skin producing 'hanging groin' lesions that may contain mobile lymph nodes, and 'hottentot apron' when the lower abdominal wall is affected. The incidence of both inguinal hernia and hydrocele is increased. Elephantiasis of legs and scrotum are rare sequels.

Unusual and geographically localised lesions:

a. *Sowda* — In Yemen and sometimes in Africa dark hyperkeratotic plaques about the ankles occur in association with prominent inguinal adenopathy. Microfilariae are scanty and the eyes are not damaged.

b. *Erisipela de la costa* — In Central America acute allergic reactions, in which facial oedema is prominent, occur in early infections. Cellulitis can be simulated, hence the name of this condition.

Onchodermatitis is diagnosed by finding microfilariae in skin snips. When they cannot be found a single tablet (50 mg base) of diethylcarbamezine may be given. Local or generalised skin reactions caused by microfilarial death occur within 24 hours; this is known as the **Mazzotti reaction**. Chemotherapy must be given under close supervision especially when there is eye involvement.

B. Loaiasis

Adult worms live for up to 15 years migrating in subcutaneous and connective tissues. Infections are sometimes clinically silent but usually recurrent acute subcutaneous swellings ('Calabar swellings') appear in response to released worm antigen. These may follow minor trauma, and the forearms and wrists are the most commonly affected sites. The skin becomes tender, reddened and indurated; the reactions last a few days and may be accompanied by systemic upset. Possibly moulting larval worms also precipitate the reactions, as the blood may be negative for microfilarae.

Loa worms are sometimes noticed wriggling immediately beneath the dermis. Their ocular manifestations (p. 150) result from migration across the orbit or beneath the bulbar conjunctiva.

C. Dipetalonemiasis

Adult *D. streptocerca* live in subcutaneous tissue. No nodules are formed but, like *O. volvulus*, the microfilariae live in the dermis and set up allergic reactions when they die. The cutaneous manifestations are always mild and consist of pruritic erythematous papules. Occasionally 'Calabar-like' swellings occur with this species as they do also with *D. perstans* and *Mansonella ozzardi*.

The chief importance of *D. streptocerca* is that its microfilariae must be distinguished from those of *O. volvulus* in skin snips.

Skin lesions due to parasitic arthropods

A. Allergic reactions to biting arthropods

Depending upon the host's state of sensitisation reactions vary from none at all, to moderate or even severe immediate or delayed hypersensitivity reactions. Most lesions are pruritic, they may be erythematous, papular or wheal-like, and can appear within minutes or up to 48 hours after the bite. Purpura can occur but is rare. Secondary vesicle formation with rupture and scabbing are common and small ulcers are a frequent sequel. Regional lymphadenopathy is minimal unless there is secondary infection. Sensitisation of an individual to a particular biting species usually follows the following sequence:

Immediate Reaction	Delayed Reaction
—	
—	+
+	+
+	—
—	—

In a few people immediate sensitivity reactions do not decline but escalate into generalised anaphylactic reactions. Specific desensitisation can be attempted. In addition to the immediate and delayed types of reaction, an intermediate Arthus-type response can occur.

Identification of the biting species is sometimes helped by the anatomical location of the lesions, their grouping and appearance, and by the time of biting.

B. True epidermal parasites

1. Scabies. The superficial burrows of *Sarcoptes scabiei* within the stratum corneum of the skin must be searched for in all patients with generalised or local pruritus. The sites of election are between the fingers, anterior surface of the wrist, elbows, axillae, belt line, genitalia and feet. The total number of mites is often between 10 and 15 and rarely exceeds 100. The sensitivity reaction comprising widespread pruritic papules coincides with the onset of the sensitivity reaction that appears two or three weeks after the infection begins; it is this allergic response that finally limits the mite population. Diagnosis can only be confirmed by finding mites within their burrows and a needle should be used to remove them for microscopy. A therapeutic trial may be justified when no burrows or mites can be found.

'Norwegian scabies' is a form of the disease occuring in very debilitated or immunosuppressed persons. The mites and their burrows are very numerous and the affected skin greatly thickened and crusted.

2. Other mites and the chigoe flea. Grain and food mites, blood-sucking mites of poultry and rodents, and the harvest mites (chiggers) can all set up temporary residence partly embedded in the human epidermis. Many pruritic dermatological conditions can be simulated. Enquiry into occupational and leisure activities may give useful clues.

The chigoe flea (*Tunga penetrans*) or jigger is a blood-feeder but the female lives almost completely embedded in the epidermis until she grows to a relatively enormous size, oviposits and finally dies *in situ*. The lesions superficially resemble verrucas but are located mainly between the toes, under the toe nails and along the sides of the feet. Occasionally they are found on the hands and buttocks. They should be removed with a sterile needle after enlarging the entrance hole.

C. Myiasis

Three types of myiasis affect the skin:

1. Wound infections. Muscid flies, screw worm flies, blow flies and flesh flies deposit their eggs (or larvae) in open wounds and sores. The diagnosis is obvious and once the maggots are found they must all be aseptically removed. Local irrigation with 15 per cent chloroform in oil anaesthetises them, facilitating their capture.

2. Faruncular form. Lesions resembling boils form around the maggot which grows *in situ* quite deeply embedded in the dermis and subcutis. Until the mature larva appears sepsis will be suspected. Dead larvae provoke unpleasant local reactions. In subsaharan Africa the usual species responsible is *Cordylobia anthropophaga* (tumbu fly). Its eggs are laid on soil, sand or clothes laid out to dry. In Central and South America, *Dermatobia hominis* is the usual species; its eggs are laid on mosquitoes and fall off the latter when they feed on man. Larvae can be extracted from farunculoid lesions by occluding the opening with petroleum jelly to block the air supply. The larvae of warble flies (*Hypoderma*) can also produce farunculoid lesions.

3. Migratory or larva migrans form. Serpentine erythematous tracks or ambulatory tumours are produced as the growing larvae migrate in the dermis or subcutis. Responsible genera are *Gastrophilus* and *Hypoderma*; lesions may simulate those caused by migrating helminths.

Morphological classification of skin lesions due to parasites

The various types of skin lesions caused by parasites are listed here under morphological headings. Brief notes are given, where relevant, on differential diagnosis and management.

A. Ulcers

1. Cutaneous leishmaniasis — Slow evolution, preceding papule or nodule.
2. *Entamoeba histolytica* — Amoebic ulcers are painful, foul smelling, and spread rapidly. They occur in perianal and genital areas, and on the abdominal wall. Amoebae are demonstrable in fresh smears.
3. *Dracunculus* (Guinea worm) — Preceding nodule and vesicle. Worm usually visible. Slow worm extraction is essential, and usually takes several days. Systemic allergic effects are common, especially if the worm ruptures. Chemotherapy is necessary for multiple lesions.
4. Wound myiasis.

B. Nodules and subcutaneous lesions

Acute inflammatory:
1. *Trypanosoma cruzi* and *Trypanosoma b. rhodesiense* — Inoculation site lesions, termed chagomas and chancres respectively.
2. *Dracunculus* (prior to vesiculation and rupture). Faruncular myiasis. Sparganosis. *Tunga* (chigoe flea). Loaiasis ('Calabar swellings'). *Dirofilaria* spp.
Chronic inflammatory:
1. Cutaneous leishmaniasis (Early lesions prior to ulceration, or diffuse cutaneous form).
2. Post-kala-azar dermal leishmanoid.
Mobile non-tender subcutaneous nodules: An excisional biopsy is commonly necessary to establish the diagnosis.
1. Cysticercosis (*Taenia solium*).
2. Onchocercal nodules.
3. Rare parasites such as *Dirofilaria* and *Spirometra*, and ectopic flukes (*Fasciola* and *Paragonimus*).

C. Papules

Persistent, very pruritic — Onchodermatitis. Scabies.

Persistent, non-pruritic — Cutaneous leishmaniasis (early lesions and diffuse form). Post-kala-azar dermal leishmanoid.

Transient, pruritic — Cercarial dermatitis. Biting arthropods. Mites other than scabies.

D. Larva migrans (Cutaneous form)

1. Hookworm — Transient lesions due to human species. Persistent lesions are usually due to the dog hookworm *Ancylostoma braziliense* which particularly affects the feet or buttocks; local or even systemic thiabendazole may be required.

2. *Strongyloides* — Rapidly moving wheal-like lesions especially around buttocks and trunk. Recurrent, often over a period of several years. Stools usually positive for larvae.

3. Creeping myiasis — *Hypoderma* and *Gastrophilus*.

4. *Gnathostoma* — Deep painful lesions with a vigorous local reaction.

5. *Loa loa* — Long worm, often visibly moving. Wheal-like reaction.

6. Ectopic flukes (*Fasciola* and *Paragonimus*) — On abdominal wall particularly.

7. *Dirofilaria* — Deep painful migratory nodule.

E. Urticaria

1. May be a systemic allergic reaction to various helminths. Common in *Ascaris* infection, the stools should be examined. Also occurs in the invasive and acute stages of schistosomiasis, and other trematode infections.

2. Trypanosomiasis — Particularly in early *T.b. rhodesiense* infections in pale-skinned persons. Appears as a circinate or annular erythema.

F. Pruritus ani

1. *Enterobius vermicularis*.

2. *Taenia saginata*.

3. *Strongyloides* — Larva migrans lesions are usually also present on the buttocks.

G. Papulo-vesicular

Vigorous sensitivity reactions or secondary infection associated with scabies and other mite infestations, insect bites, cercarial dermatitis and onchocerciasis. A large vesicle or bulla is formed by *Dracunculus* prior to rupture.

Secondary bacterial infection of skin lesions caused by parasites

This is a common sequel in scabies, reactions to biting arthropods, onchocerciasis and guinea worm, and also in lymphoedematous limbs. The primary bacterial pathogen is nearly always *Streptococcus pyogenes* but this is often followed by *Staphylococcus*, *Corynebacterium* and *Clostridium*. Non-biting flies (muscids and *Hippelates*) are very important mechanical vectors of these bacteria, transmitting them from one sore to another; in addition the bacteria are transferred by direct contact and by fomites. Although the septic lesions produced may be initially relatively trivial, the open sores often progress to local abscess formation, ascending cellulitis and septic adenitis. Other additional complications are listed below; the serious nature of most of them is self-evident.

1. *Poststreptococcal glomerulonephritis*. Epidemics have particularly been associated with infected scabies but other open sores carry the same risk. Nephritogenic strains of *S. pyogenes* are rapidly disseminated among persons with open skin lesions; prompt treatment with penicillin is essential.

2. *Tetanus*. With *Tunga* infections particularly, because of contact with soil; but may occur with any other deep septic lesion for example guinea worm.

3. *Gas gangrene*. Rare but occurs in deep myiasis and guinea worm.

4. *Cutaneous diphtheria*. *Corynebacterium diphtheriae* can often be isolated from open lesions of all kinds in the rural tropics and many of the strains are toxigenic. Clinical diphtheria is a rare sequel — when it does occur it presents as a polyneuropathy. Cutaneous infection with *C. diphtheriae* is the usual way that non-immunised children in the rural tropics become Schick negative and immune to faucial diphtheria.

5. *Exacerbation of lymphoedema*. Filarial lymphoedema is very susceptible to secondary infection by *S. pyogenes*, considerable damage is done. Lymphoedema is sometimes produced wholly by recurrent sepsis ('elephantiasis nostras').

6. *Tropical phagedenic ulcer*. These are common in many tropical countries. They usually occur on the legs below the knee and malnutrition is a contributory factor. Although the primary pathogens are the mouth commensals *Borrelia vincentii* and *Bacteroides*, the lesions always follow minor trauma. Open sores from insect bites are one source of such trauma, and perhaps an important one.

B. EYE PATHOLOGY

Onchocerciasis

This is the most important parasitic infection affecting the eye. Since it affects several intraocular structures more or less simultaneously it will be considered separately. Figure 10.3 shows how the lesions are distributed.

All eye pathology results from acute inflammatory foci around dead and dying microfilariae that have entered the globe from surrounding tissues. The process is a slow and cumulative one; significant pathology occurs only when heavy or moderately heavy infections have persisted for several years. Most microfilariae enter the eye by passing beneath the bulbar conjunctiva and penetrating the globe at the limbus; from here they enter the cornea, aqueous humour and iris. Other microfilariae pass along the sheaths of the anterior ciliary vessels to the peripheral parts of the choroid and retina.

The earliest lesion is a punctate keratitis consisting of small discrete white lesions in the corneal substance, each of which represents an inflammatory reaction around a single microfilaria; the lesions are transitory and cause no permanent damage, vision is not affected and the patient

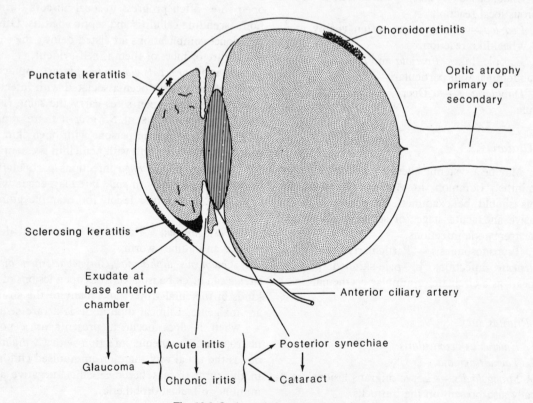

Fig. 10.3 Ocular pathology in onchocerciasis

complains only of an itchy conjunctiva. With a slit lamp living microfilariae may be seen in the aqueous humour even in early infections; when they die an inflammatory reaction is set up at the base of the anterior chamber and this progressively damages the inferior part of the iris, drawing it downwards to produce a distorted pear-shaped pupil. Episodes of acute iritis often occur and lead to posterior synechiae, chronic iritis and sometimes glaucoma or cataract. The most serious damage to the anterior part of the eye is a sclerosing keratitis, an irreversible fibrotic reaction beginning at the periphery of the cornea, near the limbus, and extending inwards with progressive visual impairment; the inferior, medial and lateral parts of the cornea are particularly affected. Choroidoretinal lesions begin peripherally as a pigmented destructive choroidoretinitis, with prominent sheathing of retinal vessels; the visual field is restricted peripherally producing tunnel vision. The optic nerve may be damaged directly by microfilariae within its substance, or secondary optic atrophy can result from the choroidoretinitis. The prevalence of posterior segment lesions is difficult to determine because they are often obscured in a heavily infected person by opacification of the cornea and lens.

The diagnosis of ocular onchocerciasis is based upon the appearance of the lesions and the presence of microfilariae in skin and conjunctival snips, and in the aqueous humour. Management is difficult because chemotherapy can produce new lesions and even blindness if acute iridocyclitis or glaucoma is precipitated. Suramin kills adult worms and can arrest or improve anterior segment lesions; unfortunately posterior lesions may progress even when the patient is parasitologically cured. Because suramin is given parenterally, and its action is slow and delayed, sensitivity reactions are dificult to control. To obviate this a course of diethylcarbamazine should be given first to destroy most of the microfilariae; steroid cover is usually necessary and supervision of treatment by an ophthalmologist is desirable. Acute anterior lesions such as iritis are best treated with diethylcarbamazine under steroid cover. Onchocercal nodules on the skull should always be removed to reduce the number of microfilariae entering the eyes.

Choroidoretinitis

1. Toxoplasmosis

A large proportion, perhaps 30–50 per cent, of cases of unexplained patchy choroidoretinitis are believed to be due to toxoplasmosis. Acquired toxoplasmosis very rarely affects the eye and nearly all examples of toxoplasmic choroidoretinitis are presumed to be isolated manifestations of congenital infection. Lesions are commonest, but by no means confined to, the anterior one-third of the retina, possibly because this is supplied by the central retinal artery which is less permeable to antibodies. *Toxoplasma* organisms proliferate within retinal cells and when these rupture an intense inflammatory reaction is set up, lesions are active at their periphery and periods of quiescence alternate with further progression. In some patients the lesions are clinically silent and discovered incidentally by ophthalmoscopy; however many patients have recurrent episodes of ocular pain and decreased vision leading to scotomata and progressive loss of vision. A vitreous haze develops during exacerbations; lesions are often in clusters containing old and recent pathology. The iris is never primarily affected although some secondary reactive damage can occur. Serological titres are low in this form of the disease but high levels of antibody are found in aqueous humour fluid; other conditions should be excluded.

Acute episodes often require steroid therapy to suppress the inflammatory response and should be given together with a course of chemotherapy, using a combination of sulphadiazine with pyrimethamine. It is doubtful whether chemotherapy often eliminates the infection completely and it may have to be repeated; alternatively long-term chemosuppression with pyrimethamine may prevent relapses.

2. Toxocariasis

The commonest manifestation of this accidental dog ascarid infection in man is an eosinophilic granuloma in the retina; a solitary larva lies at the centre of the lesion. Most patients are children between 2 and 10 years of age and nearly always there is only one lesion. The usual presentation is strabismus, or the parents may notice a white pupillary reflex. Vision can be severely impaired when lesions are near the macula; temporary impairment may be due to a vitreous inflammatory haze. The condition can closely simulate a retinoblastoma, and many eyes have been needlessly enucleated because the latter diagnosis was suspected. Rarely a more fulminant endophthalmitis is produced, especially when lesions are near the ciliary body.

Most patients with ocular involvement do not have visceral larva migrans or marked blood eosinophilia. Serology is of considerable help. Chemotherapy has not been proven to heal existing lesions but should be given to prevent other lesions developing. Steroids may be necessary to suppress acute inflammatory reactions.

Space-occupying lesions

Larval cestodes

Cysticerci (*T. solium*) may lodge in subretinal tissues; as they grow they cause retinal detachment and often perforate the retina to pass into the vitreous humour, through which they may progress to the anterior chamber. Lesions will invariably be present elsewhere. Subretinal lesions can be removed surgically without permanent damage to the eye; alternatively photocoagulation has been used. Parasites dying within the vitreous humour set up very severe inflammatory reactions. Rarely hydatids develop within the eye, originating in subretinal tissue.

Several worms have occasionally been seen in the aqueous humour, and have included adult schistosomes, a filarid worm resembling *Brugia malayi* and even larval pentastomes; intense inflammatory reactions may follow their death.

Orbital oedema and cellulitis

1. American trypanosomiasis

The conjunctival sac is the classical inoculation site for *T. cruzi*; a sleeping child scratches the site of a bug bite, contaminates his fingers with bug faeces, and then rubs his eyes. Trypanosomes proliferate locally and within a few days produce a firm unilateral orbital oedema with enlargement of the ipsilateral preauricular lymph node — the Romana sign. A few days later trypanosomes appear in the blood.

2. Trichinosis

The extraocular muscles are sites of election for lodgment of *T. spiralis*, and ocular signs appear in at least one-third of symptomatic infections. Bilateral orbital pain and oedema is produced together with some paralysis of ocular movements. Other features include scleral and retinal haemorrhages, chemosis of the bulbar conjunctiva, blurred vision, photophobia and diplopia. No permanent damage is done.

3. Loaiasis

Migrating adults or mature larvae of *Loa loa* frequently cross the orbit in subcutaneous tissue or beneath the bulbar conjunctiva, giving this worm its common appellation 'eye worm'. No damage is done to the eye itself but the worm migration is distressing to the patient, especially when a worm is seen wriggling across the scleral surface. There is intense itching and some pain and the eyelids become closed by an acute oedematous reaction that may persist for several days; the worms remain visible under the conjunctiva for less than an hour. No attempt need be made to remove the worm but a full course of chemotherapy should be given.

4. Sparganosis

Frog poultices are commonly applied to infected eyes in Thailand and Vietnam. Plerocercoid larvae of the pseudophyllidian tapeworm *Spirometra* can cross from the frog tissues to those of the patient. An intense oedema and cellulitis of the orbit follows, proceeding to nodule formation and eventually degeneration of the worms into a caseous mass. Excision may be necessary.

5. Myiasis

Flies of several genera may deposit eggs or larvae in the conjunctival sac. This occurs especially in debilitated patients, those with depressed consciousness, or with conjunctival exudates. The hatched larvae then migrate within the orbit doing considerable damage, secondary infection is common. The condition is of special importance because the globe may be entered, and the eye destroyed by panophthalmitis. *Oestrus ovis*, a parasite of sheep and goats, is perhaps the commonest species to do this but a number of other species (p. 84) may be responsible. The larvae must be removed from the orbital tissues. Fortunately *O. ovis*, which frequently 'attacks' healthy eyes, often produces only an external ophthalmomyiasis — the larvae remain in the conjunctival sac where they cause intense irritation.

6. *Larval cestodes*

The orbit is not an uncommon site for hydatid or coenurus cysts. The usual presentation is unilateral proptosis. Rupture during removal can cause severe damage.

7. *Dirofilaria repens*

This uncommon human parasite can present as a conjunctival nodule or inflammatory mass.

Keratitis

Some indolent corneal ulcers have recently been shown to be perpetuated by secondary infection with the free-living amoeba *Acanthamoeba polyphaga*; the initial lesion having perhaps been a simple abrasion. Possibly the use of local steroid applications allows these facultative parasites to gain a hold. Sulphadiazine and amphotericin B should be used locally.

Blepharitis

Some intractible cases of this condition are caused by the louse *Phthirus pubis*, and this parasite and its 'nits' should be searched for in the eyelashes, eyebrows, and also in the axillary and pubic hair.

C. PARASITES OF THE OROPHARYNX

Mucocutaneous leishmaniasis — 'Espundia'

Depending upon the infecting strain of *L. b. braziliensis* the probability of spread to the nasopharynx varies between 5 and 85 per cent. Dissemination is blood-borne and can occur even before the primary lesion has healed or as late as 20 years afterwards. The cartilaginous portion of the nasal septum is the commonest initial site, perhaps because cellular immune mechanisms cannot flourish in this avascular tissue; however lesions can begin anywhere on the palate or gums. Nasal lesions present with nasal blockage due to polypoid lesions, or as crusted destructive lesions leading to perforation of the septum. Granulomas may extend to involve the lips and eventually destroy portions of the palate and roof of the mouth. Hideous deformities can result and eating is made difficult; the larynx may be affected. Some infections become burnt out, leaving fibrous scar tissue and contractures.

Amastigotes are usually very scanty in late lesions and diagnosis is often based upon the presence of scars from primary lesions, a positive leishmanin skin test, positive serology and the exclusion of other pathologies, including blastomycosis and treponematoses. A tissue biopsy is often necessary. Chemotherapy is unsatisfactory and even three full courses of antimony may fail to halt the process. Amphotericin B is used if antimony fails.

Myiasis

The nasal cavity can be invaded by screw worms or the 'atrial' group of myiasis-producing flies (p. 84). Normal persons or those with nasal pathology may be affected. Nasal obstruction, epistaxis and severe burning sensations result, and the nose can become greatly swollen. The condition is very serious for it may extend to the air sinuses, orbit and meninges.

Leeches and pentastomes

Several kinds of aquatic blood-feeding leeches may be ingested by man when he drinks water in which they are swimming. Attachment and blood feeding is more or less painless; the leeches enter the nose posteriorly or attach anywhere in the tonsillar area, pharynx or larynx. Severe bleeding results and can continue for several days. Patients may also present with obstructive symptoms; if aware of their condition the distress is considerable. It is often necessary to narcotise the creatures to assist their removal; local applications of adrenaline or cocaine are used. Repeated leech infestation can produce anaemia and the cause is not always apparent.

Halzoun — Nasopharyngeal pentastomiasis

Halzoun is a syndrome developing a few hours after eating raw, or incompletely cooked, goat or sheep liver. The patient complains of pain and itching in the throat together with paroxysmal coughing, nasal obstruction, hoarseness and dysphagia; symptoms may continue for a week or more. The condition is commonest in Middle Eastern countries, particularly Lebanon and in North Africa; in Sudan it is known as marrara. The cause is the nymphal stages of the pentastome *Linguatula serrata*, whose adults normally live in the nasopharynx of dogs. Ingested nymphs ascend from the stomach to reach the upper respiratory tract and in man they usually attach to the tonsils or posterior nasopharynx and do not mature fully. Local oedema can be considerable and deaths have occurred from asphyxia. Previously it was believed that immature *Fasciola* flukes in raw liver could attach to the human pharynx and cause this condition, but if this ever does happen it is certainly not the usual cause. Nasopharyngeal leeches can cause similar symptoms, as can an avian trematode *Clinostomium* which has been recorded three times in the human throat.

FURTHER READING

Buck, A.A. (ed.) (1974) *Onchocerciasis. Symptomatology, pathology and diagnosis*. Geneva: World Health Organization.

Khalil, G.M. and Schacher, J.F. (1965) *Linguatula serrata* in relation to halzoun and the marrara syndrome. *Am. J. trop. Med. Hyg.*, **14**, 736–746.

Mellanby, K. (1972) *Scabies*. Middlesex, England: E.W. Classey Ltd.

11

Local effects of parasitism 5

A. NEUROLOGICAL DISEASE

Acute encephalopathy

1. Cerebral malaria — Plasmodium falciparum

Cerebral malaria is the commonest cause of death in falciparum malaria; no other form of malaria causes this syndrome in man. In highly endemic areas with unprotected populations nearly all cases occur under the age of five years before sufficient immunity has built up; in unprotected non-immunes it can occur at any age. At autopsy the brain is swollen and oedematous, the grey matter has a leaden colour due to malaria pigment, and numerous petechial haemorrhages are seen throughout the white matter. Microscopically capillaries and arterioles are packed with parasitised red cells, free pigment and fibrin; most parasitised erythrocytes lie adjacent to the endothelial surface. In the white matter the **ring haemorrhages** are seen to consist of a blocked arteriole surrounded by extravasated non-parasitised red cells, later a glial reaction produces the so-called malarial granuloma at the site of the ring haemorrhage. Some focal neuronal damage probably occurs in those who survive. Details of the mechanisms producing cerebral malaria are still not entirely clear but local anoxia and increased capillary permeability are the final common pathways; the relative roles of vascular plugging by sludged parasitised erythrocytes, disseminated intravascular coagulation, and hyperthermia are still disputed.

Clinically the progress of cerebral malaria is rapid, occuring over a period of hours rather than days with signs of diffuse brain involvement manifested by headache, irritability, confusion and stupor leading to coma; in children the onset is often heralded by fits from which consciousness is not fully regained. Meningism is common in children but otherwise focal signs are rare although hyper-reflexia and positive Babinski signs are common. The occurrence and time of appearance of cerebral malaria in *P. falciparum* infections is unpredictable. Blood films normally show heavy parasitaemia unless previous therapy has been given. Lumbar puncture may be necessary to exclude other pathology, even when blood films are positive; the cerebrospinal fluid is under increased pressure and the protein level often raised, but the cell count is normal.

Parenteral chemotherapy must be given. Tepid sponging and sometimes salicylates are often required to reduce body temperature. Dexamethasone is usually given to reduce cerebral oedema, although its effectiveness is still disputed. 4 mg intravenously every 6 hours is an appropriate adult dose. The value of antiplatelet drugs such as dipyridamole and salicylates is unproven. Over-hydration, especially with intravenous saline, may aggravate and perhaps even precipitate the condition. Heparin should not be given. Response to chemotherapy is usually rapid, and most patients either show definite improvement or die within 48 hours.

2. Trypanosomiasis — T. cruzi and T.b. rhodesiense

An acute meningoencephalitis may occur in primary infections with *T. cruzi;* very young children are particularly affected and it can be a feature of congenital infection. The leptomeninges show mononuclear infiltration and perivascular inflammation occurs in the brain with petechial haemorrhages and glial proliferation. Trypanosomes are present in the blood and amastigotes in the brain. Chemotherapy is sometimes successful.

Unlike Gambian sleeping sickness, patients with *T.b. rhodesiense* frequently die before there is marked neurological involvement. When the latter does occur it is heralded by headache, irritability or drowsiness; the cerebrospinal fluid will be abnormal and blood films always show parasites. The pathology and management is the same as for late *T.b. gambiense* infection.

3. Toxoplasmosis

Encephalitis is the most serious manifestation of toxoplasmosis in the immunologically compromised host: it may occur alone or in conjunction with hepatosplenomegaly, myocarditis or pneumonitis. It is also a rare feature of primary acquired toxoplasmosis. In either situation *Toxoplasma* organisms multiply within neuronal cells and inflammatory foci are set up when these rupture; the process is repeated until the host immune defences arrest it and thick-walled cysts are formed. Diagnosis will usually be serological and by exclusion of other conditions; the organism can rarely be isolated by mouse inoculation from the cerebrospinal fluid, which may show a moderate lymphocytosis. Chemotherapy should be given even if the diagnosis cannot be proven.

4. Trichinosis — Trichinella spiralis

Invasion of the brain is an important feature of very heavy *T. spiralis* infections. The larvae do not encyst but they do set up multiple acute inflammatory foci. Other features of the disease and eosinophilia will invariably be present. Neurological features include headache, drowsiness, hemiparesis and cranial nerve lesions. Steroids should be given together with chemotherapy.

Chronic encephalopathy

1. African trypanosomiasis

The onset of neurological involvement may be delayed for several years in Gambian trypanosomiasis, but in the Rhodesian form it normally appears earlier during the systemic phase of the infection. Once neurological signs appear death is inevitable within a year, even in the Gambian type, unless treatment is given. Pathologically there is a chronic meningoencephalitis, the dura is adherent to the brain surface and the ventricles are dilated, the brain is congested and small haemorrhages are seen within its substance. The meninges are heavily infiltrated with lymphocytes, plasma cells and scanty atypical plasma cells called **morula cells** that contain a mulberry-shaped cytoplasmic mass of IgM. The infiltrate extends into the brain substance as a vasculitis, with perivascular cuffing within which scanty trypanosomes may be seen. Later the brain substance, particularly the frontal lobes and hypothalamus, becomes infiltrated and there is neuronal degeneration and microglial proliferation. Similar changes occur in the spinal cord, and the cranial and spinal nerve roots.

The clinical presentation varies, some patients develop headache or irritability, others psychological problems including psychosis, hallucinations, mania or depression; and some develop the classical diurnal lethargy. As the process continues other neurological abnormalities appear. Frontal lobe damage produces progressive dementia. Extrapyramidal involvement produces rigidity, chorea, athetosis and hypersalivation. Hypothalamic damage probably explains the increased appetite and obesity sometimes seen in the earlier stages of the Gambian form of disease; it may also explain impotence and amenorrhoea. Muscle fibrillation is common, but pyramidal signs are not. Incessant scratching is a frequent feature. The level of consciousness declines and eventually the patient becomes stuporose and emaciated.

Lumbar puncture must be performed on all patients with known trypanosomiasis because neurological involvement necessitates the use of toxic arsenical compounds. The earliest change in the cerebrospinal fluid is a raised IgM level and this is followed by a raised total protein, a lymphocytosis and the presence of trypanosomes. In patients presenting with neurological disease the differential diagnosis includes tuberculous meningitis, neurosyphilis, psychosis and extrapyramidal disorders. Blood films will be positive in *T. b. rhodesiense* infections, but only rarely in those due to *T.b. gambiense*; in the latter trypanosomes will usually be demonstrable in lymph node aspirates.

Some patients deteriorate neurologically five to ten days after starting treatment with arsenicals; it is believed that an allergic immune-complex mediated cerebral vasculitis is often responsible, and steroids have been found useful. Parasitological cure can be achieved in about 90 per cent of patients but some survivors have irreversible neurological damage, although this is much less than would be expected when treatment is begun

2. Congenital toxoplasmosis

Mild congenital infections may present in later childhood as mental defect or epilepsy without the other classical manifestations (p. 174).

Focal and space-occupying lesions

Several parasitic diseases may present with, or be complicated by one or more focal lesions in the brain and spinal cord. They include larval cestodes *Echinococcus* (hydatid), *Multiceps* (coenurus) and *Taenia solium* (cysticercosis); ectopic trematodes (*Paragonimus*, *Schistosoma*, and rarely *Fasciola* and *Heterophyes*); migrating nematodes (*Gnathostoma, Loa, Toxocara, Angiostrongylus*), and amoebic brain abcesses (*E. histolytica* and *Acanthamoeba*). Congenital toxoplasmosis is considered elsewhere (p. 174).

Many clinical presentations are possible and these can be grouped into (1) headache and other features of raised intracranial pressure, (2) focal or grand mal epilepsy, (3) other focal neurological signs including monoplegia and hemiplegia, visual disturbances, transverse myelitis and cranial nerve lesions.

The presumptive diagnosis will often depend upon epidemiological features, the presence of known infection with one of these parasites elsewhere in the body, and in some cases relatively specific features. A blood eosinophilia will suggest any of the helminthic infections, but particularly the migrating nematodes. Intracranial calcification occurs in congenital toxoplasmosis; and also in cysticercosis (*T. solium*) when the cysts begin to degenerate, and thus usually only after symptoms

have appeared. If lesions are near the brain surface eosinophils may be found in the cerebrospinal fluid but this is unusual; serological tests to detect parasite antigen in the cerebrospinal fluid would be of great value in this context.

1. Larval cestodes

Between 2 and 4 per cent of all hydatid cysts occur in the nervous system. Most of them are primary and located in one or other cerebral hemisphere; they are commoner in children. Rarely multiple secondary cysts arise from rupture of a primary cyst on the left side of the heart. Two sites of election for bone hydatids may secondarily involve the nervous system; cysts in the vertebral bodies may compress the spinal cord, and cysts in the base of the skull may involve the basal cisterns. Most cerebral hydatids eventually produce raised intracranial pressure. Cranial osteoporosis and thinning can occur over the lesion and produce a 'cracked pot' percussion note. The relatively rare coenurus cysts usually produce lesions in the brain stem and cerebellum, uncommon sites for hydatid cysts. Cysticercosis most commonly presents as focal epilepsy, but alternatively there may be focal signs, including spinal cord compression, or raised intracranial pressure if internal hydrocephalus is produced by critically located cysts. Brain cysticerci are almost always multiple; when very numerous, dementia may be produced.

Surgery is always necessary for hydatid and coenurus cysts of the nervous system. Focal epilepsy due to cysticercosis can occasionally be corrected surgically, but most patients do well with anticonvulsants. If cysticerci cause internal hydrocephalus, the obstructive lesion must be excised or a bypass shunt inserted; excision of spinal cysts gives good results.

2. Ectopic trematodes

Cerebral paragonimiasis is an important medical problem in some endemic areas. The mature worms die in the brain and set up granulomas, mainly in the cerebral cortex, but also in the cerebellum and medulla elongata. Chemotherapy is of no avail but surgical management sometimes succeeds.

In schistosomiasis affecting the nervous system focal masses of eggs have been found surrounded by granulation tissue. Although adult worms have never been seen in sections it is presumed that ectopic worms have produced the egg masses. In *S. mansoni* and *S. haematobium* infections the lesions are usually in the lower part of the spinal cord or corda equina which the worms have reached via the paravertebral veins; a transverse myelitis may result and chemotherapy is often successful. In *S. japonicum* the lesions are in the brain and focal epilepsy is the common sequel; symptoms may begin three weeks after infection and it is presumed that schistosomulae reach the brain in arterial blood and develop *in situ*; sometimes a diffuse encephalopathy is produced.

Focal egg granulomas and also the adult worms of the minute intestinal fluke *Heterophyes* have occasionally been found in the brain and spinal cord. Ectopic *Fasciola* flukes are very rarely found in the brain.

3. Migrating nematodes

Gnathostoma larvae produce very injurious tracks in neuronal tissues, the spinal cord is sometimes affected; the meninges may also be involved, with consequent changes in the cerebrospinal fluid. *Toxocara* granulomas can cause epilepsy, but how often this happens is disputed. Focal neurological lesions have been reported several times in loaiasis and it is believed that ectopic worms enter the brain. During therapy heavily infected patients rarely develop neurological signs or occlusion of retinal vessels; possibly ectopic worms are killed *in situ* or a vasculitis is produced when massive numbers of microfilariae die in small blood vessels. Because of these complications, some physicians recommend steroid cover when treating heavy infections; if neurological signs do develop during treatment this should be stopped and an exchange blood transfusion performed before it is restarted, to reduce the intensity of microfilaraemia. Although *Angiostrongylus* classically produces a meningitic syndrome focal cortical damage can occur as an isolated phenomenon, and epilepsy may be a late sequel.

4. Amoebic brain abscesses

Although in the past these have always been regarded as due to *E. histolytica*, it is now clear that the free-living amoebae *Acanthamoeba* can cause focal inflammatory brain lesions especially in predisposed persons. *E. histolytica* brain abscesses are relatively acute and soon rupture, in the past they have been nearly uniformly fatal; if suspected during life a combination of emetine and metronidazole should be tried as both drugs enter nervous tissue. More chronic lesions due to *Acanthamoeba* may be discovered surgically.

Meningitis

1. Angiostrongylus infection — Patients eating infected molluscs, crabs or prawns, or salads upon which molluscs have shed *A. cantonensis* larvae, may develop a meningitic illness after five to 15 days. The larval and sometimes even young adult worms, measuring 0.16 to 8 mm, are present in the meninges, subarachnoid space and sometimes also in nervous tissue. A vigorous inflammatory response of eosinophils, plasma cells, lymphocytes and neutrophils is set up. Perivascular cuffing and inflammation within the brain substance can also occur and produce local cerebral softening.

The clinical features are fever, headache, meningism and impaired consciousness. Focal neurological features include diplopia, facial nerve lesions, paresthesiae and evidence of cauda equina involvement. Lumbar puncture reveals raised pressure and a cerebrospinal fluid with increased protein and an eosinophil count up to 3000 mm^3; occasionally larval worms are found. Chemotherapy is not yet established; thiabendazole or levamisole might be effective, but it is possible that worm death might aggravate the condition.

Some patients develop myositis before or simultaneous with neurological involvement; this manifests as muscular pain and weakness. Larval worms are believed to enter the central nervous system along nerves from striated muscle.

2. Meningonema peruzzi infection — This filarial worm of African monkeys may accidentally infect man; previous reports of *D. perstans* microfilariae found in human cerebrospinal fluid possibly refer to this species. In monkeys this worm inhabits the leptomeninges of the brain stem. Neurological illness in man has been attributed to this species in Zimbabwe.

3. Primary amoebic meningoencephalitis — This is an acute necrotising amoebic infection involving mainly the basal cisterns, olfactory bulbs and adjacent brain substance. The illness begins two to 14 days after swimming or diving in fresh water. All acute infections are probably due to one species of free-living amoeba, *Naegleria fowleri*, and these are believed to pass from the roof of the nose, through the cribriform plate to the olfactory bulb. Microscopy reveals a profuse neutrophilic exudate extending into the grey matter from the subarachnoid space; amoebae may be found some way ahead of the advancing edge of the lesions. The brain substance shows petechial haemorrhages, neuronal degeneration and demyelinisation.

Mild upper respiratory symptoms and headache sometimes precede the acute meningitic illness, localising neurological signs are uncommon. The disease progresses very rapidly and death usually occurs within two to five days. The cerebrospinal fluid changes resemble those of acute bacterial meningitis; red blood cells are often present. Live amoeba should be looked for in fresh wet preparations of centrifuged deposit. Culture is necessary to confirm the amoebic species but too slow for clinical diagnosis. Treatment should be attempted with amphotericin B by intravenous infusion and intrathecal injection.

B. MUSCULO-SKELETAL DISEASE

Muscle

1. Trichinosis

Muscle symptoms appear seven to 14 days after infection. Muscles become tender and oedematous. The fibres swell, lose their cross striations and become more basophilic; interstitial inflammatory cells are prominent. The larvae become encapsulated after five weeks and can live for many years. The capsules calcify after a few months but are too small to be seen on normal radiographs.

Systemic symptoms and eosinophilia accompany the myositis; the former include fever, orbital oedema and subungual haemorrhages. Severe muscle involvement can affect locomotion, respiration and mastication. Serum levels of muscle enzymes are high. As inflammation subsides, so gradually does the myalgia and weakness, although these may persist for up to a year. Diagnosis is based upon serology and muscle biopsy. All early and heavy infections should be treated with thiabendazole; steroids may be necessary.

Many light infections are symptomless and cysts may be found in routine autopsy material.

2. Cysticercosis

Cysticerci of *T. solium* are very common in striated muscles especially those of the limb girdles and thighs. Transient muscle pain occurs in heavy infections but otherwise no local damage is done. Muscle cysts, unlike subcutaneous ones, are not palpable except those in the tongue which may be both palpable and visible. Muscle cysts die over a period of years, calcify and become easily recognisable radiologically as dense elongated shadows about 1 cm in length. Patients with suspected cerebral cysticercosis should have a radiological survey for muscle cysts.

3. Toxoplasmosis

Striated muscle is one of the favoured sites for the proliferation of *Toxoplasma* during the acute phase of the infection. This could account for the fatigue and general muscular discomfort often noted in this disease, and perhaps also for the profound lethargy that follows it.

4. Sarcocystis infection

S. lindemanni is a rare parasite of man usually discovered fortuitously in muscle tissue. However the acute phase of heavy infections is associated with polymyositis and eosinophilia. More examples are likely to be found.

5. Angiostrongyliasis

After penetrating the gut, larvae of *A. cantonensis* are disseminated by the blood to muscle, and it is from here that they ascend, along peripheral nerve trunks, to the meninges. Local muscle damage occurs and it is now being recognised that the onset of nervous system involvement with this infection in man is commonly preceded by muscle pain and local weakness.

Bone

Hydatid cysts

This is the only parasitic disease affecting bone directly. Between 2 and 3 per cent of all *E. granulosus* cysts occur in this tissue and the results are always serious. The commonest sites are long bones especially the femur, tibia and humerus, the ilium and the vertebral column and the skull base; neurological sequelae from the latter sites have been mentioned (p. 155). Bone lesions do not encyst, and they grow in a multivesicular form along marrow cavities. Bone is eroded and destruction of local vessels produces secondary aseptic necrosis. The usual clinical presentation is spontaneous fracture; preceding bone pain is unusual. Spontaneous union of these pathological fractures never occurs and all affected bone must be resected. Cysts in the ilium present late as masses in the iliac fossae or gluteal region. Bone cysts may secondarily involve neighbouring joints.

Joints

Guinea worm

Local tissue reactions around *Dracunculus* worms emerging near joints can do considerable damage. Joint effusions and temporary immobilisation of the joint, usually a knee or ankle, are common and may persist for several weeks. A lot of pain is caused and disability causes great economic hardship in an agricultural community. Permanent disability follows contractures of tendons, or fibrous ankylosis; the latter occurs particularly when secondary bacterial infection of the joint cavity or adjacent tissues has taken place. Worms bursting in the tissues can cause serious muscular abscesses.

Filariasis

Calabar swellings due to *Loa loa* often occur adjacent to a joint, usually the wrist. Effusions and immobility follow but these are transient and no permanent damage is done.

Episodes of unexplained acute arthritis, often affecting the knees or ankles, appear to be common in regions where *W. bancrofti* and *B. malayi* are endemic. Recurrence is common in some infected patients, and transient effusions may develop. Transient joint symptoms are also common when these infections are treated with diethylcarbamazine, and also during the chemotherapy of onchocerciasis. It is suggested that circulating immune complexes are responsible. Fleeting joint symptoms also occur in some patients infected with *Dipetalonema perstans* and *Mansonella ozzardi*.

C. URINOGENITAL DISEASE

Two parasites *Schistosoma haematobium* and *Wuchereria bancrofti* can cause extensive damage to several urinogenital structures and these will be considered first.

Urinary schistosomiasis (S. haematobium)

Adult worm pairs live in the venous plexuses surrounding the bladder and ureters. Most eggs pass through the walls of the bladder and ureters causing only transient oedema, inflammatory changes and petechial bleeding at the epithelial surface. The eggs that are retained set up egg granulomas which pass through a series of acute, chronic and finally fibrotic stages during which the eggs are destroyed or become calcified. Most retained eggs are in the subepithelial layer. The early and late lesions of this infection are shown in Fig. 11.1.

Uncomplicated egg passage through the bladder wall is associated with the typical early symptom of urinary schistosomiasis, painless terminal haematuria. Foci of retained egg granulomas are visible cystoscopically as yellow or white 'tubercles' beneath the epithelium; where these are confluent and the overlying mucosa denuded, 'sandy patches' result. Epithelial hyperplasia may be

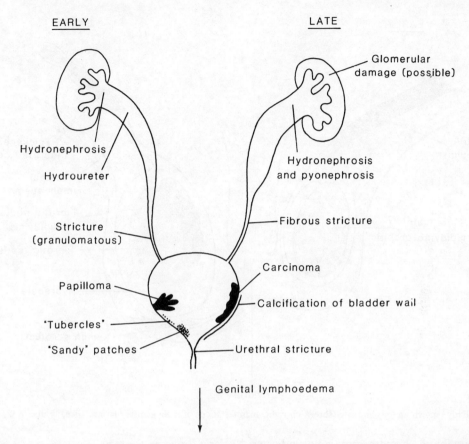

EARLY

LATE

Glomerular damage (possible)

Hydronephrosis

Hydroureter

Hydronephrosis and pyonephrosis

Fibrous stricture

Stricture (granulomatous)

Carcinoma

Papilloma

Calcification of bladder wall

'Tubercles'

'Sandy' patches

Urethral stricture

Genital lymphoedema

Fig. 11.1 Early (shown on the left) and late (shown on the right) lesions in urinary schistosomiasis (*S. haematobium*)

prominent and lead to papillomas that can bleed profusely; elsewhere there may be another epithelial change, squamous metaplasia. Early urethral lesions cause dysuria.

Early lesions in the ureters are patchy foci of granulomatous tissue whose oedema temporarily narrows or blocks the ureter. Usually no symptoms result. Ureteric papillomas may occur. Nearly all early bladder and ureteric lesions in which fibrosis has not occurred can be reversed by chemotherapy; even when the ureters have been dilated for many months, renal function may be unharmed.

Later lesions in the bladder include progressive fibrosis and contraction of the organ, especially the trigone giving dysuria, frequency and painful micturition. Bladder wall calcification may be seen on plain radiographs but is itself of no consequence since it represents only a subepithelial layer of calcified eggs, and these eventually disperse.

Squamous cell carcinomas are a late sequel and possibly also bladder stones. Damage to the trigone and base of urethra may cause urinary retention and sometimes multiple sinuses of the perineum and scrotum. Local lymphatic drainage can be affected giving genital elephantiasis. Perhaps the most important late lesions are fibrotic ureteral strictures. These may be associated with hydronephrosis, progressive deterioration in renal function and sometimes pyonephrosis. Bacteriuria and secondary bacterial urinary tract infection is associated with *S. haematobium* in some parts of its distribution but neither renal hypertension nor chronic pyelonephritis are clearly associated. Urinary carriers of *Salmonella typhi* are commoner in persons infected with *S. haematobium*.

The diagnosis of active disease depends upon the finding of viable eggs in urine specimens or in freshly examined rectal snip preparations. Unless

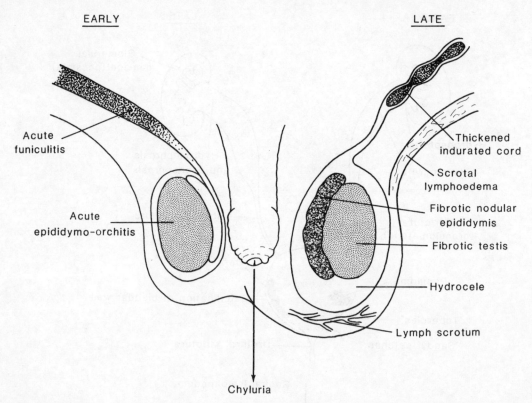

EARLY

LATE

Acute funiculitis

Acute epididymo-orchitis

Thickened indurated cord

Scrotal lymphoedema

Fibrotic nodular epididymis

Fibrotic testis

Hydrocele

Lymph scrotum

Chyluria

Fig. 11.2 Early (shown on left) and late (shown on right) manifestations of male genital filariasis (usually due to *W. bancrofti*)

live eggs are found chemotherapy is not indicated, early lesions respond extremely well to specific treatment. Cystoscopy may be necessary to detect carcinomas and to treat large papillomas locally. Intravenous and retrograde pyelography are sometimes indicated to assess the extent of the lesions and follow their progress. Surgery may be indicated for fibrotic ureteric stricture and other complications.

Immunologically mediated glomerular lesions have been suspected in this infection but never proven.

Genital filariasis

This is usually due to *Wuchereria bancrofti* although similar lesions can occur with *Brugia malayi*. It is now believed that onchocerciasis sometimes causes hydrocele but the mechanism is not clear. The early and late lesions of male genital filariasis are shown in Figure 11.2. (See also Fig. 9.2.)

Early lesions in the male.

These are the genital counterpart of acute lymphadenitis and acute lymphangitis. They often occur repeatedly during the first few years of infection, they result from acute allergic reactions to moulting larval worms, adult worm products, or dying worms. Acute funiculitis manifests as a tender fusiform swelling along the course of the spermatic cord, extending from the inguinal canal to the upper scrotum; it lasts for several days and may be associated with fever, malaise and eosinophilia. More distal lesions produce an acute epididymitis that can closely simulate gonorrhoeal infection, apart from the absence of a urethral discharge. Acute filarial orchitis is often very painful and can mimic testicular torsion so that surgical exploration may have to be performed and occasionally a needless orchidectomy. The diagnosis of filarial orchitis is difficult, microfilaraemia may be absent; the presence of other acute filarial manifestations concurrently or in the past, is of considerable diagnostic help. Small inflammatory hydroceles may accumulate around acute filarial testicular lesions; needling and the finding of microfilariae will be diagnostic.

Late lesions in the male (Frequently bilateral)

1. *Hydrocele* — This is the most important late sequel of *W. bancrofti* infection, because of its frequency and the need for surgery. Many patients give a history of past episodes of testicular inflammation progressing to permanent scrotal enlargement. The fluid accumulates because damaged lymphatics in the spermatic cord impede the drainage of the tunica vaginalis, and also because of fluid exudation from the damaged testis and epididymis. Except in early lesions the fluid is clear and straw-coloured and microfilariae are often absent. The hydroceles can reach an enormous size. Inguinal hernias are associated more often than would be expected; traction upon the cord could be the mechanism responsible.

2. *Chronic lesions of the testis* — The epididymes become hard, knobbly and irregular and the testis either firm and tense, or small and contracted. These findings may be masked by hydrocele fluid. Hydrocele patients have fewer children; sperm counts are probably reduced, mainly because of obstructive lesions in the epididymes, or autoimmune testis lesions resulting from these.

3. *Chronic lesions of the spermatic cord* — Following episodes of acute funiculitis, the cords become hard, indurated and irregular.

4. *Lymphoedema of the scrotum* — Relatively rare, results from bilateral blockage of lymphatic drainage to the inguinal nodes. It pits on pressure initially, but later it becomes indurated with secondary skin changes.

5. *Lymph scrotum* — Sometimes the lymphatics of the scrotal wall become varicose and can be felt, in the dependant scrotum, like a bag of worms. When the scrotum is elevated most of the lymph drains away and the skin becomes finely wrinkled and velvety to touch. The lesion results from bilateral valvular incompetence of lymphatic vessels and it is often associated with lymph varices in the groin. It does not appear to predispose to local lymphoedema. Minor trauma to the dilated vessels leads to persistent oozing of lymph and sometimes secondary infection; bed rest and scrotal support

is essential until healing takes place.

6. *Chyluria* — In some parts of the world this is quite a common feature of late *W. bancrofti* infections. For chyle to appear in the urine three conditions are necessary:

a. A high lymphatic block in the upper abdomen or in the thorax above the drainage of chyle from the small bowel lymphatics into the cisterna chyli.

b. Incompetence of the lymphatic system below this block so that retrograde flow is possible.

c. Communication between a dilated lymphatic and the urinary tract; this is commonest in the renal pelvis but may be into a ureter or the bladder.

The creamy-white chylous urine appears especially in early morning specimens or after fatty meals; initially blood is sometimes also present. In a flask the urine coagulates and separates into three layers: creamy chyle at the top, cellular deposit at the bottom and a middle layer of discoloured urine with clots and debris. Microfilariae can often be found, especially within the fibrin clots. Chyluria is frequently a recurrent phenomenon, each episode lasting several days or even weeks. The nutritional consequences are loss of blood, protein and fat, but these are rarely of much significance. Chemotherapy should be given and sometimes this halts the process. Pyelography with abdominal compression may demonstrate reflux into the communicating lymphatics. If a bladder communication is present this may be cauterised, otherwise surgery is very rarely necessary.

Genital filariasis in the female

Chyluria is as common in women as it is in men. Lymphoedema of the vulva is rare. Acute episodes of retroperitoneal filarial lymphadenitis and lymphangitis in women, can clinically mimic salpingitis and other forms of pelvic sepsis. Possibly the ovaries and fallopian tubes are sometimes damaged by filarial hypersensitivity reactions in adjacent lymphoid tissue, but this remains unproven.

The role of chemotherapy in genital filariasis

Recurrence of acute lesions can normally be prevented completely by drug treatment, but this should be deferred in the presence of active inflammation. The progress of late lesions can be prevented and many small and medium sized hydroceles will regress in size. Treatment of large hydroceles and scrotal elephantiasis is surgical.

Diffuse renal lesions

1. Acute renal failure — Plasmodium falciparum

In malignant tertian malaria acute renal failure is quite a common and sometimes very serious complication. Several factors are involved. Simple hypotension and reduced renal perfusion sometimes leads to temporary renal shutdown; if this is not corrected it may progress to renal tubular necrosis or even renal cortical necrosis. Immune complexes are deposited in the glomeruli during the acute illness, and sometimes produce a proliferative glomerulonephritis, but no permanent damage appears to be done. Disseminated intravascular coagulation is another contributory factor, possibly an important one.

Massive intravascular haemolysis may be followed by haemoglobinuria ('blackwater fever') and acute renal failure. In the past it was believed that tubular blockage produced renal failure, but it is now considered that reflex cortical vasoconstriction is responsible, and the mechanism is the same as in tubular necrosis. Initially the urine is red but this changes to brown and black as oxyhaemoglobin is converted to reduced haemoglobin, methaemoglobin and acid haematin. Other urinary changes in this condition are proteinuria, casts, urobilinogen and haemosiderinuria. Massive haemolysis is not necessarily a contraindication to quinine and this should be used when chloroquine resistance is suspected, unless the condition has been precipitated by previous quinine.

Management in all these situations is supportive once chemotherapy has been started. Fluid and salt overload must be avoided otherwise cerebral and pulmonary oedema can result. Peritoneal or haemodialysis may be necessary.

2. Chronic glomerular damage

Immunologically mediated glomerular disease occurs in many infectious diseases. The most clearly substantiated example among parasitic infections is *Plasmodium malariae*. Other examples are still disputed and this is an active area of current research. Renal amyloidosis may be another late result in some of these infections.

Malarial nephrosis. This is seen most commonly in African children aged 3 to 9 years and it presents as a classical nephrotic syndrome. Renal biopsies show a focal or segmental proliferative and membranous glomerulonephritis. Immunological studies have shown immunoglobulin, complement and malarial antigen on the glomerular basement membrane. The proteinuria is relatively non-selective compared with that seen in 'minimal change' disease, and the prognosis is rather poor. *P. malariae* parasitaemia may be very scanty and cannot always be demonstrated. Although malaria chemotherapy has not been proven to be beneficial it would seem appropriate to give a schizonticide and continue long-term chemosuppression in an endemic area. Response to steroids is variable and often rather poor, unless the histological changes are minimal and the proteinuria selective. Management is mainly supportive. Azathioprine has been used but results are not impressive. In older patients particularly, proteinuria may lessen and the condition progress to non-oedematous chronic renal failure and renal hypertension.

Other infections. Glomerular damage and immunoglobulin deposits have been demonstrated in hepatosplenic schistosomiasis due to *S. mansoni*, but similar deposits occur in a few patients with cirrhosis. Renal amyloid has also been associated with *S. mansoni*. There are reports of nephrotic syndrome being associated with toxoplasmosis, loaiasis and trichinosis, and of renal amyloidosis associated with visceral leishmaniasis and possibly bancroftian filariasis. In both acute *Trypanosoma cruzi* and *T.b. rhodesiense* infection there may be transitory renal damage, with cells, casts and protein appearing in the urine; possibly circulating immune complexes are responsible.

Space-occupying lesions of the kidney

1. Hydatid cysts

About 3 per cent of all hydatids occur in the kidney. They may present as loin pain, haematuria or a renal mass. Rupture through the renal capsule is unusual, and most rupture, quite early, into the renal pelvis. In the latter circumstance, secondary bacterial infection is common, and brood capsules and protoscolices may be found in the urine.

2. *The giant kidney worm (Dioctophyma renale)*

The adult stages of this enormous nematode, which occasionally infects man, live in the renal pelvis. They apparently feed upon renal tissue, and in late infections only the renal capsule remains. Infections present as loin pain, ureteric colic or haematuria; occasionally the worms are passed *per urethrum*. If both sexes are present in one kidney the characteristic eggs may be found in the urine. Treatment is surgical: usually nephrectomy is required.

Genital ulceration

1. Amoebiasis. In males, particularly homosexuals, the glans penis and prepuce may be involved in a very painful and destructive ulceration caused by *Entamoeba histolytica*. In females similar lesions occur on the vulva, vaginal wall or cervix; ascending secondary bacterial infection is common and the lesions are very foul-smelling. Cervical lesions can mimic carcinoma. Freshly examined smears will demonstrate the organism.

2. Mucocutaneous leishmaniasis. Metastatic lesions may occur on the genital mucosa.

3. Schistosomiasis. Egg granulomas, usually *S. haematobium*, can cause papillomas and ulceration of the vulva, vagina, uterine cervix or penis.

Vulvo-vaginitis

1. Trichomoniasis

This sexually transmitted infection is often symptomless in the male or produces a mild urethral syndrome. Most women with primary infections are symptomatic. The vaginal mucosa is diffusely reddened and oedematous and there is often a profuse, and sometimes frothy, greenish or yellow vaginal discharge containing numerous polymorphonuclear leucocytes and some monocytes. Vulval oedema and pruritus are common. Untreated most infections eventually subside spontaneously but they may relapse during menstruation and pregnancy. In chronic infections, the organism may be confined to the endocervix and urethral glands, and be virtually symptomless.

No serious effects are known to be produced by this parasite but its presence interferes with interpretation of Papanicolaou smears for cervical cancer. Some authorities suggest that the known association between cervical cancer and this infection could be causal. Both sexual partners must be treated. Local treatment rarely eliminates the infection, but can be useful during pregnancy.

2. Enterobiasis

Vulval pruritus is commonly caused by this infection in young girls, and results from the worm's nocturnal migrations. Sudden nocturnal perineal pain may result if threadworms become lodged in the hymen. Migration into the vagina is quite common and this infection should always be looked for as a cause of vaginal discharge before puberty. Very rarely the worms ascend the fallopian tubes and produce ectopic egg granulomas in various sites.

The association between enterobiasis and enuresis is controversial. Its role in predisposing to lower urinary tract infection in girls before puberty is better substantiated, and enterobiasis should be excluded in such patients.

FURTHER READING

Carter, R.F. (1972) Primary amoebic meningo-encephalitis. *Trans.R.Soc.trop.Med.Hyg.*, **66**, 193–208.

Spillane, J.D. (1973) *Tropical Neurology*. New York: Oxford University Press.

12

Systemic effects of parasitism

PYREXIA

Parasites contain no intrinsic pyrogenic substances analogous to the endotoxin of gram-negative bacteria that acts directly upon the temperature-regulating centre in the hypothalamus. Fever in parasitic disease results from the release of endogenous pyrogen (EP) by polymorphs and macrophages. EP is a protein with a molecular weight of about 13 000; its action upon the hypothalamus is brief because it is rapidly degraded by proteolytic enzymes. At least two distinct mechanisms underlie its release by polymorphs and macrophages. Firstly, during the process of phagocytosis, the lysosomes of both these cell types are stimulated to release EP as phagolysosomal vacuoles are formed. Secondly, antigen-antibody complexes, through the mediation of lymphokines secreted by T lymphocytes, cause the release of EP by polymorphs. Immunologically mediated EP production derives mainly from Type 3 immune complex hypersensitivity reactions and to a lesser degree from delayed cell-mediated immune reactions (CMI or Type 4).

In some parasitic diseases fever is an invariable, or at least a common feature; in others it may be evidence of·a sensitivity reaction or secondary infection. Malaria, visceral leishmaniasis, amoebic liver abscess, trypanosomiasis and toxoplasmosis regularly enter into the differential diagnosis of unexplained pyrexia. In helminthic disease fever is less common and usually results from a Type 3 sensitivity reaction; a high blood eosinophilia being a valuable diagnostic clue. In fevers caused by protozoa a relative lymphocytosis is usual and often an absolute monocytosis; the principal

exception being amoebic liver abscess, which gives a neutrophil leucocytosis.

Malaria

The febrile paroxysms of malaria, so familiar to those who have witnessed or experienced them, immediately follow the completion of erythrocytic schizogony when the parasitised red cells rupture. The reticulo-endothelial system is flooded with red cell fragments, haemozoin and other parasitic debris, and by those merozoites that fail to enter new red cells. Intense macrophage phagocytosis causes release of EP; it is because schizogony is synchronised that malaria typically produces an intermittent fever pattern with regular paroxysms. When schizogony is not synchronised, as frequently happens in falciparum malaria in non-immunes, the fever is irregular and may be either remittent or intermittent. Some of the types of fever pattern that may occur in the various forms of malaria are shown in Figure 12.1; this illustrates the difference between unsynchronised, partially synchronised, and fully synchronised parasite maturation.

A typical malaria paroxysm lasts for up to six or ten hours and comprises three stages that are usually distinct. The initial 'cold' stage lasts for one or two hours, when the patient feels very cold despite his rapidly rising temperature. Rigors and uncontrollable shivering are typical and gave malaria its old name of ague; dermal blood vessels are constricted and vomiting is common. The second or hot stage lasts for three to four hours; shivering ceases and gives way to a sensation of intense heat. The face is flushed, the pulse bounding, the headache intense and the skin dry; the tempera-

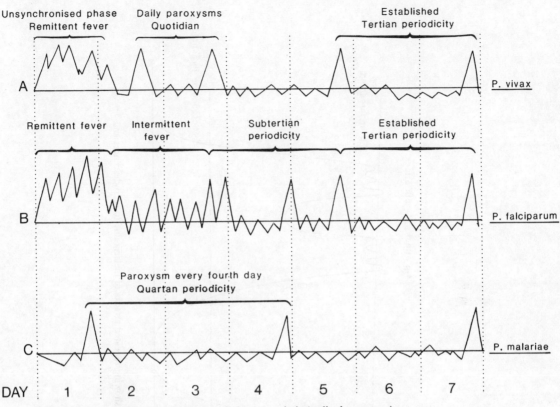

Fig. 12.1 Types of fever patterns observed in human malaria (stylised sequences)
A. *P. vivax* Initial unsynchronised phase → daily (quotidian) paroxysms → established tertian periodicity
B. *P. falciparum* Remittent fever → intermittent fever → 'subtertian' periodicity → established tertian periodicity
C. *P. malariae* Established quartan periodicity

ture continues to rise and may reach 40 or 41°C. The third or sweating stage lasts for up to four hours; sweating is profuse and may saturate the bedding. The temperature falls rapidly, sometimes to subnormal levels; the patient feels much better and sleep often follows.

a. Benign tertian malarias (P. vivax and P. ovale)

After a **prepatent period** of between 10 days and eight months parasites become detectable in blood films (Fig. 12.2), that is the number of blood parasites is great enough to be found by routine microscopical methods — the **microscopic threshold**; a commonly employed routine consists of the examination of 100 fields of a properly made thick blood film, viewed with a (x100) oil immersion objective. Parasitaemia rises and soon exceeds the level necessary to produce fever — the **fever threshold**. This marks the end of the **incubation period.** There follows a series of paroxysms that constitute the **primary attack**. Typically the paroxysms have a 48 hour periodicity but initially the fever may be remittent or two independent broods may give a daily or quotidian fever (Fig. 12.1A). The primary attack eventually terminates as host immunity controls the infection; the disease is then in remission. A series of further malarial attacks may occur later, as levels of parasitaemia rise again. Each successive attack tends to be milder than the last and to contain fewer paroxysms. The fever threshold slowly rises, an early manifestation of immunity. When new malarial attacks are derived from erythrocytic parasites they are called **recrudescenses**; they may be caused by a decline in host immunity or perhaps by the appearance of new antigenic variants. Between recrudescences the level of para-

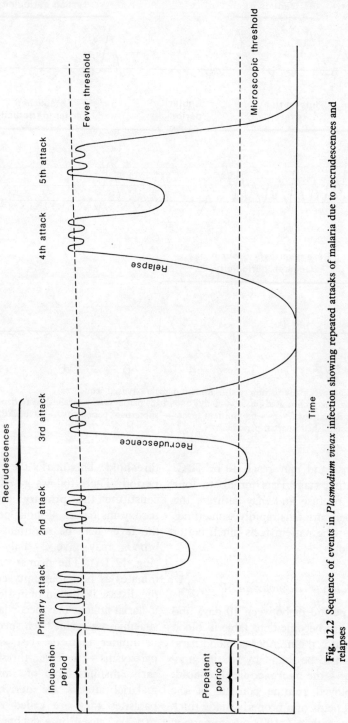

Fig. 12.2 Sequence of events in *Plasmodium vivax* infection showing repeated attacks of malaria due to recrudescences and relapses

sitaemia may or may not be below the microscopic threshold. Eventually the population of erythrocytic parasites becomes extinct. In the benign tertian malarias, however, the infection can become active once more if a true **relapse** occurs. Previously latent exo-erythrocytic schizonts in the liver rupture, reinfect the red cells, and begin the whole process once more. The total number of possible relapses is limited, and is perhaps determined by the original number of sporozoites inoculated; it is exceptional for them to continue for more than three to five years. If these two benign tertian infections are transmitted by blood transfusion, no liver schizonts are formed and relapses are impossible. In this situation all succeeding malarial attacks must be due to a recrudescence.

b. Falciparum malaria (P. falciparum) — subtertian or malignant malaria

This dangerous disease is the only type of acute malaria likely to cause death in previously healthy persons. The incubation period can be as short as eight days and primary attacks nearly always occur within three months of infection. Most deaths occur during primary attacks. The fever paroxysms are often irregular, especially in nonimmunes, and the temperature chart may initially show a remittent pattern, and then a more intermittent one usually with some tendency towards a 24 or 48 hour (subtertian) periodicity (Fig. 12.1.B). The three stages of the paroxysms may be poorly defined and constitutional symptoms are prominent. It is the lack of 'typical malarial periodicity' that often leads to this infection being mistaken for other infectious diseases. Death usually results from cerebral or renal complications or alternatively the patient may progress into a state of medical shock, so called 'algid malaria'.

In partially immune subjects a regular tertian (48 hour) pattern does emerge, and repeated malarial attacks can continue for up to 18 months. There are no persistent liver schizonts and successive attacks are entirely due to recrudescences.

c. Quartan malaria (P. malariae)

This infection is characterised by regular paroxysms every 72 hours (Fig. 12.1.C). Rigors are not usually severe and constitutional upset is relatively mild; splenomegaly may be absent. If two or more unsynchronised broods are present simultaneously, various fever cycles may result; three broods will give a quotidian pattern. Parasitaemia is usually very low even in symptomatic patients; while diligent search of many blood films may reveal parasites in symptomless persons, hence the risk of transmission by blood transfusion. The infection is very persistent and may last for 20 or even 40 years. No firm evidence exists for an exo–erythrocytic cycle, so parasites must persist at very low levels within erythrocytes; recurrent attacks are therefore recrudescences.

2. Visceral leishmaniasis

Fever is usually the first symptom in *L. donovani* infections and may precede palpable enlargement of the liver and spleen. Typically the incubation period is about three months but the extreme range extends from 10 days to nine years. The temperature pattern is irregular and fever may be intermittent or remittent; most typically there is a double rise in temperature every 24 hours. Cases with short incubation periods may run a fulminant course and can clinically resemble falciparum malaria. In more chronic cases there may be afebrile periods lasting for several weeks; appetite remains good and constitutional upset is slight despite progressive weight loss.

EP is presumably released by macrophages as they ingest amastigotes and cellular debris from neighbouring ruptured macrophages. The fever periodicity remains unexplained but may relate to intrinsic phagocytic rhythms.

3. Trypanosomiasis

In American trypanosomiasis (*T. cruzi*), fever only occurs in the acute primary illness when parasites are numerous in the tissues and the blood. Irregular fevers can continue for up to eight weeks and may coincide with recurrent episodes of inflammatory subcutaneous oedema and tender lymphadenopathy.

In African trypanosomiasis (*T.b. rhodesiense* and *T.b. gambiense*), fever may begin with the appearance of the primary chancre. In *T.b. rhodesiense* it can continue throughout the course of the relatively acute illness. In *T.b. gambiense* infection, febrile bouts are intermittent and usually coincide with the enlargement of new lymph nodes, fever may be absent for long periods especially in the later stages. Patients with neurological involvement are usually afebrile.

In all types of human trypanosomiasis, fever and constitutional upset are largely generated by immune complex reactions occurring in the tissues. Kinin release is prominent and explains the inflammatory oedemas seen in the acute forms of these diseases. In the African disease renewed bouts of fever, with a return of parasitaemia and involvement of new lymph nodes, may be related to the appearance of new antigenic variants.

4. Amoebiasis

In amoebic dysentery, fever is often low-grade or absent in contrast to the usual situation in bacillary dysentery. Amoebomas may, however, be associated with fever. In amoebic liver abscess, fever is a prominent symptom and often the presenting one; although occasionally large abscesses develop with little or no fever. Typically the fever chart in liver abscess patients shows a daily evening rise, to reach 40°C or more; rigors are brief but sweating often very profuse. Systemic upset is considerable. The erythrocyte sedimentation rate is high and there is a polymorphonuclear leucocytosis.

The fever may be generated by necrosis of liver tissue rather than by immunological mechanisms. Polymorphs around the lesion, while never numerous, probably release EP during phagocytosis of hepatocyte debris.

5. Other protozoan infections

Fever may be a feature of all forms of *Toxoplasma* infection. In the acquired form of disease it occurs in about 40 per cent of patients, and may be the only objective sign apart, perhaps, from lymphadenopathy; the fever is often low-grade but may be persistent. In *Babesia* infection the clinical features can resemble falciparum malaria. In *Naegleria* infection the high fever, systemic upset and purulent cerebrospinal fluid may mimic bacterial meningitis. In *Pneumocystis* infections fever is prominent only in the more acute cases.

6. Helminthic infections

In three conditions, particularly, fever may be prominent and cause diagnostic difficulty.

a. Trichinosis — Fever and systemic upset are common in the invasive stage and can mimic typhoid fever.

b. Lymphatic filariasis — Fever accompanies the acute inflammatory episodes in lymph nodes, lymphatic vessels, testes or spermatic cords; sometimes this is a prominent feature — hence the term 'filarial fever'. When affected nodes are not palpable, for example the intra-abdominal ones, diagnosis may be difficult. These symptoms may be precipitated by chemotherapy; antihistamines may be useful.

c. Acute schistosomiasis — Usually seen in *S. japonicum* or *S. mansoni* infections. The febrile illness 'Katayama syndrome' may be severe and prolonged; it occurs especially in heavy primary infections.

Other helminthic infections giving fever, usually low-grade, include *Ascaris* pneumonitis, invasive fascioliasis, clonorchiasis, tropical pulmonary eosinophilia, toxocariasis, and angiostrongyliasis. In all of these other features will be present. *Salmonella* septicaemia may complicate chronic hepatosplenic schistosomiasis. Steroid therapy may sometimes be necessary to control severe systemic reactions due to helminths.

WASTING AND GROWTH RETARDATION

Since many parasitic infections are either recurrent or chronic, their effects upon protein and energy metabolism are often of great significance. The metabolic disorder may manifest in several ways.

1. Loss of muscle mass and subcutaneous tissue as revealed by weight loss and by anthropometric measurements such as mid-upper arm circumference and skinfold thicknesses over the triceps and subscapular muscles.

2. Reduced ability to do physical work. In many tropical countries with an agrarian economy

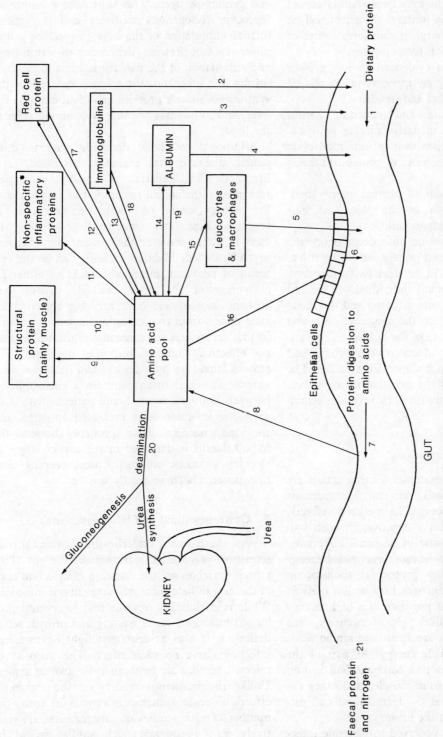

Fig. 12.3 Amino acid and protein metabolism in parasitic infections

Number key: 1 — low dietary protein because of inappetance; losses into the gut of red cells (2), immunoglobulins (3), albumin (4), leucocytes (5) and epithelial cells (6); 7 — protein digestion to amino acids, 8-amino acid absorption; muscle protein synthesis (9) and catabolism (10); synthesis of non-specific inflammatory proteins (11), red cell protein (12), immunoglobulins (13), albumin (14), leucocytes and macrophages (15) and epithelial cells (16); catabolism of red cell protein (17), immunoglobulins (18) and albumin (19); 20 — deamination of amino acids followed by gluconeogenesis and urea synthesis; 21 — faecal loss of protein and nitrogen.

* Non-specific inflammatory proteins include acute-phase reactant proteins (C reactive protein, fibrinogen, α1 antitrypsin and α1 acid glycoproteins), complement, coagulation proteins and kinin precursors.

the reduced efficiency of adults doing physical labour may be one of the most important effects of parasitism upon human welfare; the effect will be greatest when diet is marginal and normal rates of work are limited by high temperatures.

3. Growth failure as evidenced by low growth velocity or a low rating on appropriate age-related tables for normal heights and weights.

4. Hypoalbuminaemia and oedema. Serum albumin is a simple and useful marker of disordered protein metabolism as it reflects total body protein and also the net rates of protein synthesis and catabolism.

5. Other specific signs of protein energy malnutrition (PEM), such as the skin and hair changes seen particularly in children.

The effects of parasitic infections upon the metabolism of energy and protein are closely interconnected and they will be dealt with together. The clinical features in any individual will depend not only upon the parasite involved and the duration of infection but also the age, sex, diet, and previous nutritional state of the subject. The various effects of parasitic infections upon protein and amino acid metabolism is shown Figure 12.3. The overall effect is usually a negative nitrogen balance, but this can be produced by several mechanisms.

A. Febrile systemic infections

The most important examples in this group are malaria, trypanosomiasis, visceral leishmaniasis and amoebic liver abscess. The metabolic effects, namely weight loss and a negative nitrogen balance, are similar to those of bacterial infections. By elevating the metabolic rate, fever raises energy demands and increases protein catabolism; in addition up to 4 g of nitrogen may be lost daily in sweat. Anorexia in the presence of a high energy demand stimulates liver gluconeogenesis; the body's glycogen stores are small and amino acids must be used to provide energy. As part of the physiological stress reaction cortisone and insulin mobilise amino acids from muscles and other tissues, glucose is formed by deamination and nitrogen is lost as urea in the urine.

Many of the effects observed in systemic infections can be explained by the actions of a mediator released by phagocytic cells together with endogenous pyrogen. This substance is known as leucocyte endogenous mediator and its actions include stimulation of the liver to produce acute-phase reactant proteins, depression of serum iron, and stimulation of the pancreatic islets to produce insulin and glucagon; these hormones reduce the synthesis of muscle proteins and of albumin by the liver, and so increase the supply of amino acids to the liver.

Additional metabolic demands arise in individual diseases; for example, increased erythropoiesis in malaria, a greatly expanded reticuloendothelial cell population in kala-azar and the energy costs of tissue inflammation in trypanosomiasis and amoebic liver abscess. In each of these diseases the patient may become severely wasted. Malarial cachexia can be the end result of repeated untreated attacks of either *P. falciparum* or *P. vivax* malaria; patients are anaemic, wasted and have very big spleens; this state differs from tropical splenomegaly syndrome in that fevers and parasitaemias continue because no effective immune response develops. For reasons that are not understood patients with chronic kala-azar often maintain a good appetite between bouts of fever. Some patients with *T.b. gambiense* infection have increased appetites and they may become obese, probably because the hypothalamus is damaged in the earlier stages of sleeping sickness; eventually most sleeping sickness patients become greatly wasted.

B. Gastrointestinal and biliary parasites

Several mechanisms underlie the nutritional consequences of parasitic infections of the gut. Two critical variables are the duration of infection and, in the case of helminths, the intensity of infection. While it is clinically obvious that heavy and prolonged infections cause wasting and growth retardation, it is also evident that light or transient infections have no such effect. The majority of infected persons lie between these two extremes. Unlike the numerous studies on the metabolic effects of acute systemic infections in man, the number of such studies on gut parasites are relatively few. Frequently such studies would be unjustified or unethical for they would be prolonged, dietary intake must be controlled and treatment withheld; furthermore radio-isotopes are often necessary. In domestic animals the effects of gastrointestinal helminths upon growth and productivity are well-known and in recent years the mechanisms have been studied in detail using radio-isotopes. Animal studies have shown that diet critically determines the outcome in infections of moderate intensity; animals on good diets tolerate them well, while those on poor diets waste and fail to thrive. In man it is currently believed that infected persons on suboptimal diets will always be affected, except by very light or mild infections; whilst severe infections are always nutritionally harmful whatever the diet.

1. Malabsorption

The importance of malabsorption and maldigestion have in the past been given too much prominence. The functional reserve of the small bowel is enormous and local lesions will rarely affect absorption significantly. The only parasites that can produce an overt malabsorption syndrome with steatorrhoea are *Giardia lamblia*, *Isospora belli*, *Strongyloides stercoralis*, *Capillaria philippinensis* and probably acute hookworm infections. Even in these infections the direct nutritional consequences of lipid and carbohydrate calories lost in the faeces are not great and other mechanisms are more important. Protein digestion and amino acid absorption appear to be normal in most parasitic infections of the gut with the exception of heavy infections with *S. stercoralis* and *C. philippinensis*. In the absence of protein loss into the lower gut (see below) measurements of faecal nitrogen are often normal and the negative nitrogen balance seen in parasitic infections of the gut results from urea nitrogen, produced by deamination of amino acids, being lost in the urine.

2. Inappetence

Many gut parasites impair the appetite of their host by producing abdominal pain, colic and nausea; this happens especially when these symptoms follow a meal. The significance of this mechanism in man has been underestimated. An important example is children with ascariasis; they soon learn that a meal will be followed by colicky pains and possibly vomiting, and they will refuse food in consequence.

A low carbohydrate intake will deplete body proteins by stimulating gluconeogenesis to provide calories. A low protein intake reduces the synthesis of both structural protein and albumin, but catabolism continues and the amino acids entering the pool will not necessarily be used for synthesis; many will be deaminated and hence lost to the body apart from their calorific value. Low protein diets are often deficient in certain critical amino acids required for the synthesis of specific proteins; lack of these amino acids effectively blocks the synthesis of the respective proteins.

3. Loss of protein and cells into gut lumen

A damaged gut mucosa loses proteins and cells whether the lesion is local or diffuse. A leaky or denuded epithelium loses serum proteins regardless of their molecular weight; the principal protein lost is albumin but this is accompanied by immunoglobulins and other serum proteins. Mucosal damage may be produced directly by the feeding process of the parasite, or immunologically when an inflammatory exudate is produced or mast cells degranulate. Bleeding into the gut lumen produces a loss of red cell proteins and also all the serum protein components. In hookworm infection double isotope labelling of red cells and plasma proteins has shown that cells and plasma are lost more or less in proportion to their relative blood concentrations. The worms ingest a good deal of this blood but some escapes at the site of attachment and a bleeding point persists when the worms move to a new feeding site; an anticoagulant is secreted by the worm's cephalic glands. Local immune reactions probably force the worms to find new sites of attachment at least every 24 hours.

Of at least equal importance in many infections is epithelial cell loss. In the small bowel a rapid enterocyte turnover is characteristic and is evidenced by high mitotic rates, shortened and blunted villi, and sometimes crypt elongation; this phenomenon may be simply reparative but in some infections at least, such as giardiasis, it now appears to be initiated by specific immunological processes. Mucosal infiltration by lymphocytes and plasma cells is a frequent finding on jejunal biopsy in these infections and lymphocytes can be seen within the epithelium itself; it is now believed that lymphocytes cross into the gut lumen as part of the immune rejection mechanism. Lymphocytes and other inflammatory cells in the lumen form yet another source of protein loss.

Parasites living in the biliary passages cause similar effects to those in the small bowel. Sometimes bleeding due to mechanical damage can be considerable, as in *Fasciola* infection; of greater importance is epithelial denudation, local protein loss and high turnover rates of the biliary epithelial cells.

Whatever their source most of the protein and cells lost into the small bowel are digested and a large proportion of the amino acids are reabsorbed, hence the protein loss in this situation is not reflected by high levels of faecal nitrogen. In the case of damage to the colon or lower ileum the situation is very different since cells and protein cannot be reabsorbed. Examples of this type of damage are amoebic ulcers of the colon, heavy *Trichuris* infections, and intestinal schistosomiasis especially when polyposis or mucosal ulceration is present; in these conditions levels of faecal protein and nitrogen will be high.

The importance of upper gut losses is that although amino acids are reabsorbed the body cannot resynthesise all the protein that has been lost. Not only is there the energy cost of protein synthesis but for a variety of reasons relating to the infection itself, poor diet, intercurrent disease or inappetence the rates of protein synthesis are depressed. The net result is that although amino acids are reabsorbed a considerable proportion are not reutilised to make protein but are simply deaminated and lost from the body as urinary urea.

4. Increased demands for synthesis of certain proteins

The infections themselves, particularly if there is a tissue migration phase, increase the synthesis of immunoglobulins, acute-phase reactant proteins and also the multiplication of the cells involved in the various immunological and inflammatory phenomena. Red cell protein, immunoglobulin,

albumin and epithelial cells lost into the gut must be replaced.

C. Non-febrile systemic infections

There are certain parasitic diseases in which fever is not a common feature and gastrointestinal changes, if any, are insufficient to cause the observed changes in nutritional status. Three examples, in which wasting may be severe, are the tropical splenomegaly syndrome, heavy onchocerciasis, and schistosomiasis, particularly *S. japonicum* and *S. mansoni* infections. It should be noted that liver cell function remains normal in intestinal schistosomiasis until the very late stages; therefore the stunting, and sometimes even dwarfism and infantilism seen in heavy *S. japonicum* infections cannot be attributed to liver damage.

It must be presumed that in these conditions the energy cost of the inflammatory processes and the increased rates of protein synthesis exceed the host's regenerative capacity. Another factor may be release of leucocyte endogenous mediator by the phagocytes involved in the inflammatory processes, for example in the dermis in onchocerciasis; therefore the metabolic consequences may be similar to those of more acute infections.

In children between the age of six months and five years certain parasitic infections predispose to overt protein energy malnutrition. This will only happen when the child is at risk for dietary reasons. Four parasites are of special importance; these are malaria, ascariasis, giardiasis and hookworm. No special mechanisms are involved and the reason that these particular parasites are so significant, in this context, is that they are common in this age group.

IMMUNOSUPPRESSION

Several parasitic diseases are known to cause a reduced immune response to vaccines and antigens unrelated to the specific infection. The immune defect may involve both B and T lymphocytes and therefore affect both humoral and cellular responses; the mechanisms are obscure but may involve antigenic competition. Examples of diseases causing immunosuppression are malaria, African trypanosomiasis, visceral leishmaniasis, and possibly also schistosomiasis, severe onchocerciasis and lymphatic filariasis when elephantiasis is present. In visceral leishmaniasis there is also a specific immunological defect against the parasite, produced presumably by antigen excess; a similar situation exists in diffuse cutaneous leishmaniasis. In infections producing hypersplenism, particularly visceral leishmaniasis, neutropenia greatly impairs the host's defences.

In practice by far the most relevant example of parasite-induced immunosuppression is malaria because of its persistence and frequency in children. Not only are vaccination programmes adversely affected by uncontrolled malaria but such children are rendered more susceptible to other infections which may be fatal or precipitate protein energy malnutrition. Persistent hepatitis Bs antigenaemia is more common in patients with *Schistosoma mansoni* infection and prevalence rates are high where malaria is endemic; an impaired immune response to this virus could be the explanation.

The distribution of high incidence rates for Burkitt's lymphoma closely corresponds with that of high levels of malaria transmission. There is good epidemiological, clinical and experimental evidence that this tumour is usually caused by the Epstein-Barr virus in the presence of malaria; it is believed that the E-B virus can become oncogenic in the immunosuppressed host. Burkitt's lymphoma particularly affects children and often presents as a jaw tumour; the condition is most common in tropical Africa.

SYSTEMIC ALLERGIC REACTIONS

Leaking hydatid cysts can precipitate anaphylaxis. The severity of the reaction will depend upon previous sensitisation; they may be fatal if rupture occurs into the circulation or a body cavity such as the pleura or peritoneum. Mild reactions may produce only urticaria.

Systemic reactions are quite common in guinea worm infections especially when the worm dies in the tissues or has ruptured during attempted removal. Symptoms include hypotension, nausea, vomiting, intestinal colic, dyspnoea and facial oedema; an immediate sensitivity response is presumably involved.

Laboratory workers and also persons working in abattoirs quite commonly become very sensitive to *Ascaris lumbricoides* or the pig ascarid *A. suum*. Handling the worms or even proximity to them can provoke angioneurotic oedema and wheezing. For reasons that are not understood persons naturally infected with *A. lumbricoides* rarely, if ever, suffer such reactions. Any of the worm infections that cause urticaria (p. 147) can precipitate a more generalised hypersensitivity; thus facial oedema is common in *Fasciolopsis* infection.

Systemic allergic reactions to helminths may require treatment with antihistamines, steroids or even adrenaline.

PARASITISM, PREGNANCY AND THE FOETUS

Parasitic infections during pregnancy can have several important effects upon the mother and the child.

Increased maternal susceptibility

1. Malaria (In women with some immunity)

Previously immune or semi-immune women living in malarious endemic areas frequently develop patent parasitaemias during pregnancy. Very rarely, if ever, does this result in transplacental infection to the child, probably because sufficient maternal IgG malarial antibody crosses the placenta. Nevertheless the effects upon the placenta and the pregnancy itself can be serious. Primigravidae are specially affected and *P. falciparum* is the principal malaria species involved. Erythrocytic schizogony takes place extensively in the maternal blood vessels of the placenta which become filled with parasites and pigment; possibly the sticky parasitised cells adhere to the placental endothelium because of the sluggish blood flow. The frequent result of placental infection is a small placenta with multiple areas of infarction resulting from occlusion of vessels; histiocytes and other cells accumulate in the placental interstitium.

Both the prevalence and the level of parasitaemia is increased in pregnant women; haemoglobin levels fall and pyrexial episodes may precipitate abortion and premature labour. The spleen enlarges. In women who had large spleens before pregnancy but no parasitaemia, being examples of the tropical splenomegaly syndrome, the fall in haemoglobin may be very sudden and levels of parasitaemia very high. Severe malarial anaemia at the end of pregnancy contributes to maternal deaths and stillbirths.

The most important effects of *P. falciparum* in women with partial immunity result from the small infarcted placenta. The usual outcome is a low birth weight full-term child, whose chances of survival through infancy are considerably lower, because of susceptibility to malnutrition and intercurrent infection, than a normal birth weight baby. Less commonly the infarcted placenta causes stillbirths, or intrauterine and neonatal deaths.

In highly endemic areas 25 per cent or more of all placentas may show parasitisation by *P. falciparum*; some come from women without patent parasitaemia and their child's birth weight may be normal. However the mean birth weight is significantly reduced when the placenta is infected.

2. Amoebiasis

Women in the third trimester of pregnancy and in the puerperium show increased frequencies of invasive intestinal amoebiasis. Mechanisms are uncertain but by analogy with other host factors that predispose to invasive amoebiasis a depression of cellular immune mechanisms is suspected. Diagnosis and management can be very difficult in this situation, particularly when colonic perforation occurs.

3. Trichomoniasis

Previously latent *T. vaginalis* infection often reactivates during pregnancy producing a copious vaginal discharge. While there is no definite evidence that nitro-imidazoles damage the human foetus, many clinicians prefer to use local treatment of this infection during pregnancy.

Transplacental infections

1. Malaria

This is rare and occurs only in non-immune or very weakly immune mothers. Abortion and stillbirth are the more usual outcomes of acute malaria in such women. Congenital malaria infections have been recorded with all four plasmodial species that infect man. Transfer of infection is through placental tears which occur particularly during delivery; it is doubtful whether a foetus could survive for long *in utero* with parasitaemia. However in congenital *P. vivax* infection the malaria may not become apparent for several weeks.

2. Toxoplasmosis

This is by far the commonest congenital parasitic infection. Only women experiencing a primary acute infection can transfer the organism to their baby; pregnancy does not reactivate latent infection in humans and toxoplasmosis does not cause recurrent abortion or stillbirth. In Europe and North America between 0.5 and 1 per cent of women have evidence of primary infection during pregnancy and it is believed that about 40 per cent of these infections are transferred to the foetus. Between half and two-thirds of infected foetuses are normal at birth and infection is only demonstrable by finding raised total IgM or specific *Toxoplasma* antibody in cord blood. More severely affected foetuses are presumed to be infected early in pregnancy; the outcome may be abortion, stillbirth or the live birth of an infant who develops features of infection within a few weeks or months. Infected placentas show areas of necrosis and inflammation especially on the foetal side. In the systemic forms of congenital infection, fever, a rash, pneumonitis, jaundice and hepatosplenomegaly will be prominent but ocular and brain damage will often be present also and manifest as microphthalmia, microcephaly, mental retardation and epilepsy. The foetal brain shows necrosis, glial infiltration and the accumulation of perivascular lymphocytes. In infants who survive, the affected brain tissues, which are located principally around the third ventricle, become calcified; aqueductal obstruction is common in those with milder disease and these can present later with hydrocephalus and high ventricular protein levels. In some children the infection becomes apparent several years later as mental retardation, epilepsy or choroidoretinitis.

All detected congenital infections should be treated to prevent further damage; if the mother's infection is asymptomatic after delivery she need not be treated. All pregnant women with serological evidence of recent infection should be treated whether or not they are symptomatic; however therapeutic abortion is the preferable alternative on medical grounds.

Nearly all cases of toxoplasmal choroidoretinitis in later life are due to congenital infection which has remained latent in the retina; latent cysts are probably also present in the brain in these patients but are of no clinical significance.

3. American trypanosomiasis

Foetuses can be infected by asymptomatic or symptomatic maternal infections; the true frequency of congenital infection is uncertain. Affected babies are small and may show hepatosplenomegaly and generalised oedema; sometimes with jaundice and petechial rashes. Meningoencephalitis is an important manifestation.

4. Other infections

A few examples of congenital infection with *Leishmania donovani*, *Trypanosoma b. gambiense* and *Gnathostoma* have been described.

Transmammary infection

Several nematodes of veterinary importance are transferred via maternal milk; two examples are a dog hookworm, *Ancylostoma caninum*, and a dog roundworm, *Toxocara canis*. In humans patent hookworm infection with *A. duodenale* has been reported in very young infants and it must be assumed that milk-borne transmission has occurred; however the infections are light and of no clinical importance. In contrast *Strongyloides fuelleborni* has been proven to be milk-borne in Zaire and this is probably the mechanism by which infants in Papua New Guinea develop very heavy and sometimes fatal infections with this worm.

Abortion

Many acute infections can precipitate abortion and by far the commonest parasitic disease to do this is *Plasmodium falciparum* malaria in non-immune mothers. Chemoprophylaxis is essential in such women, the risks of abortion far outweigh possible drug-induced foetal damage. Visceral leishmaniasis and African trypanosomiasis usually lead to abortion when they become symptomatic during pregnancy.

FURTHER READING

Chandra, R.K and Newberne, P.M. (1977) *Nutrition, Immunity and Infection. Mechanisms of Interactions*. New York: Plenum Press.

Feigin, R.D. and Beisel, W.R. (1977) Symposium on Impact of Infection on Nutritional Status of the Host.

Am.J.clin.Nutr., **30**, Part 1, pp. 1203–1431; Part II, pp. 1439–1568

Scrimshaw, N.S., Taylor, C.E. and Gordon, J.E. (1968) Interactions of Nutrition and Infection. WHO Monograph Series No. 57.

13

Diagnostic methods

MICROSCOPIC EXAMINATION OF BODY FLUIDS AND EXCRETA

Skilful use of the microscope is of paramount importance in the diagnosis of parasitic disease. Clinicians working in this field must be familiar with several basic techniques, which are mostly very simple; they should themselves be able to give diagnostic opinions at the microscope. Constant practice is essential.

Whenever parasites are being searched for in body fluids and excretal specimens the diagnostic sensitivity of the method must be considered. This depends primarily on the volume of material examined and this will often be proportional to the amount of time spent on the examination. While numerous parasites are difficult to miss, scanty ones may be of equal importance, for example the finding of a single trypanosome in a blood film. Several simple methods of concentrating specimens are available and should be used when indicated. The size of many parasites is often of great diagnostic importance and the microscope must be equipped with a micrometer eye piece.

A. Parasites in blood specimens

1. Stained blood films

Both thin and thick blood films should always be made simultaneously when blood parasites are suspected. They should be stained with one on the Romanovsky dyes such as those of Giemsa, Leishman or Wright, which stain the nuclear chromatin of protozoa red and their cytoplasm blue; for the rapid staining of thick films, Field's method is of great value and takes only a few minutes to complete. Thin blood films are made in the same way as those used for haematological studies; they allow observations to be made on red cell morphology and show the structure of intra-erythrocytic parasites in full detail. Thick blood films are made by placing a large drop of blood in the centre of a slide and spreading it over a round or oval area about 1–1.5 cm across. After complete drying the red cells are lysed in water before staining; when Field's method is used the two processes proceed simultaneously. With experience protozoan parasites can be recognised quite easily in thick films although most of the changes within the red cells are lost. The use of thick blood films is a powerful method of parasite concentration as evidenced by the fact that when 100 fields of a thin film are examined with an oil immersion objective (x100), the volume of blood being scanned is 10–20 μl; the same number of fields on a thick film represents 100–200 μl, so that the concentration factor is about 10 to 20.

The following parasites can be found in blood films:

a. *Malaria parasites*. Morphological details of the four species of *Plasmodium* infecting man are given on p. 33 and illustrated in Figure 2.15. Species recognition is usually fairly easy in thin films but is more difficult in thick films because the shapes of some of the parasites are different and most red cell structure is lost. Details of thick film appearances should be sought in diagnostic manuals; of key importance in recognising an object as being a malaria parasite is the combination of blue cytoplasm with the bright red nuclear chromatin and sometimes the presence of malaria pigment in the cytoplasm. When specific identity

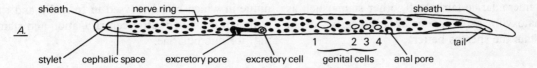

A. B.

Species	Sheath	Length (mean µm)	Width (mean µm)	Habitat*	Tail
Wuchereria bancrofti	Present	260	8	Blood (nocturnal or diurnally subperiodic)	clear of nuclei
Brugia malayi	Present	220	6	Blood (nocturnal or nocturnally subperiodic)	two terminal nuclei
Loa loa	Present	275	7	Blood (diurnal)	terminal nuclei
Dipetalonema perstans	Absent	195	4.5	Blood (non-periodic)	terminal nuclei (crowded)
Mansonella ozzardi	Absent	200	4.7	Blood (non-periodic)	clear of nuclei
Onchocerca volvulus	Absent	290	7	Dermis	clear of nuclei pointed tail
Dipetalonema streptocerca	Absent	210	3	Dermis	terminal nuclei tail hooked and blunt

Fig. 13.1 A. Microfilaria of _Wuchereria bancrofti_ (semi-diagrammatic) showing some of the morphological details used for identifying microfilariae of human or animal origin; the relative position of many of these structures down the length of the microfilaria is constant for each species
B. Tabulation of the microfilarial species found in man
* The periodicity of the blood–dwelling microfilariae is given in parentheses

is in doubt the thin film can always be referred to. In heavy malaria infections, particularly _P. falciparum_, malaria pigment is often seen within monocytes and neutrophils.

b. Trypanosomes. Normally easily recognisable in either thin or thick films. The two African parasites _T.b. gambiense_ and _T.b. rhodesiense_ are morphologically indistinguishable (Fig. 2.17 and p. 35); however the patient's geographic history will be diagnostic. In South America, _T. cruzi_ must be differentiated from _T. rangeli_ (Fig. 2.18 and p. 40), since the latter is probably non-pathogenic.

c. Piroplasms (Babesia). These uncommon human parasites can closely resemble _Plasmodium falciparum_, but no pigment is formed. Several parasites may be present within an infected red cell, often in pairs.

d. Leishmania donovani. In the Indian form of kala-azar scanty amastigotes may be found within blood monocytes. Buffy coat preparations are usually used (see below).

e. Microfilariae. The microfilariae of five species of filarial worm may be found in the blood. Their characteristics are given in Figure 13.1. Since several species have a circadian periodicity, blood must be taken at the appropriate time when a particular parasite is being searched for. Levels of microfilaraemia are not usually high enough for the parasite to be easily found in thin films and the whole of the thick film should be scanned under low magnification. To increase diagnostic sensitivity thick films for microfilariae are usually made with larger volumes of blood; when a standard volume e.g. 20 mm³ is used the parasites can be counted (see below). Although Romanovsky dyes stain microfilariae fairly well, other stains such as haematoxylin give greater morphological detail and stain the sheaths better.

2. Wet blood films

This extremely simple technique, merely a small drop of blood spread beneath a cover slip, can be used to detect trypanosomes and microfilariae. The method has comparable sensitivity to a thick film but has the obvious disadvantages of being unstained and non-permanent. Wet films, incubated in a warm humid chamber, can also be used to demonstrate the remarkable phenomenon of exflagellation by male *Plasmodium* gametocytes, a process which begins about 20 minutes after the preparation is made.

3. Buffy coat preparation

In centrifuged blood, trypanosomes are concentrated among the leucocytes at the top of the red cell column. The simplest technique is to use capillary tubes and a microhaematocrit centrifuge; the tube can then be broken near the buffy layer which is allowed to flow onto a slide. The specimen can either be examined wet under a coverslip, or dried and then stained.

Stained buffy coat films are a useful diagnostic method in Indian kala-azar, amastigotes being found in the monocytic cells.

4. Blood filtration for microfilariae

Membrane filtration of microfilariae is a powerful concentration method. Between 1 and 10 ml of blood, anti-coagulated with sequestrene or citrate, is passed through a 25 mm diameter membrane mounted in a Swinnex adaptor, using an ordinary syringe. Either a 3 micron pore size nucleopore membrane, or a 5 micron pore size millipore membrane can be used; in the latter case the blood must be lysed beforehand with a 15 per cent solution of teepol. After several washes with saline the membranes are either examined wet, after passing air through them, or fixed and then stained with haematoxylin.

Membrane filtration has largely replaced previous concentration methods such as Knott's technique in which blood is lysed in formalin and the sediment examined, after centrifugation and staining, for microfilariae.

B. Parasites in stool specimens

1. Wet preparations of unconcentrated stool

To make fresh wet preparations small quantities of stool are emulsified in normal saline, 1 per cent aqueous eosin or Lugol's iodine solution (4 per cent potassium iodide with 2 per cent iodine in distilled water) and examined under a coverslip. The three methods serve different purposes.

The primary purpose of the saline preparation is the detection of the live trophozoites of *Entamoeba histolytica*, *Balantidium coli* and *Giardia lamblia*, the former two species being sought particularly in portions of stool showing blood or exudate, while *Giardia* trophozoites are most likely to be found in loose stools whose appearances suggest malabsorption. Trophozoites of several other amoebic species may be seen in saline preparations but those of invasive *E. histolytica* are the only ones that can be positively identified. They are the largest and most active amoebae to be seen in human stool specimens and the presence of ingested host red cells is pathognomonic (p. 22). The identity of other amoebae can only be confirmed in fixed stained preparations or by the cysts that may accompany them (see below). However this is of little consequence because the bowel amoebae other than *E. histolytica* are either completely harmless or of low pathogenicity (*Dientamoeba fragilis*). The appearances of *Balantidium* trophozoites are unmistakable (Fig. 2.8 and p. 22). In addition to the characteristic *Giardia* trophozoites (Fig. 2.6), the trophozoites of four other flagellate species may be found in human stools; they are probably all non-pathogenic. One of them, *Trichomonas hominis*, bears an axostyle and an undulating membrane; it closely resembles *T. vaginalis* (Fig. 2.9). Another, *Chilomastix mesnili* (6–24 μm in length) is pointed posteriorly, has only a cytostome and bears three anterior flagellae and one recurrent one. The other two are small obscure ovoid organisms, less than 10 μm in length and bear either three flagellae anteriorly (*Enteromonas hominis*) or only one (*Retortamonas intestinalis*).

Eosin preparations are useful for detecting protozoan cysts or coccidial oocysts in fresh stools. Provided the preparations are thin enough these stand out as round or oval white objects against a pink background. Nuclear structure cannot be seen but the chromatoid bodies, found in some amoebic cysts, can be made out. Having detected cysts in eosin preparations their specific identity can be confirmed in the iodine preparation.

The iodine preparation is used to confirm the identity of protozoan cysts since the nuclei and some other structures are stained. This preparation is also often used to find helminth eggs and larvae (*Strongyloides*) although no staining is really necessary for these. The identification of all these parasites will be considered below when wet concentrated preparations are described. The relatively low sensitivity of simple stool smear preparations must always be remembered; when the numbers of cysts, eggs or larvae are low, infections are easily missed. However for the three commonest intestinal helminths, *Ascaris*, hookworm and *Trichuris*, this does not matter since significant infections nearly always have moderate or high egg counts and these will be detected on simple smears provided the whole preparation is scanned.

2. Permanent stained stool preparations

These are usually used to positively identify the trophozoites of certain intestinal amoeba and flagellates in unconcentrated stools; for example it is the only way of confirming the presence of *Dientamoeba fragilis*. The most used method is fixation in Schaudinn's solution and staining with Gomori's trichrome or Heidenhain's iron haematoxylin. These techniques are rather complex and lengthy and are not used much for routine diagnosis. They can also be applied to preserved specimens kept in polyvinyl alcohol fixative.

3. Concentration methods

Stool parasites can be concentrated by a variety of sedimentation and flotation methods; the most widely used are the modified Ritchie formol-ether sedimentation technique, and the zinc sulphate centrifugal flotation method. These methods destroy protozoan trophozoites and kill most parasites; whichever is used the concentrate is stained with Lugol's iodine and examined under a coverslip. The parasitological findings will be considered under five headings.

A. Protozoan cysts. The principal characters of the seven species most likely to be found are given in Figure 13.2; for *Balantidium coli* cysts see page 22. Although not all of these are pathogenic it is essential that one should be familiar with the various forms of all the species otherwise the pathogens may be misidentified. Multiple infections are common and the finding of a non-pathogen should increase the efforts made to find a pathogen. It will be seen that the only clear distinction between *E. histolytica* and the closely related non-pathogen *E. hartmanni* is one of size; this emphasises the importance of using an eyepiece micrometer. Glycogen vacuoles stain reddish brown with iodine; the chromatoids are highly refractile and appear pale brown in colour.

B. Coccidian oocysts and sporocysts. The morphology of the two species *Isospora belli* and *Sarcocystis hominis* are shown in Figure. 2.12. They may appear in the stool as unsegmented oocysts, oocysts containing sporoblasts or sporocysts, or as free sporocysts. Unsegmented oocysts are immature and cannot be identified unless allowed to mature in a Petri dish containing a 2 per cent solution of potassium dichromate for two to three days. Coccidia are often missed because their very low specific gravity makes them float up under the coverslip, out of the normal focal plane. Spurious infections occur when food containing cysts of various species are ingested; these will be transient.

C. Helminth eggs. The rather numerous kinds of helminth eggs found in human faeces fall into nine groups (Fig. 13.3 and Fig. 13.4); several groups contain more than one species and size is often very important, as is the patient's geographic history. The hookworm group is one of the more difficult since the degree of embryonic segmentation will depend upon the bowel transit time and the freshness of the stool specimen. Thus with hookworm itself eggs usually appear in the faeces at the eight cell stage, or less often with four or 16 cells; however segmentation may continue and produce morula and then 'tadpole' stages and

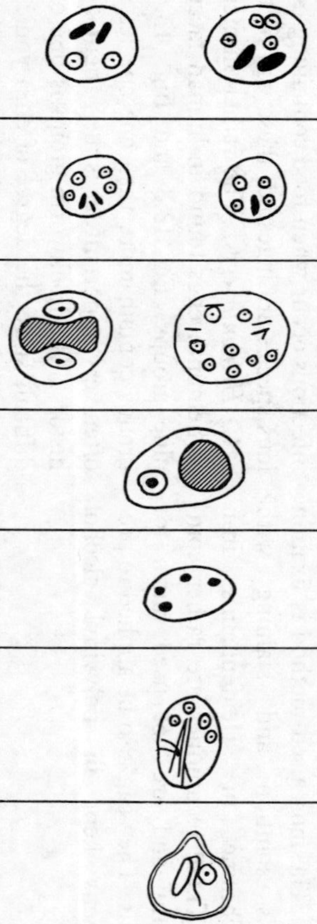

	Size	Shape	Nuclei	Chromatoids	Other features
Entamoeba histolytica	10—15 μm	Spherical	4, if immature 1 or 2 Small central endosome Fine peripheral chromatin	Thick and blunt	None
Entamoeba hartmanni	5—10 μm	Spherical	4, if immature 1 or 2 Small central endosome Coarse peripheral chromatin	Small, thick and blunt	None
Entamoeba coli	10—30 μm usually 14—20 μm	Nearly spherical	8, if immature 1 or 2 Larger slightly eccentric endosome Coarse peripheral chromatin	Fine and pointed	Prominent glycogen vacuole when immature
Iodamoeba buetschlii	6—15 μm	Oval, somewhat irregular	1, very large endosome	None	Large glycogen vacuole
Endolimax nana	6—12 μm	Oval, variable	4 (rarely 2), large endosomes	Minute or absent	None
Giardia lamblia	8—12 μm x 7—10 μm	Oval	4 (rarely 2)	None	Axonemes Median bodies
Chilomastix mesnili	7—10 μm x 4.5—6 μm	Pear or lemon	1	None	Thick wall Cytostome

Fig. 13.2 Protozoan cysts found in faeces. The cysts of the two small flagellates *Enteromonas hominis* and *Retortamonas intestinalis* have been omitted; they resemble small *E. nana* cysts but are usually overlooked and are of no importance.

1. *Hookworm type*
   (Order Strongylida)   Very thin uncoloured shell. Contain embryos at varying stages of maturity.

Developmental stages

	4 cell	*Ancylostoma duodenale* *Necator americanus*	64—76 μm x 36—42 μm Indistinguishable, embryo often at 4 or 8 cell stage, sometimes more mature
	8 cell	*Trichostrongylus* spp.	73—94 μm x 40—53 μm Embryo usually a morula
	Morula	*Ternidens deminutus*	70-94 μm x 47—55 μm Embryo usually at 8 cell stage
	'Tadpole stage	*Oesophagostomium* spp.	60—63 μm x 27—40 μm Embryo similar to hookworm
	Larva (L₁)	*Strongyloides fuelleborni*	48—61 μm x 30—40 μm Fully embryonated to first stage larva

2. *Schistosome type*   Light brown transparent shell with spine or tubercle, no operculum, contains fully embryonated miracidium.

S. mansoni	*S. haematobium*	*S. japonicum*	*S. intercalatum*
114—175 μm x 45—68 μm	112—170 μm x 40—70 μm	70—100 μm x 50—65 μm	176 μm x 61 μm

3. Operculate and embryonated Contain miracidium

Clonorchis sinensis	28—35 μm x 12—19 μm	Opercular lip
Opisthorchis spp.	30 μm x 12 μm (mean)	Lip not prominent
Heterophyes and *Metagonimus*	30 μm x 15 μm (mean)	No lip
Dicrocoelium dendriticum	38—45 μm x 22—30 μm	No lip

4. Operculate and non-embryonated. Ovum lies with mass of vitelline (yolk) cells

Fasciolopsis buski	130—140 μm x 80—85 μm	
Fasciola hepatica	130—150 μm x 60—85 μm	
Paragonimus westermani	80—110 μm x 50—60 μm	Flat operculum with small lip
Echinostoma spp.	100 μm x 70 μm (mean)	
Gastrodiscoides hominis	127—160 μm x 62—75 μm	Rhomboidal shape. Small operculum.
Diphyllobothrium latum	55—80 μm x 40—60 μm	

Fig. 13.3 Helminth eggs found in the stool (1)

finally a first stage rhabditiform larva within the thin shell. In really stale faeces, free larvae may be found and these could be confused with those of *Strongyloides*. Differentiation by larval culture is often used in the hookworm group.

It should be noted that the general shape of all helminth eggs, except *Enterobius*, is perfectly symmetrical; this feature alone distinguishes them from various other objects found in stools.

D. *Helminth larvae. Strongyloides stercoralis* is the only human helminth that normally appears in the faeces in the larval stage (Fig. 13.5). Depending upon the bowel transit time and the patient's condition these may be either rhabditiform larvae (L1 or L2) or filariform larvae (L3); much more commonly they are rhabditiform larvae. Rhabditiform larvae of *S. stercoralis* differ from those of hookworm, which may be found in stale faeces, by having a much shorter buccal cavity and a larger genital primordium. The filariform larvae of *S.*

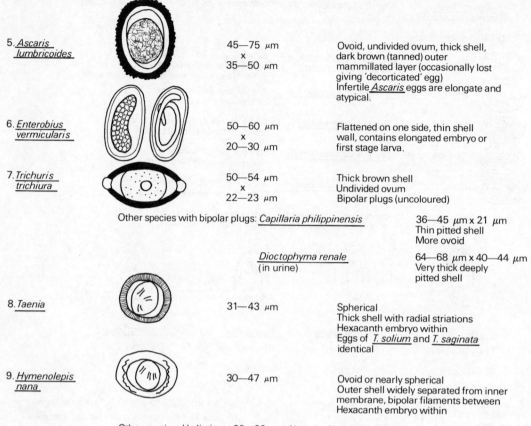

5. *Ascaris lumbricoides*	45—75 μm x 35—50 μm	Ovoid, undivided ovum, thick shell, dark brown (tanned) outer mammillated layer (occasionally lost giving 'decorticated' egg) Infertile *Ascaris* eggs are elongate and atypical.
6. *Enterobius vermicularis*	50—60 μm x 20—30 μm	Flattened on one side, thin shell wall, contains elongated embryo or first stage larva.
7. *Trichuris trichiura*	50—54 μm x 22—23 μm	Thick brown shell Undivided ovum Bipolar plugs (uncoloured)

Other species with bipolar plugs: *Capillaria philippinensis*   36—45 μm x 21 μm Thin pitted shell More ovoid

Dioctophyma renale (in urine)   64—68 μm x 40—44 μm Very thick deeply pitted shell

8. *Taenia*	31—43 μm	Spherical Thick shell with radial striations Hexacanth embryo within Eggs of *T. solium* and *T. saginata* identical
9. *Hymenolepis nana*	30—47 μm	Ovoid or nearly spherical Outer shell widely separated from inner membrane, bipolar filaments between Hexacanth embryo within

Other species: *H. diminuta* 60—80 μm. No polar filaments.

Fig. 13.4 Helminth eggs found in the stool (2)

stercoralis have three minute but distinctive teeth at the tip of the tail; those of hookworm usually have a sheath, and the tail is simple.

4. Adult worms

The only worms likely to be found in ordinary faecal specimens are *Ascaris*, *Enterobius* and tapeworm proglottids; the two former are easily recognised as are tapeworm proglottids when flattened between two slides (Fig. 3.9). To obtain adult worm specimens of other species post-treatment faecal specimens should be washed through a sieve, or repeatedly allowed to sediment in a bucket using several changes of water. To make permanent stained slide preparations of helminths, special techniques are necessary.

C. Parasites in urine

The eggs of *Schistosoma haematobium* (Fig. 13.3) are the principal parasitological finding in urine. Preferably specimens should be obtained between mid morning and mid afternoon as the number of eggs in the urine is greatest about noon; they are also more numerous at the end of the urinary stream hence 'terminal urine' can be collected. Infections of significant intensity are unlikely when there are no red cells in the urinary deposit.

Other parasites sometimes found are *Trichomonas vaginalis* and the microfilariae of *Wuchereria bancrofti* in the presence of chyluria or those of *Onchocerca volvulus* during chemotherapy. Occasionally eggs of *Dioctophyma renale* are found, or the protoscolices and brood capsules of

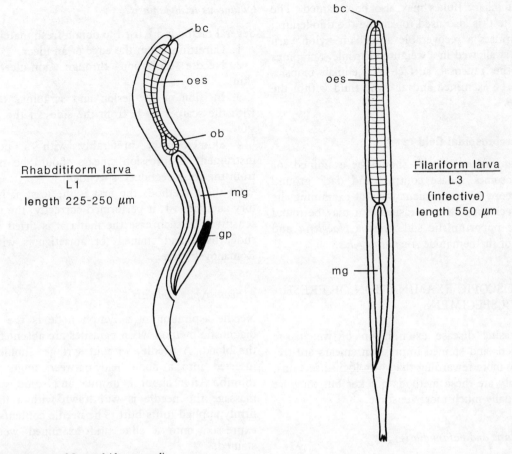

Rhabditiform larva
L1
length 225-250 µm

bc
oes
ob
mg
gp

Filariform larva
L3
(infective)
length 550 µm

bc
oes
mg

Fig. 13.5 Larvae of *Strongyloides stercoralis*
Abbreviations: bc — buccal cavity; gp — genital primordium; L1 — first stage larva; L3 — third stage larva; mg — midgut; ob — oesophageal bulb; oes— oesophagus

Echinococcus granulosus from a ruptured renal hydatid cyst.

D. Parasites in perianal swabs

This is the usual method of diagnosing *Enterobius* infection. A transparent adhesive tape is normally used and eggs are viewed through it after it has been stuck onto a glass slide. Alternatively a moistened bacteriological swab is used; this is shaken well in saline, which is then centrifuged. Eggs of *Taenia saginata* are quite common on perianal skin.

E. Parasites on vaginal swabs

Trichomonas vaginalis and rarely trophozoites of *Entamoeba histolytica*; both may be cultured.

F. Parasites in sputum

The eggs of *Paragonimus* may be found and sometimes larvae of *Strongyloides* and *Ascaris*, or even protoscolices and brood capsules from a ruptured hydatid cyst. Amoebae in sputum may be *E. histolytica*, in cases of pulmonary amoebiasis, but the mouth commensal *E. gingivalis* can easily contaminate the specimen. Occasionally adult specimens of the nematode *Syngamus laryngeus* may be found, or alternatively the ovoidal sculptured eggs of this species.

G. Duodenal fluid

The aspirates from the duodenum may contain trophozoites of *Giardia* or the larvae and sometimes even the eggs of *Strongyloides stercoralis*. The eggs of biliary flukes may also be obtained. The 'string test' is also used to sample the duodenum; it comprises a recoverable absorbant nylon yarn that is swallowed in a weighted capsule. Scrapings from the mucosal surface of jejunal biopsies should be examined and also the fluid within the capsule.

H. Cerebrospinal fluid

The centrifuged deposit should be examined for trypanosomes; phase contrast and dark ground microscopy are convenient ways of examining the wet specimen. Other parasites that may be found are the opportunistic soil amoeba *Naegleria* and larvae of the nematode *Angiostrongylus*.

MICROSCOPIC EXAMINATION OF FRESH TISSUE SPECIMENS

In parasitic disease examination of wet tissue specimens and stained impression smears are frequently more rewarding than histological sections. Not only are these methods quicker but they are also usually much more sensitive.

Amoebiasis and balantidiasis

Mucosal lesions seen during proctoscopy or sigmoidoscopy should be scraped or curetted and the material examined wet, with added saline if necessary, for haematophagous trophozoites of *E. histolytica* or more rarely those of *Balantidium coli*. Cutaneous ulcers, particularly those of the perineum or perianal region, should be examined in a similar way, as should suspicious ulcers of the uterine cervix. When liver abscesses are aspirated the amoebae are most likely to be found in the last portions obtained.

Visceral leishmaniasis

Smears should be made of aspirates from bone marrow, spleen or lymph nodes. After fixation they are stained with one of the Romanovsky dyes and examined for amastigotes of *L. donovani*. Marrow aspirates are generally preferred because of their safety; however the parasites are often more numerous in splenic material.

Cutaneous leishmaniasis

Several methods are used to obtain fresh material:
1. Curettings from the edge of an ulcer.
2. Needle aspiration through non-ulcerated skin.
3. Incision of the lesion and scrapings taken with the scalpel blade from the sides of the incision.
4. Skin biopsy, preferably with a punch instrument. Impression smears should be made from the fresh sectioned specimen.

Of these methods the first is the least satisfactory and the last, if performed correctly, the most sensitive. In each case the material is dried on a slide, fixed and stained for amastigotes with a Romanovsky dye.

African trypanosomiasis

Needle aspiration of a lymph node is the best diagnostic method when parasites are absent from the blood. A needle, without syringe, should be inserted into a node held between finger and thumb. After about a minute and some gentle massage the needle is withdrawn with a finger firmly applied to its butt. The needle contents are expressed onto a slide and examined wet or stained.

Pneumocystosis

Transbronchial or open lung biopsy specimens are now generally recommended, rather than percutaneous needle biopsy of the lung. Whichever method is used, impression smears should be made and stained with Giemsa to demonstrate the intracystic sporozoites, and also with either methenamine silver nitrate or the periodic acid — Schiff reagent, which both show the outer wall of the cyst. Sputum specimens are of very little value.

Schistosomiasis

Rectal biopsies or 'snips' are a useful method when no eggs are found in the stool. Normally three specimens are taken, using a proctoscope and a curette whose blade is drawn back into the mucosa bulging over the distal end of the endoscope. The biopsies should be examined for eggs as fresh squash preparations between two slides. In addition to the eggs of the intestinal species, those of *S. haematobium* may be present in the rectal mucosa, although they are almost never found in the stool.

Filariasis

The microfilariae of *Onchocerca volvulus* and *Dipetalonema streptocerca* are normally found in the upper dermis. Superficial skin 'snips' are taken using a scalpel blade and a pinched-up fold of skin, or alternatively a conjunctival biopsy punch may be used. The snips should measure 2–3 mm in diameter and not be contaminated with blood. After incubation in saline for 30 minutes beneath a coverslip, the microfilariae will have emerged and can be identified in the wet preparation. Normally three 'snips' are taken from each side of the body; two from the scapular region, two from the upper buttocks and two from the calves. See Figure 13.1 for the differentiation of these species.

Trichinosis

Muscle biopsies are taken from the deltoid or gastrocnemius. A simple squash preparation, between two slides, can be made from part of the specimen. If this shows no larvae the remainder of the specimen is digested in an acid-pepsin mixture and the centrifuged deposit examined for living larvae.

QUANTITATIVE TECHNIQUES

In helminthic infections the intensity of infection, that is the number of worms in a host, is an important determinant of morbidity. Since most worms do not multiply in the body and since the output of eggs or larvae per worm is relatively constant, it is possible to estimate intensity by counting eggs and larvae. The output per worm is not greatly affected by worm load. Quantitative methods are useful in chemotherapy since the percentage reduction in worm load can be estimated.

Faecal egg counts

These have been applied particularly to *Schistosoma mansoni*, *S. japonicum*, hookworm, *Ascaris* and *Trichuris* infections. Counts are expressed as eggs per gramme of stool. It has been demonstrated that eggs are randomly distributed in a stool specimen. Currently used methods include:

1. Modified Kato thick-smear technique using 50 mg of stool cleared on a slide beneath a glycerine-soaked cellophane disc.

2. Stoll dilution technique whose counts measure 10 mg of stool.

3. McMaster egg counting chamber gives counts in 20 mg of stool, by flotation in saturated saline beneath a squared grid on the roof of the chamber.

4. Sedimentation-filtration technique (Bell); used particularly for *S. mansoni* infection, it employs 1 ml aliquots from an emulsified 24-hour stool specimen made up to a total volume of one litre. Eggs are stained on the filter paper with ninhydrin.

Urine egg counts

Counts of *S. haematobium* eggs are made after filtration of a 10 ml specimen. The eggs can be stained before or after filtration.

Microfilarial counts

Blood microfilaria counts are made using:

1. Thick films made from measured volumes of blood, for example 20 mm³.

2. Membrane filtration using 1 ml of blood, or more.

3. A counting chamber in which 50 mm³ of blood is lysed in water, and the microfilariae counted immediately as they lie on the floor of the chamber.

Skin microfilariae are counted using snips of standard size or measured weight.

Trichinella larval counts

The number of larvae, obtained by digestion, can be expressed as the number per gramme of tissue. Either biopsy or necropsy material is used.

CULTURAL METHODS

Although many human parasites can now be maintained in culture, sometimes continuously, this remains largely a research procedure partly because many of the methods are complex and require considerable skill and experience. However there are some useful applications in the diagnostic field.

Leishmaniasis

Leishmania of all species will grow readily on a blood-agar slope medium called N.N.N. after its orginators Novy, MacNeal and Nicolle. The parasites grow, at 28°C, as promastigotes in the small liquid phase of the medium. A positive result may not be obtained for 14 or 21 days; bacteriological sterility is essential. Trypanosoma cruzi can also be grown on N.N.N. medium or modifications of it.

Amoebae

Most of the species of amoebae, flagellates and ciliates of the large bowel can be readily grown in simple bacteria-associated media such as those of Robinson. The method is sensitive but little used for routine work. Of the amoebae E. histolytica grows the most readily, but fixed stained preparations of the cultured trophozoites are necessary for positive identification. Dientamoeba infections can be recognised by this method.

'Free-living' amoebae, for example Naegleria or Acanthamoeba in cerebrospinal fluid specimens, are cultured upon a confluent growth of Escherichia coli on agar plates.

Strongyloides stercoralis

The larvae of this species are sometimes very scanty in stool specimens. The free-living cycle can be established in charcoal cultures using 1 gramme or more of faeces. A very small number of larvae in the original specimen generate many adults and larvae within 7 or 10 days.

Larval cultures of hookworm and related species

A portion of faeces is smeared on the middle of a long strip of filter paper, which is placed in an upright test tube with a small volume of water at the bottom (Harada-Mori technique). The width of the filter paper strip should equal the diameter of the test tube and cultures should be kept in the dark. The paper remains wet because of capillarity and hatched larvae migrate down into the water. Within 10 days at 28°C, filariform larvae can be found and identified; the larvae are infective and care is needed in handling them. Species are separated by differences in their length, sheaths, buccal cavities, tails and the length of the oesophagus. In this way infections by the two major human hookworms, N. americanus and A. duodenale, are distinguished, a matter of some importance because their response to therapy, by some drugs, differs. The larvae of Ternidens, Trichostrongylus and Oesophagostomium can also be identified; as well as Strongyloides, which also grows in these cultures.

ANIMAL INOCULATION

Used relatively little for diagnosis although many human parasites will grow and develop in suitable mammal hosts. The diagnostic applications are:

1. Leishmania donovani

Aspirates of marrow, liver, spleen or lymph node are inoculated intraperitoneally into hamsters. Even a single amastigote can establish an infection which is demonstrable, after a period of several weeks, in splenic smears. Other species of Leishmania are more difficult to establish in laboratory rodents and they must be inoculated into mouse or hamster footpads.

2. Toxoplasma gondii

Animal inoculation is usually the only way of demonstrating the organism in this infection, as tissue impression smears and histological sections are almost invariably negative. Biopsy material, such as lymph nodes or muscle, should be injected intraperitoneally into Toxoplasma-free mice. After seven to ten days smears are made of peritoneal fluid and stained with Giemsa; if negative the peritoneal fluid should be passaged into another animal. Animals surviving more than three weeks should be sacrificed and brain smears made to detect cysts; their serum should be tested for seroconversion.

3. Trypanosomiasis

Blood from patients with suspected *T.b. rhodesiense* can be injected intraperitoneally, or intravenously into the tail veins of either mice or rats. Patent parasitaemia appears within two weeks. *T.b. gambiense* is very much more difficult to establish in laboratory animals. The same methods are used in *T. cruzi* infections, and in this infection cultures grown in N.N.N. or similar media for one to two weeks can also be inoculated into animals.

4. Babesiosis

Mild or subclinical infections in man, particularly those due to the rodent parasite *B. microti*, can be detected by inoculating blood into splenectomised hamsters. These infections are probably commoner in man than is currently suspected; serology is a useful screening test.

XENODIAGNOSIS

This method employs an intermediate host or vector, within which the parasite multiplies, to detect low levels of parasitism. Its only practical diagnostic application is the use of Reduviid bugs to detect low levels of parasitaemia in *Trypanosoma cruzi* infection. This is a very sensitive method and is often the only way to demonstrate the parasite in chronic infections. 40 clean bugs of the appropriate species, usually *Triatoma infestans* or *Rhodnius prolixus*, are allowed to feed upon the patient and 30 days later live flagellates are sought in their faeces, using wet mounts.

HISTOLOGY

Detection of protozoa in tissue section is often difficult as the whole organism, particularly its nucleus, cannot often be seen. Impression smears

and scrapings examined fresh are nearly always preferable. The larger tissue cysts due to *Trypanosoma cruzi*, or *Sarcocystis* in muscle, are more easy to demonstrate in sections.

The identity of larval or adult helminths seen in tissue sections can often be determined with considerable accuracy. Situations where this method is useful include visceral larva migrans due to nematodes and other parasites, and larval cestode infections. This is a specialised field and expert help should be sought.

SEROLOGICAL DIAGNOSIS

Serological tests have been applied to most of the commoner parasitic infections in man and also to some of the less common ones such as *Babesia* and *Anisakis*. Parasite antigens are prepared from parasites grown in culture, or those obtained from naturally infected or experimentally infected animals. Virtually all the available immunological tests have been tried. The most sensitive tests include indirect haemagglutination, the enzyme-linked immunosorbent assay (ELISA) and countercurrent immunoelectrophoresis; tests of intermediate sensitivity are indirect immunofluorescence and the complement fixation tests; while those involving simple precipitation in gel, or agglutination of antigen–coated particles (latex, bentonite or lecithin-cholesterol crystals) usually have a lower sensitivity.

The obvious advantages of slide agglutination tests with coated particles is that they are simple to perform and can be made commercially. One disadvantage of the complement fixation test is that some sera in certain parasitic diseases are anti-complementary due to immune complexes.

Whichever technique is used it can usually be made sufficiently sensitive. The two major difficulties are lack of specificity and the inability of serologic tests to distinguish current from past infection. Lack of specificity results partly from the crude nature of the antigens normally used and their chemical complexity, and also because some antigens are shared by different organisms. Cross reactions are a much greater problem in helminthic infections and occur to a variable degree between parasites within the major groupings of trematode, cestode and nematode. Sometimes reactivity even crosses these zoological boundaries; for example *Trichinella* and *Schistosoma* cross-react with some tests. Even with a fairly specific test it may not be possible to distinguish between true infection and exposure to non-human parasites, thus patients with a recent history of cercarial dermatitis due to an avian schistosome may give positive results with some standard schistosome serological tests. Attempts have been made to distinguish active from past infection by looking for IgM antibodies in the former. This can be done most simply with the indirect immunofluorescence test; considerable success has been achieved in toxoplasmosis and probably also in amoebiasis. Another method of achieving this aim is to look serologically for parasite antigen and future developments can be expected in this field.

While serology is often a valuable tool in the hands of the epidemiologist (Chapter 15) the applications in the diagnosis of individual patients are more limited. When levels of transmission are high, a large proportion of 'normal' adults may be seropositive. In several infections serology serves as a useful screening test that may lead to more detailed parasitological studies, or as a test of exclusion; in neither of these situations does low specificity invalidate the method. Serology finds its greatest use in those parasitic diseases where the parasite and its infective forms cannot be found in excreta or body fluids. These include the tissue protozoans without vectors such as toxoplasmosis, the larval cestodes and zoonotic nematode infections.

The particular immunologic test used is often not of critical importance and the choice will sometimes depend upon the equipment available and the expertise of the pathologist and his staff. Currently, the useful applications of serology are:

Malaria. Sensitive but most tests show cross reactivity between *Plasmodium* species. Useless for the diagnosis of acute malaria because antibodies persist for at least two years after cure. A negative test excludes malaria as a cause of unexplained recurrent pyrexia. Useful for screening blood donors.

Trypanosoma cruzi. Sensitive and often the only method of diagnosing chronic infections; however many symptomless adults will be positive in endemic areas. Useful for screening blood donors.

Trypanosoma brucei. Sensitive and a useful screening test. A positive result should lead to further efforts to find the parasite.

Leishmania donovani. Probably sensitive. Cross-reacting antibodies to *T. cruzi* can be absorbed out. Probably a useful screening test. The acid–fast Kedrowsky bacillus can be used as antigen but this test is less sensitive and less specific. Serology is also useful in mucocutaneous leishmaniasis due to *L. braziliensis*.

Amoebiasis. At least 95 per cent of patients with liver abscess due to *E. histolytica* are seropositive. In invasive bowel disease the figure is 60 to 70 per cent but these can be diagnosed parasitologically. Useful in amoebomas. In endemic areas many persons, some of them infected carriers, will be positive but few at the high titres seen in liver abscess.

Pneumocystosis. Specific but insensitive. Many proven cases are negative and a significant proportion of normal persons are positive. With current tests only seroconversion is diagnostic.

Toxoplasmosis. Specific and moderately sensitive. The Sabin-Feldman dye exclusion test is the most sensitive but requires living organisms for its performance; parasites fail to take up the dye in the presence of antibody. Positive dye tests and indirect immunofluorescent tests appear one to two weeks after infection, while the complement fixation test becomes positive three to six weeks after infection; dye tests remain positive for life. A serologic diagnosis is based upon either a high titre, a rising titre, or IgM antibody. In adults with isolated choroidoretinitis, titres are usually low and often only the dye test is positive; however high levels of antibody can be detected in aqueous humour. IgM antibodies in cord blood indicate congenital infection.

Schistosomiasis. Possibly useful as a screening test. A positive result by itself is never an indication for chemotherapy but further efforts must be made to find the parasite.

Fascioliasis. Probably sensitive. May be diagnostic in early infections before eggs appear in the faeces, but only in highly suggestive clinical situations. Since man is an abnormal host for this parasite eggs may never appear, hence serology is probably of special importance in this trematode infection.

Filariasis. Moderately useful as a screening test. Diagnostic in the context of diffuse filarial lung disease (tropical pulmonary eosinophilia), in which very high titres are obtained.

Trichinosis. Serology often diagnostic especially when there is seroconversion. The simple bentonite flocculation slide test and the complement fixation test become positive about four weeks after infection, or sometimes earlier. The indirect immunofluorescence test becomes positive at an even earlier stage.

Toxocariasis. Sensitive but usually rather nonspecific. Most tests cross-react with *Ascaris* and other nematodes. Titres are much higher when this parasite causes visceral larva migrans rather than isolated retinal granulomas.

Larval cestodes. Serology is moderately sensitive and specific in hydatid disease. Either a crude or a purified antigen can be prepared from the fluid of *Echinococcus* cysts in sheep, but a scolex antigen is probably the best. Patients with small or nonleaking cysts may be seronegative; some cross-reaction occurs with cysticercosis. Several different serological tests for hydatid should preferably be performed on the same specimen. To diagnose cysticercosis serologically, fluid should be obtained from living cysticerci of *T. solium* in pig carcases.

Obscure eosinophilia. A battery of helminth serological tests can be applied in this context, the geographic history being of some help. The tests chosen should include at least one trematode and one nematode, and also hydatid serology. When all tests are negative a helminth cause is unlikely. Positive results should renew efforts to find the parasite. *Ascaris* serology is of some value because it is very sensitive and cross reacts with many helminths, including *Toxocara* and *Strongyloides stercoralis*; the latter species often gives a positive result with some filarial serological tests.

SKIN TESTS

Diagnostically, these are valuable in very few situations. They have been applied to many parasitic diseases; they are often as sensitive as serology, but even less specific. Positivity is usually lifelong, hence the use of skin tests in epidemiology. Only two tests are currently useful for individual diagnosis.

Leishmanin test. This is sensitive and specific. It is a delayed sensitivity test that becomes positive in cutaneous leishmaniasis at about the time the primary papule ulcerates. It remains negative in diffuse cutaneous leishmaniasis, and is negative in *L. donovani* infections until after recovery when reactivity is greatest after one or two years and then fades. Performed by injecting 0.1 ml of a suspension of killed promastigotes, 10^6 organisms per ml in 0.5 per cent phenol saline intradermally, and read after 48–72 hours. A papule exceeding 5 mm in diameter indicates a positive reaction. The different species of *Leishmania* cross-react.

Casoni test. Crude or refined hydatid cyst fluid is used; 0.2 ml is injected intradermally and this produces a wheal and flare reaction within 20 minutes. A saline control must be used. The test is probably very sensitive but positive reactions are often given by patients with schistosomiasis.

RADIOLOGY AND SCANNING TECHNIQUES

The following helminths may calcify in the tissues to produce characteristic dense opacities on ordinary radiographs: Guinea worm (*Dracunculus*), usually in the pelvis, perineum, or leg especially near hip or knee joints; *Loa loa*, fine coiled shadows often in forearms, wrists or hands; *Echinococcus*: many hydatids do not develop calcification of their adventitial coat, those that do are usually in the liver, bone hydatids are osteolytic; *Taenia solium*, elongate or oval shadows up to 1 cm long especially in muscles of shoulder and hip girdles, thighs and chest wall, but they may also calcify in the brain; *Armillifer armillatus* (pentastomiasis), typical horseshoe shaped shadows in abdomen, chest or chest wall; *Paragonimus*, dead worms may be demonstrable as irregular peribronchial shadows. Calcified dead eggs of *Schistosoma haematobium* in the bladder submucosa may outline the bladder giving a 'foetal head' appearance.

It should be noted that although larvae of *Trichinella* become calcified they are too small to show on ordinary films. Similarly although dead *Wuchereria bancrofti* do calcify, they are so thin as to be almost never visible on X-ray films. Old amoebic abscesses of the liver sometimes leave bizarre calcific shadows in fibrous scar tissue.

Scanning techniques are of particular value in demonstrating amoebic abscesses of the liver or larval cestodes in many tissues.

FURTHER READING

Chitwood, M.B. and Lichtenfels, J.R. (1972) Identification of parasitic metazoa in tissue sections. *J. Parasit.*, **32**, 407–519.

Fife, E.H. Jr (1971) Advances in methodology for immunodiagnosis of parasitic diseases. *Experimental Parasitology*, **30**, 132–163.

Kagan, I.G. (1973) Parasitic diseases. In: *Serological Epidemiology*, eds Paul, J.R. and White, C. New York and London: Academic Press.

Robinson, G. L. (1968) Laboratory diagnosis of human parasitic amoebae. *Trans. R. Soc. trop. Med. Hyg.*, **62**, 285–294.

Taylor, A.E.R. and Baker, J.R. (1968) *The Cultivation of Parasites* in vitro. Oxford: Blackwell Scientific Publications.

[See also Belding (1965) and Faust, Russell, and Jung (1970) as cited on p. 11]

14

The chemotherapy of parasitic infections

INTRODUCTION

Antiparasitic agents were among the first specific remedies to be used in medicine. A number of plant alkaloids act as vermifuges and expel worms from the gut when given by mouth; some of these have been used since antiquity. The Ebers papyrus of 1550 BC records the use of pomegranate bark to eliminate tapeworms and Theophrastus in 300 BC recommended male fern (*Aspidium*) for the same purpose: the latter has considerable toxicity but has only recently been replaced by synthetic compounds. Applications containing sulphur were advocated by the Roman physician Celsus in AD 25, for what appears to have been scabies; preparations of sulphur are still used for this purpose. Two alkaloids are also still in use; crude cinchona bark had been used for malaria since 1630, and its active principle quinine was isolated in 1820; emetine, an extract of ipecacuanha was first used for amoebiasis in 1912.

The antiparasitic drugs in current use, together with their toxic effects on man, are listed in Tables 14.1, 14.2, 14.3 and 14.4. Several compounds have a wide range of activity against parasites that are zoologically unrelated. As an indication of recent progress in this field, only six of the listed synthetic drugs were introduced before 1940; these were suramin in 1920, tryparsamide in 1921, potassium antimony tartrate in 1924; tetrachlorethylene in 1925, mepacrine in 1930 and di-iodohydroxyquin in 1936. The search for new compounds continues as many problems remain unsolved and new ones are generated by drug resistance. The situation can only be regarded as reasonably satisfactory for the intestinal nematodes, the intestinal cestodes, the lumen-dwelling protozoa and drug-sensitive malaria. Currently used drugs for African trypanosomiasis are very toxic and those for American trypanosomiasis are both toxic and relatively ineffective. New safe drugs are required to kill the adults of several species of filarial worms, in particular *Onchocerca volvulus*, and the treatment of the hermaphroditic flukes is unsatisfactory. Safer, more effective, drugs are still needed for schistosomiasis and leishmaniasis and there are at present no established drugs for larval tapeworms.

Indications for chemotherapy

The potential toxicity of many antiparasitic drugs implies that their use must be based upon accurate diagnosis. Parasitological findings must always be considered in the context of the patient's clinical state, and should not delay the search for other, perhaps more important, diagnoses. For example, the presence of *E. histolytica* in the stool in no way excludes a co-existent colonic carcinoma, nor does the finding of *P. falciparum* in the blood film from a comatose patient eliminate the possibility of meningitis.

The decision to treat must be based on the severity of the condition. Thus, life-threatening infections such as amoebic liver abscess, falciparum malaria, African trypanosomiasis and visceral leishmaniasis must always be treated with the safest available drug. At the other extreme, treatment of very light infections with hookworm, *Ascaris* and *Trichuris* is usually unnecessary and symptomless *Giardia* infection or threadworm may only require treatment to prevent spread within a household. Most infections occupy an intermediate posi-

Table 14.1 Currently used antiparasitic drugs, their activity and toxicity

Drug class	Drug name	Antiparasitic effect	Toxicity
Heavy metals			
Antimonial compounds (trivalent)	Antimony potassium tartrate i.v. / Antimony sodium dimercaptosuccinate i.m. }	*Schistosoma*	Cough. Vomiting. Muscle pains. Bradycardia. Occas. myocardial damage, jaundice, renal failure.
Antimonial compounds (pentavalent)	Sodium stibogluconate (Pentostam) i.v. or i.m. / Meglumine antimoniate (Glucantime) i.m.	*Leishmania*	As above. Much less toxic.
Arsenical compounds (trivalent)	Melarsoprol i.v.	*Trypanosoma brucei*	Vomiting. Neuropathy. Myocardial damage. Reactive encephalopathy. Occas. shock.
Arsenical compounds (pentavalent)	Tryparsamide i.v.	*Trypanosoma brucei*	Vomiting. Fever. Occas. optic neuritis, exfoliative dermatitis.
Plant alkaloids			
Emetine	Emetine hydrochloride i.m. / Dehydroemetine hydrochloride i.m. }	*Entamoeba. Fasciola (Paragonimus)*	Diarrhoea. Vomiting. Muscle weakness. Occas. precordial pain, arrhythmias, myositis (local or systemic).
Quinine	Quinine sulphate p.o. / Quinine dihydrochloride i.v. }	*Plasmodium*	Cinchonism — tinnitus, deafness, nausea, and visual disturbance. Occas. arrhythmias, abortion, haemoglobinuria.
Dyes and derivatives			
Acridine	Mepacrine p.o.	*Giardia. Taenia. (Plasmodium)*	Dizziness. G.I. disturbance. Yellow skin. Occas. psychosis. Red stools.
Cyanine dye	Pyrvinium pamoate p.o.	*Enterobius*	Vomiting. nausea, abdominal cramps.
Azo dye (colourless analogue)	Suramin i.v.	*Trypanosoma brucei Onchocerca*	Vomiting. Paresthesiae. Urticaria. Occas. collapse, renal damage.

Parasite names given in parenthesis indicate that drug is not normally used for this purpose.
Abbreviations: i.m. — intramuscular; i.v. — intravenous; p.o. — per os (oral)

Table 14.2 Currently used antiparasitic drugs, their activity and toxicity

Drug class	Drug name	Antiparasitic effect	Toxicity
Antibiotics			
Polyene	Amphotericin B. i.v.	*Leishmania donovani* *L. braziliensis* *Naegleria*	Renal damage. Fever. Phlebitis. Occas. neuropathy, anaphylaxis.
Aminoglycoside	Paromomycin p.o.	*Entamoeba. Balantidium.* *Taenia. Hymenolepis.* *Diphyllobothrium*	G.I. disturbance. Occas. auditory nerve, renal damage.
Tetracycline	Tetracycline p.o. or i.v.	*Entamoeba. Balantidium.* *(Plasmodium)*	G.I. disturbance. Stained teeth. Occas. liver damage, enterocolitis.
Macrolide	Spiramycin p.o.	*Toxoplasma*	G.I. disturbance. Occas. allergic reactions.
Antifolates			
Biguanides	Proguanil p.o. Cycloguanil pamoate i.m.	*Plasmodium.* *Leishmania mexicana* *(Plasmodium)*	Mild G.I. disturbance. Local pain. Occas. blood dyscrasias.
Diaminopyrimidines	Pyrimethamine p.o.	*Plasmodium.*	Toxic in children (overdose).
combined with para-amino benzoic acid analogues	Pyrimethamine + sulphadoxine (Fansidar) p.o.	*Plasmodium.*	Occas. sensivity reactions and blood dyscrasias.
	Pyrimethamine + dapsone (Maloprim) p.o.	*Plasmodium.*	Folic acid deficiency.
	Pyrimethamine + sulphadiazine p.o.	*Toxoplasma. Isospora*	Occas. megaloblastic anaemia
	Trimethoprim + sulphamethoxazole p.o. (co-trimoxazole)	*Pneumocystis. Isospora* *(Plasmodium)*	Sensitivity reactions.
Diamidines	Pentamidine i.m.	*Leishmania.* *Trypanosoma brucei* *Pneumocystis. Babesia.* *(Trypanosoma brucei).* *Babesia.*	Hypotension. Vomiting. Occas. diabetes mellitus, liver damage.
	Diazoaminobenzene (Berenil) i.m.	*Babesia.*	As above

Parasite names given in parenthesis indicate that drug is not normally used for this purpose.
Abbreviations: i.m. — intramuscular; i.v. — intravenous; p.o. — per os (oral)

Table 14.3 Currently used antiparasitic drugs, their activity and toxicity

Drug class	Drug name	Antiparasitic effect	Toxicity
Quinoline derivatives			
4-aminoquinolines	Chloroquine p.o. or i.v. (or i.m.) (amodiaquine p.o.)	Plasmodium. Entamoeba. Clonorchis. Opisthorchis Fasciola. Paragonimus	G.I. upset. Pruritus. Hypotension. Ocular accommodation. Occas. corneal and retinal deposits (if total dose > 100 g).
8-aminoquinolines	Primaquine p.o.	Plasmodium vivax and P. ovale (exo-erythrocytic stage in liver)	Abdominal cramps. Haemolysis and methaemoglobinaemia in G-6-PD-deficient persons.
Hydroxyquinolines	Di-iodohydroxyquin p.o.	Entamoeba. Balantidium. Dientamoeba	Rashes. Diarrhoea. Anal pruritus. Occas. optic atrophy.
Tetrahydroquinoline	Oxamniquine i.m.	Schistosoma mansoni	Dizziness. Local pain.
Imidazole and thiazole derivatives			
Nitroimidazoles	Metronidazole p.o. (or i.v.) (tinidazole, nitrimidazine and ornidazole)	Entamoeba. Balantidium. Trichomonas. Giardia. (Dracunculus)	Dizziness. Metallic taste in mouth. G.I. upset. Antabuse-like effect with alcohol.
	Benznidazole p.o.	Trypanosoma cruzi	Nausea. Dizziness. Weight loss. Occas. neuropathy, exfoliative dermatitis, purpura.
Nitrothiazole	Niridazole p.o.	Schistosoma mansoni. S. haematobium. Dracunculus. (Entamoeba)	Dizziness. Vomiting. Occas. psychosis, epilepsy, coma.
Benzimidazoles	Thiabendazole p.o.	Strongyloides. Capillaria. (Other gut nematodes) Toxocara. Trichinella Cutaneous larva migrans	G.I. upsets. Occas. leucopenia, jaundice, sensitivity reactions.
	p.o. or topical		
	Mebendazole p.o.	Enterobius. Trichuris. Ascaris. Hookworm. (Trichinella)	Minimal. Because of possible mutagenic effect not used in pregnancy or children <2 years.
	Levamisole p.o.	Ascaris. (Hookworm)	Occas. G.I. upsets, dizziness.

Parasite names given in parenthesis indicate that drug is not normally used for this purpose.
Abbreviations: i.m. — intramuscular; i.v. — intravenous; p.o. — per os (oral)

Table 14.4 Currently used antiparasitic drugs, their activity and toxicity

Drug class	Drug name	Antiparasitic effect	Toxicity
Halogenated diphenyl compounds			
Salicylamide	Niclosamide p.o.	*Taenia. Diphyllobothrium. Hymenolepis.* (As above)	Occas. nausea, abdominal pain.
Diphenylmethane	Dichlorophen p.o.		Nausea, Colic. Occas. jaundice.
Diphenylsulphide	Bithionol p.o.	*Paragonimus. Fasciola.* (*Taenia*).	G.I. disturbance. Urticaria. Photosensitivity.
Piperazine compounds			
Parent compound	Piperazine p.o.	*Ascaris. Enterobius.* Intestinal flukes.	Nausea. Abdominal pain. Occas. ataxia, hypotonia.
Carbamyl derivative	Diethylcarbamazine p.o.	Filarial worms, see Table 14.7 *Toxocara.* (*Ascaris*)	Mild G.I. disturbance. Allergic reactions to worm death.
Quaternary ammonium compounds	Bephenium hydroxynaphthoate p.o.	Hookworm (*Ancylostoma*) Intestinal flukes.	Nausea. Occas. hypotension.
	Bitoscanate p.o.	Hookworm (*Ancylostoma* and *Necator*)	G.I. upsets. Dizziness.
Thioxanthone	Hycanthone i.m.	*Schistosoma mansoni*	Vomiting. Occas. liver damage (severe).
Pyrimidine	Pyrantel pamoate p.o.	*Ascaris.* Hookworm. *Enterobius.*	Occas. dizziness and G.I. upset.
Organophosphorus compound	Metrifonate p.o.	*Schistosoma haematobium*	Mild G.I. upsets. Depressed cholinesterase levels in blood.
Dichloracetamide	Diloxanide fuorate p.o.	*Entamoeba*	Flatulence. Nausea.
Chlorinated hydrocarbons	Tetrachlorethylene p.o.	Hookworm (*Necator*). Intestinal flukes.	Epigastric burning. Vomiting. Occas. collapse, jaundice.
	Hexachloroparaxyjol p.o.	*Clonorchis. Opisthorchis.* (*Paragonimus*)	Vomiting. Vertigo.
Nitrofurans	Furazolidine p.o.	*Giardia*	Occas. diarrhoea, rashes.
	Nifurtimox p.o.	*Trypanosoma cruzi* } *Leishmania braziliensis* } *Trypanosoma brucei*	Diarrhoea. Sensitivity. Haemolysis in G-6-PD-deficient persons.
	Nitrofurazone p.o.		Occas. neuropathy, psychosis.

Parasite names given in parenthesis indicate that drug is not normally used for this purpose.
Abbreviations: i.m. — intramuscular; i.v. — intravenous; p.o. — per os (oral)

tion and in these risks of therapy must be weighed against the anticipated benefits. Important determinants will be the severity of current pathology, the prognosis without therapy, the risk of further exposure, and for most helminthic infections, the intensity of infection.

Failure of chemotherapy

1. Acquired drug resistance. The widespread use of antiprotozoan drugs acts as a selective force when drug-resistant mutants appear spontaneously. Since 1960 resistance of *Plasmodium falciparum* to chloroquine has emerged as a major problem in Southeast Asia and South America. In a sensitive strain asexual parasitaemia disappears within seven days of starting the standard course of chloroquine. Three grades of resistance are recognised: in Grade I, asexual parasites all disappear within seven days but this is followed by a recrudescence, in Grade II there is a considerable reduction of asexual parasitaemia but no clearance, while in Grade III there is no reduction in asexual parasitaemia. Some clinical improvement can usually be expected in Grades I and II resistance, and it is fortunate that Grade III resistance is relatively uncommon. Partial resistance of this parasite to quinine has also been noted in Southeast Asia, creating a potentially very dangerous situation. No resistance of the other *Plasmodium* species to chloroquine has been reported in man but resistance of both *P. falciparum* and *P. vivax* to pyrimethamine and proguanil, which are widely used as prophylactics, is now widespread in several continents.

African trypanosomes (*T. brucei*) develop resistance fairly rapidly to most agents to which they are exposed, and tryparsamide which was previously widely used for late cases of sleeping sickness is now useless in many areas. A few partially drug-resistant strains of *Trichomonas vaginalis* and *Entamoeba histolytica* have now been isolated *in vitro* but these have not yet posed clinical problems.

Resistance of *Schistosoma mansoni* to hycanthone has been produced in laboratory animals, but so far there are no known instances of human infections with helminths showing acquired resistance.

2. Geographic parasite variants. Another problem is the variable responses to drugs of strains of *Leishmania donovani* and *L. braziliensis* in different parts of their distribution. This phenomenon is related to intrinsic genetic forms of the parasite and it is not due to drug exposure. As an example, *L. donovani* infections in Sudan may require four times as many doses of antimony as those in India. Analogous problems are the response of different geographic forms of *S.mansoni* to oxamniquine and the poor response of New Guinea strains of *P. vivax* to primaquine.

3. Host differences. It is suspected that genetically determined defects in drug metabolism in the body may affect the clinical response. Thus the rate of acetylation of sulphonamides and sulphones by the liver affects the blood levels of these drugs. Acetylator status is a genetic trait and it probably affects the response of malaria to these drugs; similar genetic differences in drug metabolism are being sought with chloroquine and primaquine.

The patient's immunological status affects the outcome of treatment in leishmaniasis and toxoplasmosis. Chemotherapy alone probably never entirely eliminates these parasites and when the host's immune competence is impaired, a cure may in certain circumstances be impossible.

MODE OF ACTION OF ANTIPARASITIC DRUGS

The biochemistry of drug action has been studied using whole parasites and parasite homogenates. Radio-isotope-labelled drugs can be used to follow distribution in the host's body and the uptake by the parasite. Sometimes several effects are identified and it is uncertain which plays the primary or predominant role. The active form of a drug may be a metabolite produced in the host or even within the parasite. The action of a drug may not be the same in different parasites. None of the peptide antibiotics, such as the penicillins, that act upon cell wall synthesis have any action upon parasites for they are animals and have no cell wall. Activity can be grouped under several headings.

1. Nucleic acid synthesis. Chloroquine molecules intercalate between the base pairs in DNA and thereby prevent it acting as a template. Mepacrine, quinine and primaquine probably act in a similar way, although primaquine and its metabolites also directly damage mitochondria and inhibit protein synthesis. Erythrocytes parasitised by *Plasmodium* concentrate chloroquine one hundred-fold. Diamidines also bind to nuclear DNA but they do not intercalate with it; in addition these drugs become attached to and directly damage the kinetoplastic DNA of trypanosomes.

2. *Protein synthesis*. The antibiotics paromomycin, tetracycline and spiromycin probably act against parasites as they do against bacteria by binding with ribosomal subunits to block polypeptide synthesis. Emetine also inhibits polypeptide elongation but the receptor site is unknown; mammalian cells are similarly affected and there is secondary inhibition of DNA synthesis. Diloxanide is structurally not unlike chloramphenicol and it appears to block protein synthesis.

3. *Carbohydrate metabolism*. Arsenicals and antimonials bind rather non-specifically to the sulphidryl groups of many enzyme proteins of both the parasite and the host, hence their therapeutic indices are low. In trypanosomes, the main target enzyme for arsenicals is pyruvate kinase, and in schistosomes trivalent antimonials bind strongly with phosphofructokinase. *Leishmania* are only damaged by pentavalent antimonials after their reduction to the trivalent form, within host macrophages. The arsenical melarsoprol and the trivalent antimonial sodium dimercaptosuccinate both have the chelating agent BAL incorporated in the molecule and this considerably lessens toxicity.

Several anthelminthics act more specifically. Thus, pyrvinium and mebendazole both block the uptake of glucose into the worm; while thiabendazole and levamisole selectively block the enzyme fumarate reductase that is essential for anaerobic glycolysis; and niridazole inhibits glycogen phospholyase leading to depletion of glycogen stores. Niclosamide inhibits, at an unknown site, the production of ATP from anaerobic carbohydrate metabolism.

4. *Inhibition of hydrogen production*. Metronidazole acts upon anaerobic bacteria and the anaerobic protozoa that inhabit the gut and vagina, by trapping electrons by virtue of its very low redox potential. The generation of H_2 from pyruvate is halted and the organism soon becomes depleted of NADH and NADPH. The nitro ring of metronidazole becomes cleaved in the process, producing a toxic substance that hastens cell death.

5. *Antifolates*. As in bacteria these compounds can act at two points in the folic acid pathway. Thus, the sulphonamides and the sulphones compete with para-aminobenzoic acid in the synthesis of dihydrofolic acid, a process that is circumvented in the mammal by the active transport of folic acid into the cell. Pyrimethamine and trimethoprim bind selectively to the enzyme dihydrofolate reductase of some protozoan species, preventing the synthesis of tetrahydrofolic acid and thereby arresting nucleic acid synthesis. The biguanides are inactive until metabolised in the host liver to the active dihydro-triazine derivative that binds, like pyrimethamine, to the dihydrofolate reductase of the parasite but very little to that of the host. Drug combinations that act at both sites have a very strong synergistic action and can be very valuable.

6. *Neuromuscular blockade*. Piperazine rapidly produces a temporary flaccid paralysis of the intact *Ascaris* worm. The drug is an analogue of the natural inhibitory neurotransmitter and so hyperpolarisation is produced; this action is antagonised by acetylocholine. Mammals presumably have a different receptor as they are very rarely affected by the drug which is freely absorbed from the gut. Pyrantel is also paralytic upon nematodes but in this case there is depolarisation and a spastic contracture of the worm; this drug is not absorbed from the gut. Bephenium is structurally similar to acetylcholine and is believed to act as an analogue producing contraction and detachment of the worm. Metrifonate is an organophosphorus anticholinesterase compound with a special affinity for the tissues of certain helminths including *Schistosoma haematobium*, the cholinesterase levels of host red cells are reduced for several weeks after therapy but the compound appears to be safe in man. Hycanthone blocks acetylcholine receptors allowing intrinsic serotonin to over-stimulate the worms. Altered peristalsis and incoordinated movements can then prevent

the worms feeding properly; the drug also damages the tegument directly.

7. *Other known and unknown effects.* The antibiotic amphotericin interacts with sterols in the cell membrane of some protozoa and thereby alters permeability. The hydroxyquinolines appear to act upon intracolonic amoebae by chelating Fe^{++} ions that are essential for their metabolism. Suramin is a very acidic compound that binds firmly to serum proteins but does not normally enter mammalian cells; it does however enter trypanosomes by pinocytosis and combines non-specifically with several enzyme proteins. Tetrachlorethylene temporarily paralyses hookworms, probably by damaging the lysosomes of the gut epithelial cells. The antiparasitic actions of bitoscanate, oxamniquine, dichlorophen, bithionol, diethylcarbamazine (see p. 99) and the nitrofurans are unknown; however, bithionol has potent bactericidal and antifungal activity.

CHEMOTHERAPY OF PROTOZOAN INFECTIONS

1. Amoebiasis, giardiasis, balantidiasis and trichomoniasis

Amoebiasis

Most patients with invasive amoebiasis can be successfully treated with a five or eight day course of oral metronidazole, using 800 mg three times daily for adults and 35–50 mg/kg daily in three divided doses for children. However, some patients tolerate the drug rather poorly; and a few drug failures have occured in patients with a liver abscess when this has not been drained. Metronidazole and certain other nitroimidazoles are the only drugs that act upon *E. histolytica* both within tissues and in the gut lumen, that is they have both systemic and luminal amoebicidal activity. The only other systemic amoebicides are emetine, its synthetic analogue dehydroemetine, and chloroquine; the latter only being active in the liver. Intramuscular emetine (1 mg/kg daily to a maximum of 60 mg) is the most potent and rapidly acting amoebicide. Dehydroemetine is more rapidly excreted in the urine, it appears to be as effective as emetine and less toxic; the daily dose is 1.25 mg/kg to a max-

imum of 90 mg. Both emetine and dehydroemetine have an appreciable cumulative cardiac toxicity, they are not used in patients with cardiac disease. In children dehydroemetine is well tolerated. If emetine or dehydroemetine is used for amoebic liver abscess a 10 day course is required, but three to five daily doses are usually sufficient for bowel disease. In either situation, unless metronidazole is also being used, a three week course of oral chloroquine should also be given, using in adults 600 mg base for two days then 300 mg daily and in children 10 mg/kg daily to a maximum of 300 mg daily. Tetracycline is useful in severe bowel disease, especially in children or when there is bowel perforation; but this must be combined with oral chloroquine to protect the liver, unless metronidazole is also being used. The recently available parenteral metronidazole promises to be useful in very ill patients unable to take oral medication.

Symptomatic patients who are not treated with metronidazole must be given a luminal amoebicide, otherwise a recurrence of tissue invasion is quite likely.

Symptomless *E. histolytica* infections normally need to be treated only in food handlers or when the risk of reinfection is low, the objectives being to prevent transmission or future tissue invasion. Of the available luminal amoebicides the most satisfactory is a 10 day course of diloxanide using in adults 500 mg three times daily and in children 20 mg/kg daily in three divided doses. The alternatives are a five to 10 day course of paromomycin using 25–35 mg/kg daily in three divided doses, a 20 day course of di-iodohydroxyquin using in adults 650 mg three times daily and in children 30–40 mg/kg in three divided doses to a maximum of 2 g daily, or an eight day course of metronidazole using the same daily dose as in invasive disease.

Giardiasis

Cure rates of up to 90 per cent can be achieved with either mepacrine or metronidazole. The usual schedule for mepacrine is a five day course using 100 mg three times daily in adults, and 2 mg/kg three times daily in children to a maximum of 300 mg daily. Metronidazole is given for five to eight days using 400 mg three times daily in adults and 5 mg/kg three times daily in children. Retreatment is sometimes necessary but some apparent relapses are due to reinfection from the patient's family. Furazolidine appears to be an effective alternative but has not been widely used.

Balantidiasis

For symptomatic infections tetracycline is probably the drug of choice; a 10 day course is required using in adults 500 mg four times daily and in children 10 mg/kg four times daily to a maximum of 2 g daily; alternatives are ampicillin (2 g daily for adults), or paromomycin or metronidazole using the dosages employed in amoebiasis. Symptomless infections are probably self-limiting but can be treated with either metronidazole or di-iodohydroxyquin (dosages as for amoebiasis).

Trichomoniasis

Vaginal infections can usually be eliminated with a seven day course of metronidazole using 200 mg three times daily in adults and 5 mg/kg three times daily in children. The male consort should also be treated simultaneously or advised to use a condom for a month. Topical treatment by vaginal pessaries and douches has been extensively used but cure is unlikely. In the male topical treatment cannot be used, and he is likely to cause reinfection. Some authorities recommend topical treatment for pregnant women.

Some of the newer nitroimidazole compounds may eventually replace metronidazole in these four infections. However, at the present time, metronidazole remains the best of these drugs for amoebiasis although reports of tinidazole, using single daily doses of 50–60 mg/kg for three to five days in children, are encouraging. Similar regimens of tinidazole have also been successfully used in giardiasis and trichomoniasis; other drugs in this group are nitrimidazine (nimorazole) and ornidazole. Because of their possible teratogenic effects on the foetus, all the nitroimidazoles should, when possible, be avoided in early pregnancy; however the risk is probably very small and it has never been demonstrated in humans.

2. Malaria

Drugs for malaria suppression and chemoprophylaxis

Several drugs are available for this purpose; the choice will sometimes be determined by personal preference and drug tolerance. For visitors to an endemic area medication should begin on the day of entry and continue for four weeks after leaving the area; the latter ensures that any pre-erythrocytic infections acquired just before departure are destroyed when they invade the blood stream. Chloroquine has a bitter taste which many people dislike, but it is available as a flavoured syrup for children; the tasteless pyrimethamine is also available in syrup form. The alternative schedules are shown in Table 14.5.

Table 14.5 Drug dosages for the prevention of malaria

	Adults	< 1 year	1–3 years	4–7 years	8–12 years
Proguanil (Paludrine) (daily dose)	100–200 mg	25 mg	50 mg	75 mg	100 mg
Pyrimethamine (Daraprim) (weekly dose)	25 mg	6.25 mg	8 mg	12.5 mg	19 mg
Chloroquine (weekly dose — base)	300 mg	50–75 mg	75–125 mg	125–200 mg	250 mg
Maloprim* (tablets taken weekly)	1	¼	¼	½	¾
Fansidar** (tablets taken every two weeks)	2	¼	½	1	1½

* Maloprim tablets contain 12.5 mg pyrimethamine and 100 mg of dapsone
** Fansidar tablets contain 25 mg pyrimethamine and 500 mg sulphadoxine

Whenever possible proguanil or pyrimethamine should be used; however *P. falciparum* and *P. vivax* show resistance to one or both of these drugs in many areas, especially tropical Africa. Patchy resistance of *P. falciparum* to chloroquine is present in many parts of Asia from Assam and Nepal eastwards, and in Central and South America; in addition a few instances have recently been confirmed in East Africa. In areas of possible chloroquine resistance the drug of choice is Maloprim, but proguanil may sometimes still be effective; Fansidar is reserved mainly for the treatment of chloroquine-resistant *P. falciparum* infections but it may be used as a prophylactic for periods that should preferably not exceed six months.

Apart from areas of known or suspected *P. falciparum* resistance the most reliable prophylactic will be chloroquine, but Maloprim is apparently an effective alternative. In areas of intense transmission, such as tropical Africa, it is now recommended that higher doses of chloroquine be used for the first three months to allow adequate blood levels to build up; chloroquine has a very long half-life in the body. The higher dose of chloroquine now recommended in such areas is 75–100 mg base daily for adults; this dosage should never be continued for more than three years because of the risk of permanent retinopathy.

In the doses recommended none of these drugs have been shown to be teratogenic; their use in pregnancy is therefore strongly recommended.

None of these drugs prevents later relapses of *P. vivax* or *P. ovale* malaria; but taking them appears to reduce the probability of their occurrence.

Treatment of acute attacks

Drugs used to treat malarial attacks are known as blood schizonticides and they act directly upon the asexual erythrocytic stage of the parasite. Chloroquine and quinine are the most rapidly acting schizonticides and both have, in addition, anti-inflammatory properties that increase their therapeutic effect especially in cerebral malaria. The gametocytes of *P. falciparum*, unlike the other species, are unaffected by these drugs and they may be found in blood films for up to three weeks after treatment. Mepacrine is another relatively strong schizonticide but it is rather toxic.

Uncomplicated attacks due to all plasmodia, except chloroquine-resistant *P. falciparum*, should normally be treated with the standard course of oral chloroquine (total adult dose 1.5 g base over 3 days, given as follows: 600 mg stat. then 300 mg after six hours, and then 300 mg daily for two days; in children the dosages are 10 mg/kg stat., then 5 mg/kg after six hours, and then 5 mg/kg for two days). Mild illness however in persons who are presumed to be partially immune, such as unprotected older children and adults living in a stable endemic area, may be treated with smaller doses of chloroquine or with the more slowly acting schizonticide pyrimethamine which has the advantage that *P. falciparum* gametocytes are rendered non-infective to mosquitoes.

Patients with severe *P. falciparum* infections must be treated with parenteral chloroquine or quinine. Many clinicians believe that quinine has a more rapid effect than chloroquine in cerebral malaria. In general, however, chloroquine is the simpler drug to use as it is less toxic, especially in the presence of liver damage, and a shorter course is required. The two drugs should not be used together as they are apparently antagonistic. Serious toxicity may occur with either drug when given parenterally; the safest route is by slow intravenous infusions given over four hours and repeated every 12 hours, the drug dose of either chloroquine base or quinine dihydrochloride should be 5–10 mg/kg body weight for each infusion; oral medication should be substituted as soon as possible. Chloroquine (5 mg base/kg, repeated 12-hourly) is also effective by intramuscular injection but this may unfortunately occasionally cause cardiac arrhythmias and even sudden death, especially in children.

Patients severely ill with suspected chloroquine-resistant *P. falciparum* malaria must be treated initially with quinine dihydrochloride by intravenous infusion, as already described, changing to oral quinine sulphate when their condition improves. In such situations, and also in uncomplicated attacks, quinine should be combined with one of the following three alternatives: pyrimethamine plus sulphadiazine; tetracycline; or mefloquine. Oral quinine sulphate should be given

THE CHEMOTHERAPY OF PARASITIC INFECTIONS 201

as a 10–14 day course using 650 mg three times daily in adults and 25 mg/kg in three divided doses for children. Pyrimethamine should be given for three days using 25 mg twice daily in adults and in children a daily dose of 6.25 mg if weight less than 10 kg, 12.5 mg if weight between 10 and 20 kg, and 25 mg if weight greater than 20 kg. Sulphadiazine should be given for 5 days using 500 mg four times daily in adults and 120 mg/kg daily in four divided doses for children. Tetracycline should be given for seven days using 500 mg four times daily in adults and 10 mg/kg four times daily in children. Mefloquine may be given to adults as a single dose of 1.5 g. Patients with very light infections can often be cured with a single dose of Fansidar (each tablet contains 25 mg of pyrimethamine and 500 mg of sulphadoxine), the adult dose being three tablets.

Radical treatment to prevent relapses

Primaquine is the only currently used drug for the elimination of the secondary liver schizonts of *P. vivax* and *P. ovale*. A 14 day course of treatment is needed using 7.5 mg base twice daily in adults and 0.15 mg base/kg twice daily in children. The drug is relatively toxic; in persons with glucose-6-phosphate dehydrogenase deficiency, there may be significant haemolysis and sometimes methaemoglobinaemia. The drug fails to cure up to 10 per cent of *P. vivax* infections; it should only be used in persons leaving an endemic area or as part of an eradication campaign. If the patient is to be re-exposed to infection and intends to continue suppressive treatment, it is pointless to give primaquine.

3. Leishmaniasis

Visceral leishmaniasis due to *L. donovani* should be treated with a course of daily intravenous injections of the pentavalent organic antimonial sodium stibogluconate using 600 mg daily in adults and 10 mg/kg daily in children. Strains differ in their susceptibility, for example in India six injections may be sufficient while in the Sudan up to three courses of ten injections may be required. If necessary, the drug can be given intramuscularly; in Latin America, a pentavalent antimonial called

glucantime is used. When antimonials fail or are contraindicated, then up to 15 doses of pentamidine should be given intramuscularly at a daily dosage of 2–4 mg/kg; if side effects are troublesome, doses should be spaced at three or four day intervals. When both of these drugs fail, then amphotericin B should be used at a dosage of 0.25 to 1 mg/kg by slow infusion in 5 per cent dextrose daily for up to eight weeks. Cutaneous relapses of *L. donovani* (post-kala-azar dermal leishmanoid) can be successfully treated with sodium stibogluconate.

Lesions of Old World cutaneous leishmaniasis due to *L. tropica* can, if they are single and relatively small, often be allowed to heal spontaneously using local antiseptics and antibiotics when necessary. In more severe cases, a course of six to ten injections of sodium stibogluconate should be given, or alternatively up to 2 ml of the drug can be injected locally at weekly intervals. Many other local treatments are sometimes used; these include intralesional injection of 0.5 ml of 15 per cent mepacrine or 2 per cent berberine sulphate, and heating the lesion to 50°C with coned infra-red rays. Berberine is a plant alkaloid used by traditional healers in India. Intralesional steroids have been used in leishmaniasis recidivans to suppress the exaggerated T-cell lymphocyte response, but this must be combined with parenteral stibogluconate. The diffuse cutaneous form seen occasionally in Ethiopia does not respond to antimonials, and either pentamidine or amphotericin B must be used.

In the New World, lesions due to *L. mexicana* or *L. peruviana* can often be left untreated or alternatively a single intramuscular injection of the repository drug cycloguanil pamoate in oil can be given using a dose of 350 mg base (140 mg base in infants under 1 year, and 280 mg base in children aged 1–5 years). All patients with primary *L. b. braziliensis* lesions should receive a full 10 day course of a pentavalent antimonial to prevent metastatic spread; an alternative drug that is currently being evaluated is nifurtimox. When metastases have occurred then up to three 14-day courses of an antimonial should be given, with three-week intervals between; pentamidine is of no value in this form of the disease, and if antimonials fail amphotericin B should be tried. The diffuse cutaneous form is sometimes caused by two subspecies of *L. mexicana*, and should be treated in the same way as the Ethiopian disease.

4. Trypanosomiasis

Patients with early African trypanosomiasis, without neurological signs and with a normal cerebrospinal fluid, should be treated with a course of five intravenous injections of suramin; following a test dose of 100–200 mg a 1 g dose should be given to adults on days 1, 3, 7, 14 and 21; the paediatric dose is 20 mg/kg for each of the five injections. The alternatives to suramin are a course of 10 intramuscular injections of pentamidine, 4 mg/kg for each dose, given over a period of 10–20 days; or possibly a course of three injections of melarsoprol. When neurological involvement is present melarsoprol offers the only real hope of cure; if the patient's condition permits, a few injections of suramin should be given first as this reduces the likelihood of an allergic encephalopathy, which may appear five to ten days after starting arsenical therapy. Melarsoprol is given intravenously as an irritating 3.6 per cent solution in polyethylene glycol; the full dosage for each injection is 3.6 mg (0.1 ml)/kg to a maximum of 5 ml. A suitable schedule for an adult would be 2.5 ml on days 1 and 3, 5 ml on day 5, then a rest of one or two weeks followed by three more injections of 5 ml at two day intervals, a further rest of one week and then three further injections of 5 ml at two day intervals. Follow up should be for at least one year and if there is further evidence of active neurological involvement another full course of melarsoprol should be given, together with oral nitrofurazone at an adult dose of 500 mg, six hourly for five days. Nitrofurazone is a toxic drug but the course should be repeated on two or three occasions.

Some strains of *T. b. gambiense* are still sensitive to tryparsamide and patients with neurological involvement due to these strains can be treated with 12 injections of tryparsamide (each dose 30 mg/kg intravenously) at five day intervals, together with 12 injections of suramin (each dose 10 mg/kg intravenously) at five day intervals.

In American trypanosomiasis due to *T. cruzi* there are two alternative drugs, nifurtimox and benznidazole, that will eradicate parasitaemia but it is doubtful whether either destroys all intracellular parasites as in some patients parasitaemia reappears. Both drugs are toxic and their main indication is early acute disease; it is not known whether these drugs arrest further progress in more chronic infections. The schedule for nifurtimox is 8 mg/kg by mouth daily for 120 days; benznidazole is given orally at a dosage of 5 mg/kg for 60 days.

5. Miscellaneous protozoan infections

Toxoplasmosis

Many patients with the more benign forms of acquired toxoplasmosis do not require specific chemotherapy unless the primary infection occurs during pregnancy. The most effective treatment is a three or four week course of pyrimethamine with sulphadiazine. Adults should be given 75 mg pyrimethamine on the first day followed by a daily dose of 25 mg; 4 g of sulphadiazine should be given daily in divided doses. Because this drug combination may cause marrow toxicity a daily parenteral dose of folinic acid, 6 to 10 mg for adults, should be given as well. Infants with congenital infection should be given pyrimethamine 1 mg/kg for the first three days followed by 0.5 mg/kg for the remainder of the course; the daily dose of sulphadiazine in infants is 100 mg/kg. Because of the possible toxic effects of high doses of pyrimethamine on the foetus, it is sometimes recommended that infections acquired during pregnancy be treated with spiramycin.

Chemotherapy does not destroy the cystic form of the parasite. In adults with persistent active toxoplasmic choroidoretinitis a weekly suppressive dose of 25 mg pyrimethamine has been found useful.

Babesiosis

Human infections with *Babesia* have sometimes been treated with chloroquine, the results have been poor despite some reduction in the level of parasitaemia. Pentamidine, by daily intramuscular injections of 4 mg/kg, is probably the drug of choice in severe infections, but the related compound diazoaminobenzene (Berenil) could be tried as it is very effective in non-human babesiosis.

Pneumocystosis

For several years *Pneumocystis* pneumonia has been treated, with moderate success, using a 12 to 14 day course of intramuscular pentamidine (4 mg/kg each dose). More recently co-trimoxazole has been found effective and much less toxic, if necessary an intravenous preparation can be used; a 14 day course is given using trimethoprim 20 mg/kg plus sulphamethoxazole 100 mg/kg each day in four divided doses.

Isosporiasis

Symptomatic infections with *I. belli* can be treated with either co-trimoxazole, or a combination of pyrimethamine with sulphadiazine. No controlled trials have been done and optimal drug dosages remain uncertain. Nitrofurantoin may be an effective alternative.

Infections by free-living amoebae (Naegleria, Acanthamoeba)

The drug of choice for *Naegleria* meningoencephalitis appears to be amphotericin B intravenously according to the usual schedule, together with intrathecal administration of the same drug in the doses used for cryptococcal meningitis. Sulphadiazine can be used to supplement amphotericin and may be of particular value if the invading amoebae are *Acanthamoeba*. The antifungal drug clotrimazole is active against *Naegleria in vitro*. Topical amphotericin can be used for corneal ulcers caused by *Acanthamoeba*.

CHEMOTHERAPY OF HELMINTHIC INFECTIONS

1. Schistosomiasis

The most widely used drugs for schistosomiasis are the trivalent antimonials and niridazole; the latter is usually the safer alternative but it may be less effective, particularly for *S. japonicum* infections. Niridazole (25 mg/kg/day in three divided doses) is given orally for ten days but should not be used if there is a history of psychosis or epilepsy, and must be used with care when there is liver damage or porto-systemic anastomosis due to portal hypertension; the drug causes a brownish discolouration of the urine. The safest antimonial appears to be sodium dimercaptosuccinate, given as five weekly intramuscular injections at a dose of 8 mg/kg each week. However, for *S. japonicum* infections, satisfactory results can really only be obtained with the much more toxic antimony potassium tartrate given intravenously according to a complex schedule. Two alternatives for *S. mansoni* infections are hycanthone and oxamniquine; hycanthone is given as a single intramuscular injection (3 mg/kg to a maximum of 200 mg) that often produces vomiting and very occasionally severe liver damage, oxamniquine is given orally as a single dose of 15 mg/kg, but should not be given to patients with a history of epilepsy. The anticholinesterase drug metrifonate appears to be safe and effective for *S. haematobium* infections, three doses of 7.5 mg/kg are given orally at two-weekly intervals.

2. Hermaphroditic flukes

Bithionol is the drug of choice for paragonimiasis and fascioliasis, it is much less effective in clonorchiasis and opisthorchiasis, 10–15 doses (30–50 mg/kg each dose) of the drug are given orally every other day. Alternatively, for fascioliasis, a 10-day course of dehydroemetine hydrochloride (each dose 1 mg/kg intramuscularly) may be used, combined with a three-week course of chloroquine (adult dose 150 mg base thrice daily). For clonorchiasis and opisthorchiasis, chloroquine should be used alone (adult dose 150 mg base thrice daily) for six or even eight weeks, parasitological cure is unlikely but a significant reduction in egg count will be obtained; paragonimiasis may also be treated in this way. Hexachloroparaxylol appears to be effective for clonorchiasis, opisthorchiasis and paragonimiasis, and to be relatively non-toxic; however, the drug is rarely available outside China and Russia.

Intestinal flukes (*Heterophyes, Metagonimus, Fasciolopsis, Echinostoma, Gastrodiscoides*) have been treated with many drugs but results are poorly documented. Bephenium appears to be the drug of choice, but if unsuccessful piperazine may be tried or the more toxic tetrachlorethylene; the doses of these drugs being the same as those used for gut nematodes.

3. Gut cestodes

Niclosamide is now the treatment of choice for most patients with tapeworm infections of the gut; the tablets must be chewed thoroughly and given on an empty stomach. Toxicity is minimal and an 80–90 per cent cure rate can be expected after a single dose (for adults give 2 g, children 11–34 kg give 1 g, children over 34 kg give 1.5 g) for *Taenia* and *Diphyllobothrium latum* infections or five daily doses for *Hymenolepis nana*. Dichlorophen is somewhat more toxic and must be given for two days to achieve an 80 per cent cure rate in *T. saginata* and *D. latum* infections; the daily dose for adults is 6 g, for children 1 to 5 years 0.25 to 1 g, for children 6 to 12 years 1 to 4 g. Another alternative is paromomycin given for one day in *T. saginata* and *D. latum* infections (adults 1 g every 15 minutes for 4 doses, children 11 mg/kg every 4 hours for 4 doses) and five days in *H. nana* infections (45 mg/kg each day); however, this drug can produce side effects, including vomiting in up to 50 per cent of patients. With all of these drugs, the worms usually disintegrate before they appear in the faeces so that the scolex of the large species is rarely found; the patient must therefore wait four months before the therapeutic result is known. Another possible disadvantage of this disruption of the proglottids is that eggs of *T. solium* may be released into the bowel to cause the serious complication of cysticercosis especially if vomiting occurs. For this reason pretreatment antiemetics and post-treatment laxatives are recommended when this infection is treated with niclosamide. The patient and his attendants should also be warned of the infectivity of post-treatment stools.

An alternative therapy for hospital patients with *Taenia* or *D. latum* is mepacrine (adult dose 1 g in 100 ml warm water) given by intraduodenal tube after a 48-hour fast and followed by a magnesium sulphate purge. This rather drastic treatment may give a higher cure rate than niclosamide and has the advantage that the scolex of the worm can be identified. If mepacrine is given orally or through an incorrectly positioned duodenal tube vomiting may occur. However, properly administered this form of therapy is the safest way to treat *T. solium* infection.

4. Larval cestodes

The treatment of these conditions, when indicated, remains surgical. However a few recent reports suggest that the germinal membranes and proloscolices of hydatid cysts are killed in patients receiving prolonged courses of mebendazole or the related fluoromebendazole.

5. Gut nematodes

Several alternative drugs are available for some of these infections (Table 14.6); the choice will often be determined by cost and availability. As most of these infections are relatively benign, it is essential to use compounds with low toxicity. Mixed infections are common and for these wide-spectrum anthelminthics are particularly useful. Although thiabendazole has a wide spectrum of activity, side effects are relatively common so that other drugs are preferred when alternatives are available. Complete elimination of *Trichuris* and hookworm is never necessary, similarly light *Ascaris* infections have a very low morbidity. Coproculture may be useful for distinguishing the two main species of hookworm, as these may require different treatment.

For hookworm infections a daily dose of pyrantel, or mebendazole twice daily, for three days are the least toxic of the effective drug regimens. Like bitoscanate (three doses given at 12 hour intervals), which causes more gastrointestinal upsets, these drugs are effective against both *Ancylostoma* and *Necator*; although mebendazole appears to be slightly more effective against *Necator* than *Ancylostoma*. Bephenium (one dose daily for three days) is a useful alternative for *Ancylostoma*. A single dose of tetrachlorethylene, if used carefully, is safe and effective against *Necator*; patients should be fasting and no food is taken for three hours after the medication; better results are obtained if the dose is repeated twice at four-day intervals. Tetrachlorethylene must never be given to patients infected with *Ascaris*, as it causes these worms to migrate actively and this can lead to serious obstructive pathology; similarly, any drug or anaesthetic agent that causes vomiting may be dangerous in the presence of *Ascaris*.

For *Ascaris* infections piperazine (one dose daily for two days) is still regarded as the drug of choice but pyrantel (single dose) and levamisole (single dose), and perhaps also mebendazole (twice daily for three days), are equally safe and probably as effective.

For *Trichuris* infection mebendazole (twice daily for three days) is the only safe, effective and widely available drug.

In *Enterobius* infections, total elimination is the objective, as otherwise autoinfection will soon allow incompletely treated infections to build up again; threadworm is often a familial infection and it is often prudent to treat the whole family. Pyrvinium, mebendazole and pyrantel all have the advantage that single doses are used unlike piperazine which is given once daily for a week; of these four compounds pyrantel probably has the most side effects. To eliminate autoinfections the course of piperazine is repeated after a two week interval; and if the other drugs have been used the single dose is repeated after 14 and 28 days.

For *Strongyloides* infection thiabendazole (twice daily for two days) is the only really effective drug. As autoinfection regularly occurs, it is essential to achieve a complete parasitological cure; this is particularly important in the immunologically-compromised host.

Trichostrongylus infections can be treated with a single dose of pyrantel or three daily doses of bephenium.

Capillaria philippinensis infections must be completely eliminated and long courses of treatment

Table 14.6 Relative activity of drugs used for the common gut nematodes

	Ascaris	Hookworm	*Enterobius*	*Trichuris*	*Strongyloides*
Piperazine (Antepar, Entacyl) 75 mg/kg	+++	+	+++	—	—
Pyrantel pamoate (Combantrin, Antiminth) 11 mg/kg	+++	++	+++	—	—
Mebendazole (Vermox) 100 mg (> 2 years of age)	++	+++ (*Necator*) ++ (*Ancylostoma*)	+++	++	+
Thiabendazole (Mintezol) 25 mg/kg	(++)	(++)	(++)	+	+++
Levamisole (Ketrax) 5 mg/kg	+++	+	+	—	—
Bephenium (Alcopar) 5 g (> 2 years of age)	+	+++ (*Ancylostoma*) + (*Necator*)	—	—	—
Bitoscanate (Jonit) 100 mg (not children)	+	+++	—	—	—
Pyrvinium (Vanquin, Povan) 5 mg/kg	+	—	+++	—	—
Tetrachlorethylene 0.1 ml/kg (max. 5 ml)	Danger	++++ (*Necator*) ++ (*Ancylostoma*)	(+)	—	—

Proprietary names in parentheses. Size of single dose given. Activities given in parenthesis indicate that the drug is not used for that species.

are necessary. Mebendazole is the drug of choice using one to four daily doses for 10–30 days; alternatively thiabendazole 25 mg/kg is given daily, in divided doses, for one month.

Trichinella spiralis (see p. 207).

6. The filarial infections and Guinea worm

The only reasonably safe and widely used filaricide is diethylcarbamazine, whose action against the different filarial worms is shown in the Table 14.7. This is a potent microfilaricide against all the species pathogenic to man but unfortunately it has little or no action as a macrofilaricide against adult *O. volvulus*. Sensitivity reactions resulting from worm death are common. In onchocerciasis generalised reactions and serious ocular damage can occur, and steroids may have to be given by mouth or locally into the eye. Small doses of the drug must be given initially and increased to the full dose (2–3 mg/kg three times daily) which is continued for three weeks. Localised reactions may occur near to the adult worms producing lymphangitis or lymph node abscess in *Brugia* infections; and also less commonly in *W. bancrofti* infection, which responds less well to the drug. Tropical pulmonary eosinophilia responds well to diethylcarbamazine and rarely relapses, suggesting that the adult worms and their microfilariae are destroyed. *Loa loa* is the only species whose larval stages are affected by diethylcarbamazine which can therefore be used prophylactically (p. 219).

Suramin is the only currently used macrofilaricide used for *O. volvulus;* after a small test dose, adults should be given 1 g intravenously at weekly intervals for five weeks and children 20 mg/kg intravenously at weekly intervals for five weeks. Because of toxicity it is used only for patients whose vision is threatened; the drug has a slow and delayed action against both adult worms and microfilariae and unless given after diethylcarbamazine can cause severe sensitivity reactions that are difficult to control. Treatment can arrest or partially reverse lesions of the anterior segment of the eye but unfortunately retinitis and optic nerve damage can progress after treatment.

The extraction of guinea worms by traction is made considerably easier following a five or seven-day course of niridazole 25 mg/kg daily in three divided doses for seven days or metronidazole, 25 mg/kg daily, to a maximum of 500 mg thrice daily for five days. Drug treatment is usually reserved for heavily infected patients or those with significant local pathology; it is believed that the beneficial effects of both drugs results partly from their anti-inflammatory action.

7. Other tissue nematodes

Thiabendazole has a potent action against the intestinal phases of *Trichinella spiralis*, and also a

Table 14.7 Relative activity of diethylcarbamazine against filarial worm infections and the frequency of allergic reactions

	Larval stages	Adult worms	Microfilariae	Allergic reactions with treatment
Wuchereria bancrofti	0	+	+++	+
Brugia malayi	0	++	+++	++
Loa loa	++	+++	+++	+++
Onchocerca volvulus	0	±	+++	++++
Dipetalonema streptocerca	0	+	++	+
Dipetalonema perstans / *Mansonella ozzardi*	0	0	0	0
Tropical pulmonary eosinophilia	0	++	?	++

weaker effect upon larvae recently encysted in muscle; the dosage regimen is 25 mg/kg twice daily for five days. This drug is particularly useful during epidemics of trichinosis that are recognised early; recent work suggests that mebendazole may also be effective. Oral thiabendazole, 25 mg/kg twice daily for two days can be used for cutaneous larva migrans due to *Ancylostoma braziliense* but the drug is also effective in this condition when applied topically for three or four days as a cream containing 15 per cent thiabendazole powder in a hydrosoluble base.

Both thiabendazole (25 mg/kg twice daily for five days) and diethylcarbamazine (2–4 mg/kg thrice daily for 21 days) have been used with apparent good effect to treat visceral larva migrans due to *Toxocara*; however, no comparative trials have yet been published.

So far there are no reports of successful chemotherapy in infections with *Anisakis, Gnathostoma, Oesophagostomium, Dioctophyma*, or in intestinal angiostrongyliasis due to *M. costaricensis*. These conditions are usually diagnosed during surgery and managed by local excision if this is appropriate. Thiabendazole does appear to have some effect in meningeal angiostrongyliasis due to *A. cantonensis*. However, further trials are necessary as this condition is usually self-limited and worm death could increase pathology.

DRUGS FOR ECTOPARASITES

1. Pediculosis

Many formulations are available to kill lice, and may be in the form of dusts, shampoos, lotions and creams. In several countries the use of preparations containing the chlorinated hydrocarbons DDT and dieldrin is restricted. The three most commonly used compounds are lindane (gamma benzene hexachloride a relatively non-toxic chlorinated hydrocarbon), malathion (a relatively safe organophosphorus insecticide), and pyrethrins (natural substances obtained from the flower heads of certain *Chrysanthemum* species) in piperonyl butoxide. Resistance to lindane is now quite common. Body lice (*Pediculus h. humanus*) are best treated with dusts, while head lice (*P.h. capitis*) and pubic lice (*Phthirus pubis*) can be

treated with shampoos, lotions or creams; with the latter two parasites retreatment after 10 days is recommended to destroy newly hatched lice whose eggs were unaffected by the first application.

Appropriate environmental measures must be used to prevent reinfection; these include disinfection of clothes, bed linen, hair brushes and combs.

2. Scabies

Normally all family members should be treated simultaneously. The most commonly used medications are 25 per cent benzyl benzoate application, 10 per cent crotamiton cream (Eurax), 1 per cent lindane cream, 5 per cent sulphur in lanolin, and 25 per cent monosulphiram lotion (Tetmosol) diluted just before use with two or three parts of water. Following a bath the medication should be applied to the whole body surface below the chin; it may be washed off the following day. One or two retreatments at weekly intervals are commonly recommended. Laundering of underclothes and bedding is essential.

3. Repellants for biting arthropods

Most proprietory insect repellants contain either dimethylphthalate or diethyltoluamide; lotions or creams may be applied to the skin, or aerosol sprays used for application to skin and clothing. Diethyltoluamide can be used to impregnate clothing to repel fleas. Another compound, ethyl-hexanediol, is repellant against insects and chiggers, and when combined with dimethylcarbamate and butopyronoxyl (Indalone) can be used to impregnate clothing against ticks and fleas. Another formulation used to impregnate clothing against ticks and chiggers contains butylethyl-propandiol, butylacetanilide and benzyl benzoate; this mixture is used by the United States army as formula M-1960.

4. Repellants for land leeches

Several compounds can be applied to skin and clothing, and give moderate protection; they include dimethylphthalate, ethyl-hexanediol and Indalone. Alternatively clothing can be impregnated with M-1960.

FURTHER READING

Cavier, R. and Hawking, F. (eds) (1973) *Chemotherapy of helminthiasis*. Vol 1, Section 64 of the International Encyclopedia of Pharmacology and Therapeutics. Oxford: Pergamon Press.

Davis, A. (1973) *Drug treatment in intestinal helminthiases*. Geneva: World Health Organization.

Hall, A.P. (1976) The treatment of severe falciparum malaria. *Trans.R.Soc.trop.Med.Hyg.*, **70**, 367–379.

Jopling, W.H. (1968) *The Treatment of Tropical Diseases*. Bristol: John Wright and Sons Ltd.

Knight, R. (1980) The chemotherapy of amoebiasis — a review. *J. antimicrobial Chemotherapy*, **6**, 630–648.

The Medical Letter on Drugs and Therapeutics (1978) Drugs for parasitic infections, **20**, No. 4. New York: Medical Letter, Inc.

Pratt, W.B. (1977) *Chemotherapy of infection*. Part III (p. 305–407): Drugs employed in the treatment of parasitic disease. New York: Oxford University Press.

15

The study and control of parasites within communities

SURVEYS FOR PARASITIC INFECTION

Introduction

Hospital statistics, particularly those from developing and tropical countries, generally underestimate the importance of parasitic disease. There are several reasons for this. (1) Parasitic diseases are often commonest in the poorer sections of the community and in places remote from hospital; patients from these backgrounds are less likely to visit hospital. (2) The symptoms of several parasitic diseases are often poorly defined and only slowly progressive; thus growth failure, weight loss and poor work performance often do not prompt hospital attendance. (3) Inadequate and underused laboratories miss many diagnoses.

Community studies are therefore often necessary to establish the importance of these infections. Compared with many non-infectious, chronic or degenerative diseases, those caused by parasites are often relatively easy to control and treat at a low or moderate cost. Community studies that make only one set of observations upon the study population are described as **cross-sectional**; while those involving repeated observations, over a period of time, are referred to as **longitudinal**. Longitudinal surveys that monitor the effects of control measures are called **intervention studies**. The methodology used in surveys can be considered under the following headings.

1. Organisation and planning. The survey objectives must be clearly defined. National and local formalities must be completed to obtain permission for the survey. The study population should be chosen and the sampling methods defined; a full demographic survey is often necessary. The purposes of the study must be explained to local community leaders and their cooperation obtained; medical aid must be offered throughout the study. A proforma should be designed and printed so that all data can be recorded systematically. Staff must be trained and all survey procedures standardised. 'Lines of flow' should be worked out so that each subject passes through the same routine; this may include the recording of demographic data, anthropometric measurements, a clinical examination, collection of blood, stool or other appropriate specimens, skin tests and any other special procedures. Logistic support for the survey team and transport of biological specimens should be arranged.

2. Parasitological. The usual diagnostic methods will normally be used (Ch. 13). Some procedures will have to be carried out in the field. But preservation methods can be used for stool and urine specimens; in addition microfilariae in lysed blood, or skin snips in water, can be temporarily stored in the wells of sealed plastic microtitre plates. Blood films can be fixed in the field and stained later prior to their examination.

3. Clinical. In addition to height and weight, other anthropometric measurements can be taken; these include the triceps or subscapular skinfold thickness, mid-upper arm circumference, head circumference and a record of tooth eruption. Signs of malnutrition should be recorded. Some parasitic diseases show reasonably specific signs: splenomegaly in malaria, hepatosplenomegaly in intestinal schistosomiasis, lymphadenopathy and other signs in lymphatic filariasis, cervical lymphadenopathy in African trypanosomiasis, and characteristic skin and eye lesions in onchocerciasis. When work performance is being assessed the appropriate ergometric tests can be applied, and also the change in heart rate in response to a standard exercise.

Relevant haematological and biochemical tests might include haemoglobin level, eosinophil count, serum iron and ferritin, serum albumin etc.

4. Immunological. Both serology and skin tests are often of a greater value in epidemiological studies than they are for individual diagnosis. This is because they remain positive for long periods, sometimes for life in the case of certain skin tests. Hence these tests act as markers of both past and current infection, and so indicate a subject's total exposure to infection. However, it must always be remembered that poor test specificity usually renders these applications invalid.

Other immunological tests might include estimation of serum immunoglobulin levels, and the detection of parasite antigens or immune complexes in the serum.

5. Vectors and intermediate hosts. When the life cycle of the parasite includes vectors and intermediate hosts, the population sizes and infection rates of these species can be estimated. Entomological studies may also include biting rates and estimation of insect longevity using various age grading methods.

The purpose and objectives of the various types of survey can now be considered.

1. Measurement of prevalance and intensity of infection

This is the simplest and most commonly performed type of epidemiological survey, being simply a cross-sectional study at one point in time. Results can be analysed in relation to various epidemiological variables such as age, sex, occupation, ethnic group, household clustering or local topography.

Measurement of the intensity of helminthic infections by means of egg or microfilaria counts adds greatly to the value of the study but the analysis of results needs some care. Because of the non-random aggregation of metazoan parasites among their hosts (which approximates to a negative binomial distribution, see p. 88), the calculation of the arithmetic mean of the counts is not only misleading but also erroneous if statistical comparisons are to be made; when plotted on a linear scale a set of hypothetical egg counts, for example, will show a positively skewed frequency distribution (Fig. 15.1 A). To overcome this difficulty individual counts (N) can be transformed to $\log_{10}(N+1)$ before the mean and standard deviation are calculated; this transformation will produce a frequency distribution reasonably close to a normal (Gaussian) curve (Fig. 15.1 B), one is added to N so that negative findings can be included (if $N = 0$, then $N + 1 = 1$ and $\log_{10} 1 = 0$). Another method of analysis that is valuable for graphical demonstration involves the calculation of the cumulative percentage of positive counts. To do this, the positive counts are tabulated in numerical order, starting with 1, together with their frequency; from this table the cumulative frequency of positives for each count is easily calculated and when the latter are converted into percentages of the total number of positives and then plotted, they give a sigmoid curve (Fig. 15.1C). A nearly linear plot can then be obtained by probit transformation of the cumulative percentage of positive counts (Fig. 15.1 D). From this linear plot the median positive count (M) can easily be estimated from the intercept of a horizontal line drawn through the 50 per cent cumulative percentage (equal to probit 5); the median positive count will be virtually identical with the antilog of the mean log. positive count. Similarly the percentage of the population with counts exceeding any particular value can easily be read from the linear probit plot, thus from Figure 15.1 D one can readily see that 30 per cent of the population have counts of 100 or more. This is a valuable technique when the likely morbidity is being assessed (see below). Calculation of the cumulative percentage of positives also serves to demonstrate how a small number of persons with high intensity infections often contribute a large percentage of the total infectivity of a population; thus a few adolescent boys can sometimes contribute 50 per cent of the total daily *Schistosoma haematobium* egg output of a village. This concentration of infectivity in a small number of persons underlies the potential effectiveness of targeted chemotherapy.

2. Morbidity

Assessment of the amount of disease caused by a

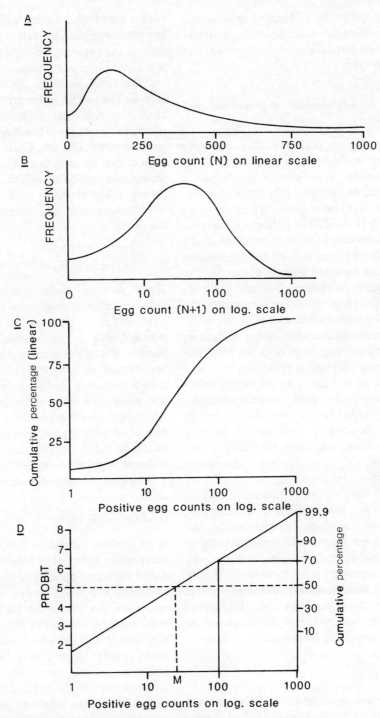

Fig. 15.1 Alternative graphical representations of helminth egg counts
A. Frequency distribution on linear scale showing skewed distribution
B. Frequency distribution of log. egg count (N + 1)
C. Cumulative percentage (linear) of positive counts
D. Cumulative percentage (probit scale) of positive counts. Horizontal intercept from probit 5 gives median positive count (M), vertical intercept from egg count 100 shows that 30% of population have counts ⩾100

parasite is often the primary objective of a survey. Because epidemiological methods are relatively crude this aim is often difficult to achieve. Several methods can be used:

A. *Inference from measurements of prevalence and intensity of infection*

When dealing with an organism that is always pathogenic, such as *Trypanosoma b. rhodesiense* or *Leishmania donovani*, it is clearly justifiable to make direct inferences from prevalence figures. However with less pathogenic organisms this method may not be valid. For example if the prevalences of *E. histolytica* in two communities are 40 per cent and 20 per cent it does not necessarily follow that more amoebic disease occurs in the former. Morbidity frequently depends upon so many variables, such as the strain of parasite, the nutritional and immunological status of the host, and whether incidence is stable, rising or falling, that accurate inferences cannot be made from the prevalence rates in different populations.

Measurement of the intensity of worm infections has, however, frequently proved valuable. For example if studies in one area show a certain percentage of abnormal pyelograms in persons with *S. haematobium* egg counts exceeding a certain value, this will generally apply elsewhere; similarly in *Ascaris* infections the probability of acute intestinal obstruction is closely related to worm loads. The probit method of analysis, described above, allows the proportion of the population with egg counts over a certain value to be readily estimated and this may therefore be used to define the number of persons at risk of serious disease. Unfortunately inferences of this kind cannot be made in hookworm infections, unless dietary iron and body iron stores are similar in the communities being compared.

B. *Population studies*

Studies of samples from whole populations will only be useful if the parasite being studied is relatively common. Comparisons can be made between persons with and without infection or between those with different intensities of infection. The method will be inefficient when the preval-

ence is very high, as there will be too few controls; or very low, giving too few infected persons. Similarly if the intensity of infection is very uniform few conclusions can be drawn.

Either cross-sectional or longitudinal surveys may be used. The latter are more expensive and carry the risk that high defaulting rates may invalidate the study. However longitudinal studies have the great advantage that changes within each subject can be recorded. Thus growth rates and weight loss can be measured, as may the changes in any other variable, such as the haemoglobin level, serum iron and serum albumin in hookworm infection.

C. *Case control studies*

These can be more precisely controlled but require preliminary surveys to find suitable subjects. The method allows controls to be accurately matched with infected subjects, and enables the number of cases required for statistical analysis to be planned in advance. This method is nearly always necessary for low prevalence infections. It also allows the effect of intensity of infection to be studied more efficiently, using similar numbers of subjects at each level of intensity; the latter feature is rarely found in natural populations.

As in population studies, either cross-sectional or longitudinal methods can be used.

D. *Intervention studies*

If an infected population can be divided into two comparable groups and effective control or eradication measures applied to one of them, the total morbidity and mortality due to the parasite can be estimated. An alternative method is to study one population before and after the parasite has been eliminated; this is less satisfactory because the study population may have been subject to other influences which cannot be controlled. Unless chemotherapy is the method of control, intervention studies often take several years to complete, because of the long duration of many parasite infections. The use of intervention studies to measure the harmful effects of a parasite has the great advantage that it demonstrates both direct and indirect effects. Thus in two African studies, nearly complete malaria control reduced infant mortality rates by 30 per cent and 50 per cent respectively, and crude death rates by 30 per cent and 40 per cent. Many of the excess deaths must have been due to the indirect effects of malaria, probably mainly those producing immunosuppression and impaired nutritional status; thereby increasing host susceptibility to other infections and to overt malnutrition. It is likely that a significant proportion of the harm done by many other parasites is indirect, by interaction with other diseases and poor nutritional status.

Intervention studies employing chemotherapy can be very simple in design. Thus the effect of *Ascaris* infection upon child growth can be measured by repeatedly deworming one group. Similarly regular malaria chemoprophylaxis can be given to one group of children, and their haemoglobin levels, school absenteeism and antibody responses to vaccinations compared with those of an unprotected group.

3. Measurement of incidence and the level of transmission

Knowledge of these parameters is required to monitor control programmes, and also to detect natural changes so that future trends in prevalence can be forecast. They are also of key importance in the understanding of the dynamics of an infection, and in the construction of mathematical models whose main practical function is to predict the outcome of control programmes.

Incidence measures the number of new infections generated in a known period of time. In helminthic infections one can regard incidence either in terms of conversion from a non-infected state to an infected one, or as the acquisition of one more worm; the former is obviously more practical but the latter is more directly related to the level of transmission.

Under steady-state conditions when prevalence is constant and the number of new infections is exactly balanced by loss of infection it is evident that, on average, one infection will generate one new infection in another subject. Similarly in bisexual worm infections, at equilibrium, one reproductively active female worm will in the course of her lifetime produce, on average, one new reproductively active female worm. The average number of new infections generated by one infective host is termed the **net reproduction rate** (NRR). When prevalence is rising, as during an epidemic, NRR will be greater than 1. In a steady state the value of NRR will be 1, or just above it, to take into account host deaths and emigration. If NRR remains below 1, an infection must eventually die out; hence this is the target that control measures must achieve, it is known as the **break point** in transmission.

In endemic infections the observed reproduction rate is usually much less than the maximum number of new infections that could, under the existing environmental conditions, be generated by one infection; this maximum is known as the **basic reproduction rate** (BRR). The main reason for the discrepancy between the NRR and the BRR is acquired host immunity which limits the entry of new infections and sometimes also the infectivity of the infected host; an example of the latter being the suppression in malaria of gametocytaemia before asexual parasitaemia, during the earlier stages of acquired immunity. In asexual infections superinfection probably has the same effect as immunity, although it is possible that multiple infections in non-immunes can coexist independently. In bisexual worm infections superinfections are essential for reproduction and it is the unmated worms, that occur mainly in light infections, which contribute to the discrepancy between the NRR and the BRR. When an asexual infection is introduced into an uninfected population the BRR may be achieved and an epidemic results; introduction of a sexual worm infection gives an initially delayed response due not only to the longer prepatent period but also the fact that many of the earlier infections will be light and reproductively non-viable.

A useful concept is the **force of infection** (h) which is defined as the number of effective contacts to which a host is exposed in unit time; an effective contact being one that generates a new infection in a susceptible host. One can divide a population into the infectives, which in most situations will be equivalent to the prevalence of infection (P, expressed as a proportion of the whole population), and the susceptibles (1–P). In many discussions and simple mathematical models of infection one can assume uniform mixing of infectives and susceptibles; at least this is generally true in most parasitic infections except when prevalence is very low. It is fairly self-evident that the force of infection (h) is the product of two components: the number of infectives (P); and the mean infectivity of each infective (K). K is the **transmission constant**, and is defined as the number of contacts, in unit time, between any two persons sufficient to produce infection if one is an infective and the other is a susceptible. Thus if one infective is introduced into a population of susceptibles the maximum number of new infections in unit time is K. Thus h = PK.

The two simplest models of transmission can be represented by very simple diagrams; they are sometimes called catalytic models because of their similarity to chemical reactions.

Model 1

This describes a non-reversible process in which susceptibles become infected at a rate equal to the constant force of infection (Fig. 15.2 A). It may be represented by the differential equation:

$\frac{dP}{dt} = h(1-P)$, which is equivalent to the incidence of infection, t being the time interval.

When integrated this expression gives $P = 1-e^{-ht}$, under the initial conditions P=0 when t=0. Given enough time (P) will always reach 1 (ie. 100 per cent prevalence) whatever the value of (h); however the magnitude of (h) determines the shape of the curve, becoming steeper as its value rises (Fig. 15.2.B).

MODEL 1

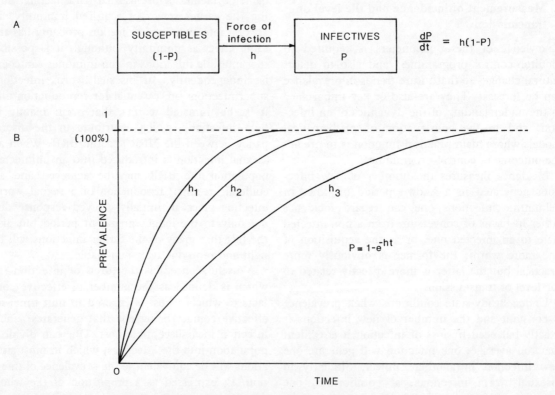

Fig. 15.2 Model 1, a non–reversible infectious process. A. diagrammatic representation with differential equation. B. relationship between prevalence and time for different values of h, the force of infection (h₁>h₂>h₃)

Model 2

This describes a reversible process and introduces a new constant (r) for the recovery process (Fig. 15.3.A). We define (r) as the probability that one infective will lose infection and revert to the susceptible state in unit time; hence loss of infection in unit time is (Pr). The model may be represented by the differential equation:

$$\frac{dP}{dt} = h(1-P) - Pr$$

When integrated this expression gives

$$P = \frac{h}{h+r}\left[1-e^{-(h + r)t}\right]$$

under the initial conditions P = 0 when t = 0.

This equation for (P) leads to an equilibrium value or limiting prevalence (P_L), whose value is given by $\frac{h}{h+r}$. Clearly the higher the value of (h), for a given value of (r), the greater will be the limiting prevalence (Fig. 15.3.B). This model assumes that superinfection does not affect the duration of infection. Other equations can be derived to describe true superinfections, which do occur in malaria infection among non-immunes.

There are three methods of measuring incidence; two of them utilise the two simple models which have just been described.

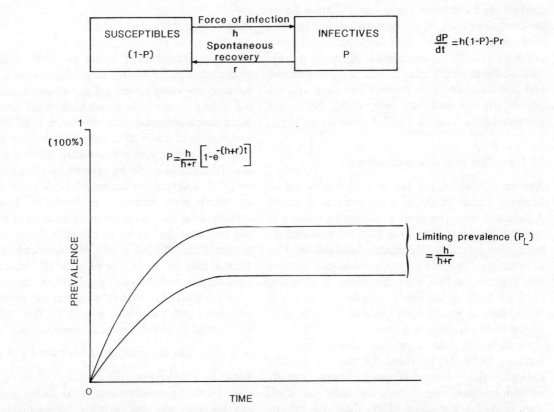

MODEL 2

Fig. 15.3 Model 2, a reversible infectious process. A. diagrammatic representation with differential equation. B. relationship between prevalence and time for different values of h (force of infection) and r (spontaneous recovery); curves reach an equilibrium value (limiting prevalence)

A. Direct method

A preliminary survey is used to detect non-infected persons and these are examined again after an appropriate time interval. The incidence is then the number of new infections expressed as a proportion of the initial non-infected population. This method is appropriate in infections of long duration such as schistosomiasis and hookworm but cannot be used for short infections, such as malaria, because infections may be gained and lost between the two surveys.

B. Frequently sampled cohort method

A non-infected population is identified and then resurveyed at frequent intervals; persons becoming positive are not re-examined. The cumulative time-related incidence is then calculated; this will correspond to the integral of model 1, i.e. $P = 1 - e^{-ht}$. Simple mathematical manipulations convert the cumulative curve for (P) into a linear function and enable (h) to be estimated. Incidence is then the product of (h) and the initial uninfected population $(1 - P)$. A convenient study group for this method are newborn infants, who are non-infected and non-immune. This method has been applied particularly in malaria, each child being re-examined once a month until it becomes positive.

C. Estimation from cross-sectional studies

Age prevalence curves for many parasitic infections are similar in shape to the integral of model 2; infection rates rise until a limiting prevalence is attained corresponding to a state of equilibrium when new infections are exactly balanced by loss of infection (Fig. 15.3B). Age prevalence curves of this type imply that the same force of infection applies at all ages. Fairly simple mathematical manipulations enable both (h) and (r) to be estimated from curves of this type.

Immunodiagnostic data may also be used to estimate incidence, provided the tests are specific enough. Since immunodiagnostic tests usually remain positive longer than the infection itself they have a lower value of (r) than that of the infection; they therefore record both current and past infection, or what is sometimes called period prevalence. With some skin tests positivity may be more or less life-long in which case $r = 0$ and model 1 applies. Similarly for infections with high incidence rates, such as malaria, one may use the age prevalence of seropositivity in infants and young children, among whom the conversion rate positive to negative is virtually nil. As with skin tests, seropositivity curves in children can be applied to the integral of model 1 and the value of (h) estimated.

If we return once again to the concept of the basic reproduction rate (BRR) it is evident that if one infective, or one reproductively active female worm, is introduced into an uninfected susceptible population the number of new infectives (BRR) will be the product of the transmission constant (K) and the duration of infection. If (r) is the recovery rate in unit time, then the duration of infection is its reciprocal $\dfrac{1}{r}$.

Hence $BRR = \dfrac{K}{r}$

For most infections it is not possible to give a quantitative value to (K) from observational data because one cannot measure the number of infective forms — amoebic cysts, hookworm larvae or schistosome cercariae, that enter each host, nor the proportion of these that actually produce infection. Sometimes one can measure relative exposure risks, for example by repeatedly sampling soil or water and making counts of hookworm larvae or schistosome cercariae respectively; however even here no very accurate measurement of exposure risks can be made, as infective forms are so unevenly distributed in the environment. Sometimes it may be possible to estimate (K) indirectly; for example model 2 can be applied to amoebiasis, which appears to behave as a simple reversible infectious process. Since $h = KP$, this may be substituted in the differential equation and it can be shown that the limiting prevalence $P_L = \dfrac{K-r}{K}$; hence if (r) is known, (K) is easily estimated.

In vector-borne infections the situation is different because one can, using entomological data, give a quantitative maximum value for the transmission constant in a particular ecosystem. In this context the transmission constant is termed the **vectorial capacity** and one day is its unit of time. Vectorial capacity is defined as the maximum number of secondary cases distributed by the vector population from one infective on one day. The concept of vectorial capacity has been used very successfully in malaria to predict the effects of control measures applied to the adult or larval mosquito population; this is worth describing in some detail as it illustrates the usefulness of relatively simple mathematical models. It is necessary to define four variables:

m = Mosquito density relative to man; in other words the total vector population in an ecosystem divided by the number of humans.

a = Average number of persons bitten by one mosquito on one day, since mosquitoes feed every two, three, four or more days, the value of (a) is always < 0.5.

p = Probability that a mosquito will survive through one day; values range from 0.5 to 0.95.

n = Time taken for completion of extrinsic cycle of malaria parasite in mosquito; values will be 11 or more days.

The mathematical expression for vectorial capacity can now be built up in the following way: on any one day the infective subject will be bitten by (ma) mosquitoes, this being the product of the mosquito population relative to man and the frequency with which each mosquito feeds on man. Of these mosquitoes the proportion that survive long enough to become infective at the end of the extrinsic incubation period is p^n. The longevity of a mosquito is $\dfrac{1}{-\log_e p}$. Since deaths in mosquitoes, as in most invertebrates are random the expectation of life is the same on each day, whether this be day one or day (n); during each day of its infective life span $\dfrac{1}{-\log_e p}$ each mosquito will feed (a) times on man.

Hence vectorial capacity

$$= ma \times p^n \times \frac{1}{-\log_e p} \times a$$

$$= \frac{ma^2 p^n}{-\log_e p}$$

Each of the four variables, m, a, p and n can be estimated from entomological observations. Different control measures modify one or more of these variables; however because of the structure of this formula the effects are very different (p. 222).

By incorporating two further variables into the vectorial capacity an expression for the basic reproduction rate is obtained. Firstly the variable (b) is introduced and defined as the proportion of biting mosquitoes with sporozoites in their salivary glands which actually transmit infection. Secondly the duration of infectivity of the human subject is given by $\dfrac{1}{r}$, where r is the recovery rate.

Hence the basic reproduction rate

$$= \frac{ma^2 b p^n}{r(-\log_e p)}$$

If one substitutes known values for the different variables in this expression, estimates of the basic reproduction rate may reach 100 or more, the highest values being 3000 in parts of West Africa where malaria is holoendemic. These high values emphasise the difficulty of malaria eradication in these circumstances, since the BRR must be reduced below the break point of 1 before success is possible. Even when the BRR is very high it must be remembered that under stable conditions, such as in holoendemic malaria where the highest values are observed, the actual or net reproductive rate is only just above 1. The enormous discrepancy is accounted for by acquired immunity and superinfection; the former reduces the prevalence and intensity of gametocytaemia to very low levels so that very few subjects, usually the youngest children, are actually infectious to mosquitoes. Furthermore mosquitoes infected by blood with low gametocyte counts have themselves, after the extrinsic incubation period, very few sporozoites in their salivary glands; hence their infectivity (b) is low.

In discussions on malaria control it is simpler to use the expression for vectorial capacity rather than that of the basic reproduction rate, as the former contains only entomological variables, which can be measured. The two parasitological variables (b) and (r) are either difficult to estimate, as in the case of the recovery rate (r); or are subject to variation (b), since the number of sporozoites in the salivary glands is altered by immunity in the infective human host.

In vector-borne infections one can also calculate the force of infection (h), or inoculation rate, to which each susceptible is exposed. Thus if (s) is the proportion of mosquitoes with sporozoites in their salivary glands, then the maximum possible value of (h), each day, is (mas), since each person is bitten by (ma) mosquitoes. However when the true value of (h) is estimated from the observed incidence in a cohort of infants in a highly endemic area, the value is much lower. The difference is due to the low value of (b), the proportion of biting infective mosquitoes that actually produce a new infection. Field studies suggest that the value of (b) is often within the range one to five per cent, although the value can be much higher in heavily infected mosquitoes.

It will be noted that so far the terms **level of transmission** and **transmission rate** have not been defined. For most purposes they should be regarded as synonymous and equivalent to the force of infection (h), as this measures the amount of infective exposure to which each susceptible is exposed. Some authors, however, have regarded these terms as equivalent to incidence, the transmission constant (K), BRR or even NRR; they are often used in a very loose sense without any definition.

4. Intervention studies

For many parasitic infections there are several options available for control, for example chemotherapy, vector control or the provision of a clean water supply. These measures can be applied singly or in combination. Only carefully designed and well executed studies will reveal the cost effectiveness, acceptability and untoward effects of each measure and the synergistic or other interactions of combined control measures. Careful monitoring of intervention studies will give data applicable to other contexts, for example a nationwide control programme.

Intervention studies are often very costly and may take several years to complete. For them to yield valid data it is essential that full base-line observations are made and that rigorous efforts be made to standardise all the methods of data collection. Most intervention studies will compare two or more populations, or areas, which must be similar in as many ways as possible. Alternatively the same population can be studied before and after instituting control; this has the disadvantage that transmission levels may change for reasons other than the control measures used.

a) Monitoring of human population. The following variables can be measured, using the methods already described: incidence of infection; intensity of infection (in metazoan infections); prevalence of infection and morbidity. Except when chemotherapy is the control measure, the first observed change will be incidence and the last will be morbidity; in helminthic infections, such as filariasis, it may be many years before morbidity is reduced. Children born after the institution of control provide a very useful measure of its effectiveness, for if transmission has been completely interrupted they will remain uninfected and seronegative.

b) Monitoring of vectors. The four variables included in the expression for the vectorial capacity can be measured, together with the prevalence and intensity of infection in the vectors and the estimated entomological inoculation rate.

c) Monitoring of intermediate hosts. Measurements can be made of size and age structure of the intermediate host population, for example snails in schistosomiasis control programmes. The prevalence and intensity of infection can be measured.

d) Monitoring of environment. In life cycles with free-living stages, standardised methods can be used to count parasites in the environment. Thus soil samples will provide counts of helminth eggs and larvae, and water samples counts of schistosome cercariae.

CONTROL OF PARASITIC INFECTIONS

Parasitic infections may be controlled either by reducing the source of infection in man or a reservoir host, or by reducing the transmission between hosts (transmission constant K or vectorial capacity, see p. 214 and p. 217). Frequently there are several possible methods of control for a particular parasite. In general the more complex a parasite's life cycle, the more possible means of attack there are available. Often two or more control measures are applied simultaneously because of the synergistic effect of such combinations.

Use of drugs in man

Drugs used on a community basis must have low toxicity and few untoward effects because they will often be given with little medical supervision, and compliance with the programme will soon fall if side-effects are noted. Furthermore it is unethical to give a potentially dangerous drug unless the person is known to be infected with a serious pathogen, or has a high intensity of infection.

A. Chemoprophylaxis

1. Malaria. Apart from the antifolate drugs, such as proguanil and pyrimethamine, all antimalarials are really suppressives rather than true prophylactics; the antifolates, in addition to their schizonticidal effect upon erythrocytic forms, destroy the pre-erythrocytic schizonts of *P. falciparum* in the liver. However, in practice this makes no difference. Personal prophylaxis for non-immunes is described on page 199. The principle targets for the community use of antimalarials are children under five years and pregnant women. Whenever possible proguanil or pyrimethamine should be used, or if there is significant resistance to these, then chloroquine. If parasites are resistant to these three drugs, then the sulphone plus pyrimethamine combination (Maloprim) should be used, although the optimum dose and effectiveness of this drug is uncertain, when it is used on a community basis. Quinine and mefloquine should be reserved for the chemotherapy of chloroquine-resistant *P. falciparum* infections; as should Fansidar (sulphonamide plus pyrimethamine), except for short term personal prophylaxis (less then six months).

2. Gambian trypanosomiasis. Pentamidine at an intramuscular dose of 4 mg base/kg gives protection against this infection for six months, and it has been widely used as a prophylactic in former French and Belgian colonies in Africa. When used alone it can never achieve eradication. Suramin is a less satisfactory alternative, because it must be given intravenously, and it only gives protection for three or four months.

Chemoprophylaxis should not be used against. *T.b. rhodesiense* because resistance is common, and this results in partially suppressed infections which present at a late incurable stage.

3. Pneumocystis infection. Co-trimoxazole can be used to control outbreaks in nurseries and to protect immunosuppressed subjects who are exposed to infection.

4. Loaiasis. A monthly schedule of diethylcarbamazine 5 mg/kg body weight daily for three days gives protection against this filarial worm. This is the only example of a drug, active against the larval stage of a worm, that is safe enough to use as a prophylactic in man.

B. Chemotherapy

1. Malaria. Treatment of proven or suspected malaria in infants and children with a schizonticide has beneficial effects even when all attacks are not detected and treated. This is because the attacks become more widely spaced, and therefore better tolerated. Free availability of antimalarials in endemic areas reduces morbidity considerably, at the risk, or course, of producing drug resistance. Proguanil and pyrimethamine have the advantage that *P. falciparum* gametocytes are rendered non-infectious, an important consideration in control because gametocytes are commonest in children; however drug resistance is a problem and their schizonticidal activity rather slow.

Chemotherapy plays a vital role in the later stages of an eradication programme based upon residual insecticides. All detected infections must be treated with a schizonticide followed, in *P. vivax* and *P. ovale* infections, by a course of primaquine.

2. Gambian trypanosomiasis and Indian kala-azar. Case finding and treatment is often the most effective way of controlling these infections, which both have human sources of infection.

3. Amoebiasis. Relatively limited use has been made of repeated chemotherapy to control this infection in highly endemic areas. Diloxanide furoate is the most appropriate drug because of its very low toxicity and efficiency in cyst excreting carriers. Where appropriate, populations should be retreated every three or six months. If stool microscopy is impossible, food handlers can be treated empirically with diloxanide.

4. *Soil-transmitted nematodes*. Considerable success has been achieved by repeated chemotherapy in *Ascaris*, hookworm, *Trichuris* and *Enterobius* infections. As these infections are frequently multiple, broad spectrum drugs are particularly useful. In *Ascaris*, *Trichuris* and *Enterobius* infections, children will be the main target, and drugs can be administered in nursery or primary schools. Hookworm may affect any age group, but adult males in rural areas are often the most heavily infected. Treatment may have to be repeated two, three or even four times each year. If transmission is limited to a short season, treatment should be given immediately before, and again about two months after this period.

5. *Schistosomiasis*. When combined with other measures, chemotherapy is the most effective way of controlling this infection. Annual retreatment is sometimes necessary. Niridazole can be used for all species, but in *S. haematobium* infections, metrifonate will generally be preferred because of its very low toxicity. Oral oxamniquine can be used for *S. mansoni*, but it is expensive; intramuscular hycanthone is also effective, but produces occasional serious hepatotoxicity. *S. japonicum* is the most difficult species to treat but recent trials with praziquantel, a drug previously used in veterinary medicine, have been promising.

6. *Taeniasis*. The more recently available taenicides, such as niclosamide, have a very low toxicity and their use should provide the simplest and cheapest method of control where these infections are economically important (*T. saginata*), or a danger to man (*T. solium*). Chemotherapy is a less effective measure for the fish tapeworm (*Diphyllobothrium latum*), because of the animal reservoir.

7. *Lymphatic filariasis*. Chemotherapy of *W. bancrofi* and *B. malayi* infections with diethylcarbamazine is both safe and effective, and provides a powerful method of control. A total dose of 72 mg/kg body weight given in monthly divided doses over six or twelve months will eliminate all adult *B. malayi* worms, and a large proportion of *W. bancrofti*. Allergic reactions resulting from the death of microfilariae and adult worms occur with both species, but are more severe with *B. malayi*.

The treated population must be warned in advance of these effects, which are most pronounced in those with high levels of microfilaraemia, and symptomatic treatment should be available.

Mass treatment of onchocerciasis is not at present feasible because of the severity of allergic reactions, which can cause blindness, and the toxicity of suramin, the only currently used macrofilaricide. Similarly, the allergic reactions in *Loa loa* infections after diethylcarbamazine prohibit mass chemotherapy, except under fairly close medical supervision.

Mass, selective and targeted chemotherapy. Chemotherapy can be deployed in several ways in control programmes. If an infection is very common and the drug very safe, then the whole population may be treated regardless of whether infection is proven or not; this is known as **mass chemotherapy**. Alternatively a preliminary survey is used to identify those who are infected, and chemotherapy is offered to these; this constitutes **selective chemotherapy**. Another option in metazoan infections is **targeted chemotherapy**, which aims to treat those persons with the highest intensity of infection; these constitute the greatest source of infection to others, and are themselves liable to the greatest morbidity. Targeted chemotherapy has been applied particularly in schistosomiasis, but is also appropriate in *Ascaris*, *Trichuris* and hookworm infections. In lymphatic filariasis it is now believed that persons with low levels of microfilaraemia are important in transmission; the infectivity of persons with high counts being limited by the lethal effects upon the vector of multiple larval worms.

Vector control

A. Larviciding

1. *Mosquitoes*. This is most effective when the number of breeding sites is limited, as in urban areas, and in rural areas of arid regions. Applications of oils to form a film over the water surface which asphyxiates the air-breathing larvae and the use of Paris green, an arsenical compound, are the oldest methods and they are still used. The anti-

cholinesterase compounds difenphos and fenthion are now used for anopheline control in malaria, and also for *Culex* control of filariasis in urban areas. Chlorinated hydrocarbon insecticides are generally avoided because they encourage resistance, and cause unnecessary environmental pollution. The main disadvantage of larviciding is the necessity to repeat the applications at frequent intervals.

2. *Simulium*. Limited breeding sites such as the outfalls of dams, mountain streams and even parts of large rivers can be controlled with DDT, using for example, slow release brickettes. The current *Simulium* eradication scheme in seven West African countries employs the anticholinesterase compound abate, applied mainly by aerial spraying from helicopters and light aircraft. This onchocerciasis programme currently relies wholly upon larviciding.

3. *Chrysops* (Mango flies). The larvae of this vector of the filarial worm *Loa loa* breed in the mud of forest streams. Dieldrin can be applied to the mud and is especially useful where streams pass through partially cleared areas, such as rubber plantations.

B. Source reduction

This implies reduction or elimination of vector breeding sites.

1. *Mosquitoes*. Anopheline breeding sites can be removed by filling in pools, efficient land drainage and diking, and other engineering methods. *Culex fatigans* can be controlled by sealing cess pits and installing piped sewage disposal. *Mansonia* larvae, which depend upon aquatic vegetation for their respiration, can be controlled by weed clearance and herbicides.

2. *Sandflies*. Peridomestic species can be controlled by removal of rubble, loose masonry, and by better house construction; these methods eliminate the dark moist cracks and crevices in which larvae breed.

3. *Reduviid bugs*. Better home construction, especially the replacement of dilapidated mud and wattle homes, removes the breeding places and day time resting sites of the vectors of Chagas' disease.

4. *Tsetse flies*. The vectors of Gambian trypanosomiasis are riverine species, principally *G. palpalis*, whose populations can be reduced or even eliminated by partial or complete forest clearance beside watercourses. Similarly barrier clearings can limit fly movement.

C. Adulticiding

1. *Residual house spraying*. The spraying of indoor surfaces of houses with a residual insecticide is a very effective weapon against local vectors that enter homes (**endophilic species**), and especially those species, such as the mosquito vectors of malaria and filariasis, that rest on walls after their blood meal. DDT at a standard dose of 2 g per square metre remains the almost perfect insecticide for this purpose because of its cheapness, low toxicity and persistence on surfaces for up to six months. When resistance occurs, the alternatives such as the anticholinesterase compounds, malathion and propoxur, are much more expensive and considerably less persistent. One of the benefits of malaria control by residual spraying, has been reduction and sometimes near-extinction of urban oriental sore and Indian kala-azar; both of these leishmanial infections have endophilic sandfly vectors. Unfortunately when spraying ceases the sandflies often return. Reduviid bugs can also be controlled by residual insecticides.

2. *Space application*. Various fogging and mist blowing machines, some of them mounted on road vehicles or aircraft, are used to control adult insect populations; sometimes they have larvicidal effects as well. A recent development is the ultra-low-volume method of dispersal. Organophosphorus compounds, such as malathion and fenthion, are usually used. An important target for these methods are urban mosquito populations, especially during epidemics; another application is their use against riverine tsetse flies in Gambian trypanosomiasis. Zoonotic leishmaniasis can sometimes be controlled by insecticide aerosols, usually DDT, sprayed into sandfly breeding sites, such as the colonial burrows of gerbils in rural oriental sore, or the ventilation shafts of deserted termite hills in East African kala-azar; the residual effect will be considerable when DDT is used.

D. Protection against biting insects

These methods include the use of house screens and bed nets to protect against indoor-feeding (**endophagic**) mosquitoes, and the construction of better quality housing that provides fewer shaded resting sites for mosquitoes or hiding places for reduviid bugs. Protection against sandflies is more difficult because their very small size allows them to penetrate most nets and screens. They are however easily deterred by the air currents of a fan, and their weak flying ability means that the sometimes simple precaution, during the transmission season, of sleeping on the roof or in an upstairs room, prevents these flies reaching their human hosts.

Insect repellants, such as diethyltoluamide or dimethylphthalate, and protective clothing may be the only way of preventing sandfly bites in rural areas, such as the Central and South American rainforests. The simple measure of burning mosquito coils at night, in village huts, has a considerable deterrent and insecticidal effect.

E. Biological control

Various fish (in particular *Gambusia*) that eat mosquito larvae can be introduced into large bodies of water, such as lakes and rice paddy fields; unfortunately their effectiveness is often low. Several methods of genetic manipulation are being attempted in vector control; they include release of sterile male tsetse flies and the introduction of genes for refractoriness against *W. bancrofti* in mosquitoes. So far large-scale effectiveness has not been achieved.

Vector control and the concept of vectorial capacity

Only rarely is the objective of vector control the extinction of the target species, although this can sometimes be done, for example on small islands; it was also achieved when the notorious African malaria vector *Anopheles gambiae* was accidentally introduced into Brazil in 1930, and when the same species reinvaded Egypt in 1942.

More commonly the aim is either: (1) to reduce levels of parasite transmission so that morbidity is reduced to an acceptable level; or (2) to maintain the basic reproduction rate of the parasite below unity for a period long enough for the parasite to become extinct. It is helpful to examine how various control measures reduce the vectorial capacity (VC) (p. 217) in malaria.

$$VC = \frac{ma^2p^n}{-\log_e p}$$

Measures such as larviciding and source reduction reduce the size of the vector population (m), and so reduce VC in direct proportion. Protective measures against biting may deviate the vector species to feed on animals (**zoophagy**) rather than man (**anthropophagy**) and this will reduce the value of (a), the man-biting habit. Since in the expression for VC the value of (a) is squared a reduction to, for example, one half will reduce the VC to one quarter. Other measures can sometimes reduce (a), for example the siting of cattle stalls near houses may deviate mosquitoes to cattle; and chicken, which do not act as reservoirs for *T. cruzi*, kept peridomestically deviate the reduviid bugs away from man. No control measures affect (n) the length of the extrinsic period, since this is mainly controlled by ambient temperature; the instability or absence of malaria at high altitudes in the tropics, results from lower temperatures increasing the value of (n) from 11 to say 16 days; this has a very big effect of the VC.

Adulticiding, particularly residual house spraying against mosquitoes, has an enormous effect upon VC, the main effect being a reduced longevity (p). The most efficient malaria vectors known, *Anopheles gambiae* and *A. funestus* are both African species; they have the highest natural longevity, with (p) values of up to 0.95, indicating that 95 per cent survive through one day, and hence about 50 per cent through the extrinsic cycle, ie. p^{13}. Less efficient vectors have (p) values of about 0.75. When residual spraying is efficiently employed against an endophilic, anthropophagic species it is usually possible to reduce (p) by 20 or 30 per cent; this will be sufficient to eradicate malaria when the basic reproduction rate is not too high. However when BRR is very high (2000 or more) then one can calculate that (p) must be reduced by 50 to 60 per cent to achieve eradication; this is currently impossible and is the main reason why house spraying in tropical Africa with present methods will never achieve eradication. Residual spraying has two other effects: it reduces the adult mosquito population (m), and by its irritant effect it deviates some mosquitoes to feed on non-human hosts, hence (a) may also be reduced. The dramatic effectiveness of house spraying came initially in 1947, as a surprise to malariologists; it became readily explicable when it was realised that transmission was related to the new value of (p) raised to the power of (n). The attack phase of malaria eradication schemes normally lasts three to five years, after which house spraying is stopped and any remaining parasites eliminated by chemotherapy. The mosquitoes usually return almost to their previous population sizes, but when eradiction succeeds the result is then anophelism without malaria.

Unlike malaria eradication the present seven-country African onchocerciasis programme does aim at extinction of the vector *Simulium*, as there is no acceptible form of mass chemotherapy in this disease; the programme must therefore continue for 20 years, the limit of the life span of the onchocercal worm. Some tsetse programmes do achieve local eradication, but the borders of fly-free areas must be maintained to prevent reinvasion by the vector.

Control of intermediate hosts

A. Snail control

1. Use of molluscicides. The chemical control of snail populations has been of considerable success in schistosomiasis, and also in the veterinary field for fascioliasis. Their use for the control of the various Asian species of hermaphroditic fluke (*Clonorchis, Fasciolopsis* etc.) is far more limited because many molluscicides are toxic to fish, and some are herbicidal or toxic to man. Copper sulphate has been the most extensively used molluscicide but has now been largely replaced by Balucide (chemically identical to the anthelminthic niclosamide), Frescon (N-tritylmorpholine) and other compounds such as sodium pentachlorophenate. Some molluscicides kill snail eggs. There are many formulations of these chemicals and methods of applying them; preliminary surveys and expert guidance are essential and the

timing of the applications is often critical to achieve the maximum effect upon parasite transmission.

2. Environmental measures. These include the drainage of marshy areas, and the lining or covering of canals and water conduits. Irrigation ditches can be regularly cleaned or subjected to alternate flooding and drying. These engineering methods are often combined with the use of molluscicides. The success of snail control can in large part be attributed to the fact that snails are amplifier hosts of trematodes, one miracidium producing many hundreds or even thousands of cercariae if the snail lives long enough. Control measures reduce the size of the snail population and also the longevity of its members. The introduction of the carnivorous snail *Marisa* to destroy the *Biomphalaria* hosts of *S. mansoni* has had some success in Puerto Rico.

B. Cyclops control for guinea worm

1. Chemical. Since *Cyclops* can only transmit infections to man when ingested in drinking water, chemicals to control this microcrustacean must be non-toxic to humans. This can now be achieved by adding the anticholinesterase insecticide abate to well water.

2. Other measures. These include provision of piped water, sieving drinking water through a cloth, and also the introduction of fish. The redesigning of open wells, particularly the so-called step wells of India, so that a wall prevents contamination of the water by larvae from the open sores of infected persons, is very effective.

The other human parasites using *Cyclops* as an intermediate host (pseudophyllidean tapeworms and *Gnathostoma*) are not amenable to these forms of control, as they are usually rural and zoonotic. Furthermore they normally require a second intermediate host, usually a fish, before man is infected.

Most of the other intermediate hosts of human parasites such as fish, crayfish, crabs and domestic animals are not amenable to control methods that limit their populations, for these intermediate hosts are themselves collected or bred for human consumption.

Control of reservoir hosts

A. Destructive methods

1. *Leishmaniasis*. Infected dogs have to be killed, as chemotherapy is very difficult. The number of infected dogs can also be reduced by destroying stray animals and introducing licensing. Colonial rodents, such as gerbils, can be eliminated by trapping and fumigation of their burrows. Forest rodents are impossible to control.

2. *Trypanosomiasis*. Elimination of wild game animals will reduce the source of *T.b. rhodesiense* infection but the vector tsetse species, principally *G. morsitans*, soon diverts to domestic animals. This measure is rarely deliberately practised now, as it is undesirable on both ecological and aesthetic grounds. American trypanosomiasis has so many reservoir hosts, many of them domestic animals, that this form of control is not feasible except when armadillos or opossums are important.

3. *Trichinosis*. Rat control, especially in and near pigstyes, will sometimes have beneficial effects.

4. *Schistosomiasis*. Rats and other rodents are quite important reservoirs of *S. japonicum*. Their destruction, especially on marshy and irrigated land, is a useful control measure.

B. Therapeutic methods

Unfortunately this is only currently feasible for two important conditions that have domestic animals as a reservoir.

1. *Toxocariasis*. *T. canis* infections in dogs can be greatly reduced by regular deworming; puppies, and bitches post-partum, should be the main target. Kittens may also be treated for *T. cati*, a less important pathogen in man. Deworming of dogs can also be used to limit creeping eruption due to *Ancylostoma braziliense*.

2. *Hydatid infection*. Regular deworming of dogs, especially those on farms, to eliminate *Echinococcus granulosus* is highly effective; arecoline hydrobromide and dichlorophen are the drugs usually used. These drugs may also be used for other tapeworms of the dog that infect man; these are *E. multilocularis*, *Dipylidium caninum*, *Multiceps multiceps*, *Spirometra* and also *Diphyllobothrium latum*.

Public health hygienic measures

A. Improved domestic water supplies

1. *Water quality*. Increased water purity reduces the risk of water-borne infections; however this is a relatively unimportant source of parasitic infection. The cysts of both *Giardia lamblia* and *Entamoeba histolytica* are relatively resistant to chlorination. Several water-borne outbreaks of giardiasis have now been reported, and also a few due to *E. histolytica*; they have usually followed accidental sewage contamination of piped water supplies. Other water-borne infections are:

a. Guinea worm — the intermediate host *Cyclops*, measuring 1 mm in length, is easily removed by filtration and can be killed by chlorination.

b. Schistosomiasis — cercariae remain viable for up to 24 hours, hence storage of snail-free water for this period eliminates the risk; cercariae are very active and can penetrate some sand filters, but they are killed by chlorination.

c. Hermaphroditic flukes — unattached metacercarial cysts of, for example, *Clonorchis* and *Fasciolopsis*, may contaminate water supplies drawn from ponds or lakes; they are resistant to chlorination, but being quite large and heavy they can be removed by filtration or sedimentation.

2. *Water quantity*. An increase in the quantity of domestic water usage greatly reduces the transmission of most faeco-oral infections. The only effective method is by provision of piped water inside each home, a measure that often increases per capita water usage three or fivefold; it is only practicable in fairly dense settlements. Provision of communal stand pipes does not increase water usage very much, and vessels used to store water in the home easily become contaminated. Greater water usage encourages bathing and frequent hand washing, and facilitates more frequent laundering of clothes; in the kitchen it enables vegetables and fruit to be washed, and cooking and eating utensils to be cleaned more effectively.

Among the parasitic infections, increased water quantity will have its greatest effect upon the transmission of the intestinal protozoa (*Giardia*, *E. histolytica*, *Balantidium*, and *Isospora belli*), and the gut helminths with direct life cycles, especially *Ascaris*, *Trichuris*, *Enterobius* and *Hymenolepis nana*.

Free availability of domestic water encourages bathing and laundering within the home, and so reduces the amount of contact with surface water outside the home. This effect is important in schistosomiasis as it reduces exposure to cercariae, it also reduces the likelihood of contamination of surface water by larvae from guinea worm sores. Provision of domestic water eliminates the need to collect water from distant sources, which so often encourages promiscuous defaecation and micturition and so lead to water contamination; it also reduces exposure to insect vectors, such as *Simulium* and riverine tsetse, which bite near water.

B. *Improved disposal of sewage and wastewater*

Scattered or promiscuous defaecation not only contaminates the soil but it can also directly contaminate agricultural food crops; furthermore, following rain, faecal material is washed into rivers and pools. The provision of latrines should reduce this source of environmental contamination. Unfortunately unless they are well constructed and maintained, latrines can themselves be important foci of infection. The prevalence of *Ascaris* infection is often higher among urban latrine users than among rural non-users. The eggs of this species and also those of *Trichuris* are very resistant and they can remain viable in the latrine environment for long periods. In addition, the moist soil around a latrine favours the survival of hookworm larvae and the free-living cycle of *Strongyloides stercoralis*.

In many developing and tropical countries, even the presence of perfectly clean latrines does not remove the problem of excreta-derived infections; nor does the installation of piped sewage disposal. There are several reasons for this:

1. Human faeces, in the form of 'nightsoil', are rightly regarded as a valuable resource, and are used to fertilise crops;

2. The productivity of fish ponds is increased by adding night soil to them, or by siting latrines directly over the pond;

3. Domestic waste water, and the excreta that inevitably accompanies it, is used for irrigation; this contaminates crops and puts irrigation workers at special risk;

4. Untreated or partially-treated sewage may be discharged into lakes and rivers;

5. Some of the solid wastes from sewage treatment plants are used to fertilise agricultural land, this happens in developed countries as well as developing ones.

The first two problems can be overcome by composting which is a reliable way of killing the infective forms of parasites; it also encourages the use of all vegetable and human wastes as fertilisers. Efficient composting takes three to four months. Aerobic fermentation raises the temperature of most of the heap to 50–60°C and provided the heap is well turned all the material will reach this temperature. All parasite cysts, eggs and larvae are quite rapidly killed at temperatures of 55°C, and die within a few days at 45°C. The heap must be well maintained or its periphery will become an intense transmission focus. A possible alternative to composting, is the chemical treatment of holding tanks which retain excreta for 12–24 hours; ammonium sulphate and other substances have been used for this purpose but it is important that the final product is non-toxic to fish and plant life.

The only solution to the remaining problems are sewage treatment methods that render the final product completely non-infectious; in practice this is difficult to achieve. Sewage treatment removes or destroys parasites mainly by sedimentation and the creation of completely anaerobic conditions. The efficiency of sedimentation depends upon the size and specific gravity of the parasite, and the detention time. Septic tanks for individual homes or small institutions have detention times of 12–24 hours. The primary sedimentation tanks of community treatment plants have detention times of only two to four hours, and this is followed by secondary biological treatment, comprising activated sludge or a trickling filter, which probably has little effect on parasite removal. Neither of these methods removes all protozoa and helminths and expensive tertiary treatment, by alum coagulation and sand filtration, are necessary to achieve this. The other principal method of sewage treatment involves the use of oxidation ponds, usually arranged in a series down which the waste passes; the detention times with this method are usually at least six days and sometimes as many as 30. All protozoan cysts and helminth eggs apparently settle within six days in oxidation ponds, but there is still the problem that hookworm and schistosome eggs may hatch during the process and their larval forms appear in the final effluent. The only way to circumvent the latter problem is to include an initial anaerobic tank, with a detention time of two days, before the waste enters the oxidation ponds. The eggs of *Taenia*, and to a lesser extent *Ascaris*, are notoriously resistant and they sometimes survive in the solid wastes taken from sedimentation tanks or ponds. Solid wastes, containing eggs of *T. saginata*, can infect cattle when it is distributed on farmland.

In most developing countries, inadequately treated sewage creates fluid effluents and solid wastes, that are a serious threat to human health. When these wastes are distributed on cultivated land, or discharged into irrigation systems, lakes or rivers, they constitute a direct source of infection to agricultural workers. In addition they contaminate growing vegetables, and infect domestic animals, rodents, snails and microcrustaceans (*Cyclops*), that act as the first or only intermediate hosts of many human parasites.

C. Slaughter-houses and meat inspection

The most important hygienic measures in slaughter-houses, from the parasitological viewpoint, are the exclusion of dogs and the treatment, by cooking, of all offal before it is fed to dogs. If these precautions are strictly observed the transmission of hydatid infection (*Echinococcus granulosus*) will be greatly reduced. The lungs and livers of sheep are the greatest source of infection, but not the only ones. Sheep carcases may also contain coenurus cysts in the brain and elsewhere; these also can infect dogs which are important definitive hosts of the causative tapeworm *Multiceps multiceps*. Rats should be excluded from slaughter houses, as by gaining access to discarded meat and offal they can acquire *Trichinella* infection, which can later be passed onto pigs.

Meat inspection will detect the presence of the cysticerci of *Taenia saginata* in bovine carcases, and those of *T. solium* in porcine ones. However not all carcases can be fully examined, as this would greatly decrease their value. Similarly some light infections will be missed even if the sites of election, such as the tongue for *T. solium* cysticerci, are thoroughly examined.

The detection of *Trichinella* larvae in pork and other meats can be achieved by using a trichinoscope; this is a projection microscope that enables the larvae to be seen in small pieces of compressed muscle, taken usually from the tongue. A more sensitive method is the pooled digestion technique, in which muscle samples from several pigs are pooled, digested and then examined with the trichinoscope. Where the livers of sheep and goats are eaten raw, these organs should be inspected for larval pentastomes that cause halzoun (p. 152).

The deep freezing of carcases and meat to minus 20°C for a period of 10–14 days will destroy all parasites transmitted to man by eating undercooked meat. These include, besides those mentioned already, the protozoan parasites *Toxoplasma* and *Sarcocystis*.

Personal hygienic measures

A great deal of parasitic diseases could be prevented if it was easy to modify human behaviour. In practice this is often very difficult, especially when the advice given contradicts long established and culturally based customs. Dietary preferences and methods of preparing food are among the most difficult to change, and indeed when other methods of control are available, it is doubtful whether certain dietary practices should be interfered with. Health education can take many forms; it is perhaps most effective when given in schools. For specific diseases propaganda campaigns using the news media can be useful.

1. Personal cleanliness. Infected food handlers are important disseminators of *Giardia* and *E. histolytica* cysts. These infections often show household and family clustering. In amoebiasis it seems that children are often infected by their mother as she prepares and serves their food, while in giardiasis, children often infect one another, and commonly infect their parents in the process. The importance of personal hygiene is emphasised by the high prevalence of parasites in institutions for the mentally subnormal. The commonest species include all the intestinal protozoa, and the two helminths with simple direct life cycles; these are

Hymenolepis nana, whose eggs are fully embryonated in fresh stools, and *Enterobius* whose eggs embryonate within a few hours. Dirty clothes and dust play an important part in the transmission of both these helminths.

2. *Close contact with pets*. The embryonated eggs of *Echinococcus granulosus* commonly contaminate an infected dog's fur; fondling of dogs, especially by children, must be discouraged as it is a common source of hydatid infection; contaminaed fingers soon reach the mouth. In rural areas, particularly on farms, working dogs should not be allowed indoors; nor should they share eating utensils with man.

The sticky eggs of *Toxocara canis* require embryonation before they are infective. Children become infected, by oral contamination, while playing on soil or sand polluted with dog faeces. Cat boxes, and children's sandpits polluted by cat faeces are important sources, to man, of *Toxoplasma* oocysts.

3. *Shoes and protective clothing*. The apparently simple measure of wearing shoes as protection against infective hookworm and *Strongloides* larvae is not always practicable. The rural farmer may dislike wearing them, and under wet conditions they easily become filled with muddy water. Hookworm is common on tea and rubber estates, and under these conditions it is sometimes possible to enforce the wearing of shoes, if they are provided by the employer.

Persons dealing with composted human faeces must wear shoes, and ideally gloves as well. Protective clothing and insect repellants should be used by personnel entering the American rain forests, to reduce biting by the sandfly vectors of leishmaniasis.

4. *Bathing in schistosome-infected waters*. In hot climates, children and adolescents cannot easily be dissuaded from bathing in such water; nor, for that matter, can foreign tourists.

5. *Advice to travellers*. The risks of foreign travel are frequently ignored, sometimes deliberately, by travel agents. Simple health precautions can be very effective and malaria chemosuppression may be essential. Protective immunity to malaria declines over one or two years in the absence of continued exposure. Previously immune persons returning to the tropics after a stay in a temperate country often develop overt malaria.

6. *Food hygiene and cooking*. Simple but important measures include adequate washing of salad vegetables and fruit, frequent hand washing and cleaning of kitchen utensils.

Proper cooking of meat removes the risk of all meat-derived parasites (p. 226), but to many people this reduces palatability so that it is not practised. The preference of many peoples for uncooked, salted, dried or pickled fish is often impossible to change as it is part of their cultural tradition. Fish-derived infections include *Diphyllobothrium*, *Clonorchis*, *Opisthorchis*, *Heterophyes*, *Metagonimus*, *Gnathostoma* and *Capillaria philippinensis*. Raw or pickled crabs and crayfish are the source of *Paragonimus* infection. In the case of the trematode infections, even when these foods are properly cooked the risks are not entirely removed, as kitchen utensils or fingers can become contaminated by metacercariae during food preparation and so transferred to other foods or directly to the mouth. In Holland, herring worm disease (*Anisakis* infection) has disappeared since the introduction of deep freezing of all herrings and mackerel; larval worms are killed within 24 hours at $-20°C$.

Some molluscs are eaten deliberately and these can produce infection by *Echinostoma* flukes and the nematode *Angiostrongylus cantonensis*. In addition, when small slugs and snails contaminate salads, infection by *A. cantonensis* and *Morerastrongylus costaricensis* can result. Ants can also contaminate salads and vegetables to produce *Dicrocoelium* infections.

Avoidance of wild-grown watercress and the prohibition of sheep in the water catchment areas of commercial watercress farms will eliminate the risks of human *Fasciola* infections. Careful peeling of water calthrop nuts and washing or boiling water vegetables grown in Asian fish ponds will reduce exposure to *Fasciolopsis* and *Gastrodiscoides* infection.

FURTHER READING

Bailey, N.T.J. (1975) *The Mathematical Theory of Infectious Diseases and Its Applications*, 2nd edition. London: C. Griffin and Co. Ltd.

Barker, D.J.P. (1976) *Practical Epidemiology*, 2nd edition. Edinburgh: Churchill Livingstone.

Cruickshank, R., Standard, K.L. and Russell, H.B.L. (1976) *Epidemiology and Community Health in Warm Climate Countries*. Edinburgh: Churchill Livingstone.

Garrett-Jones, C. and Shidrawi, G.R. (1969) Malaria vectorial capacity of a population of *Anopheles gambiae*. An exercise in epidemiological entomology. *Bull. Wld Hlth Org.*, **40**, 531–545.

Harrison, G. (1978) *Mosquitoes, Malaria and Man. A History of Hostilities since 1880*. London: John Murray.

Jelliffe, D.B. (1966) The assessment of nutritional status of the community. WHO Monograph No. 53. Geneva: WHO.

Knight, R. (1975) Surveys for amoebiasis, interpretation of data and their implications. *Ann. trop. Med. Parasit.*, **69**, 35–48.

Macdonald, G. (1956) Epidemiological basis of malaria control. *Bull. Wld Hlth Org.*, **15**, 613–626.

Macdonald, G. (1973) *The Dynamics of Tropical Disease*. Eds Bruce-Chwatt, L.J. and Glanville, V.J. London: Oxford University Press.

Pampana, E.J. (1969) *A Textbook of Malaria Eradication*. London: Oxford University Press.

Southgate, B.A. (1974) A quantitative approach to parasitological techniques in Bancroftian filariasis and its effect on epidemiological understanding. *Trans. R. Soc. trop. Med. Hyg.*, **68**, 177–186.

White, G.F., Bradley, D.J. and White, A.U. (1972) *Drawers of Water: Domestic Water Use in East Africa*. Chicago: University of Chicago Press.

Appendix

A SIMPLIFIED ZOOLOGICAL CLASSIFICATION OF THE GENERA OF HUMAN PARASITES

Phylum PROTOZOA (unicellular animals)

Subphylum Sarcomastigophora (locomotion by flagella, pseudopodia or both)

Superclass Mastigophora (locomotion mainly or wholly by flagella)

Order Rhizomastigida (pseudopodia and flagella present simultaneously, or at different stages of life cycle)
Dientamoeba, Naegleria.

Order Retortamonadida (2–4 flagella; cytostome, if present, bordered by fibril)
Retortamonas, Chilomastix, and *Enteromonas* (no cytostome).

Order Kinetoplastida (bearing kinetoplast at base of flagella; the human parasites have only a single flagellum)
Trypanosoma, Leishmania.

Order Diplomonadida (bilaterally symmetrical; two nuclei and four pairs of flagella)
Giardia.

Order Trichomonadida (undulating membrane with recurrent flagellum in free margin, 4 or 5 anterior flagella; axostyle present)
Trichomonas.

Superclass Sarcodina (locomotion by pseudopodia — 'amoebae')

Order Amoebida
Entamoeba, Endolimax, Iodamoeba, Acanthamoeba.

Subphylum Sporozoa (usually form spores containing sporozoites; no cilia, flagella or pseudopodia)

Class Telosporea (with sexual phase; form spores unless vector-borne)

Subclass Coccidia (trophozoites intracellular, bear an 'apical complex')

Order Eucoccida [cycle with alternation of asexual (schizogony and sporogony) and sexual multiplication]

Suborder Eimeriina (sexual phase in gut epithelium of vertebrate; one host or alternation between two; sporozoites enclosed in 'spore')
Isospora, Sarcocystis, Toxoplasma.

Suborder Haemosporina (schizogony in vertebrate, sporogony in invertebrate vector; naked sporozoites)

Family Plasmodidae (primary exoerythrocytic schizogony; erythrocytic schizonts form pigment; insect vectors)
Plasmodium.

Family Babesidae (no exo-erythrocytic schizogony; no pigment; tick vectors)
Babesia.

Class Haplosporea (no sexual phase; spores present; single host)
Pneumocystis (form a cyst containing sporozoites).

Subphylum Ciliophora (locomotion by cilia; two dissimilar nuclei)

Class Ciliata
Balantidium.

Phylum PLATYHELMINTHES (Flatworms)

Class Trematoda (Trematodes or Flukes) (oral

and ventral suckers; bifurcated blindly ending gut)

A. *Schistosomes* (blood flukes; sexes separate; cercariae penetrate definitive host directly)

Family Schistosomatidae
Schistosoma, Trichobilharzia, Ornithobilharzia.

B. *Hermaphroditic flukes* (adults bisexual; definitive host infected by ingesting metacercariae)

Family Echinostomatidae (with a collar of spines behind oral sucker; cercariae encyst in molluscs or fish)
Echinostoma.

Family Fasciolidae (large species; cercariae encyst on aquatic vegetation)
Fasciola, Fasciolopsis.

Family Paramphistomatidae (large ventral sucker at posterior end of body)
Gastrodiscoides.

Family Troglotrematidae (testes side by side behind ovary; cercariae encyst in crustacea)
Paragonimus.

Family Dicrocoelida (testes anterior to ovary; cercariae encyst in insects)
Dicrocoelium.

Family Opistorchiidae (testes in tandem behind ovary; cercariae encyst in fish)
Clonorchis, Opisthorchis.

Family Heterophyidae (minute species; cercariae encyst in fish)
Heterophyes, Metagonimus.

Class Cestoda (tapeworms) (scolex holdfast organ with ribbon of proglottids; no gut)

Order Pseudophyllidea (scolex with dorsal and ventral grooves; genital aperture ventral; 'worm-like' larvae)
Diphyllobothrium, Spirometra.

Order Cyclophyllidea (scolex with suckers; genital apertures marginal; 'cystic' larva)

Family Taeniidae (gravid proglottids longer than broad; numerous testes; one genital pore; larva in vertebrates)
Taenia, Multiceps, Echinococcus.

Family Hymenolepidiidae (gravid proglottids transverse; 1–4 testes; one genital pore; larva in insects)
Hymenolepis.

Family Dilepidiidae (gravid proglottids longer than broad, filled with egg capsules, bilateral genital pores; larva in insects)
Dipylidium.

Phylum NEMATODA (Roundworms)

Subclass Secernentea ('Phasmidia') (phasmids present; numerous caudal papillae)

Order Rhabditida (alternation of free-living and parasitic generations; parasitic female parthenogenic)
Strongyloides.

Order Strongylida (males with copulatory bursa; mouth with no lips)

Superfamily Strongyloidea (prominent buccal capsule; with 'leaf crown' surrounding mouth)
Oesophagostomium, Ternidens.

Superfamily Ancylostomatoidea (prominent buccal capsule; with ventral teeth or cutting plates)
Ancylostoma, Necator.

Superfamily Trichostrongyloidea (inconspicuous buccal capsule; no intermediate host)
Trichostrongylus.

Superfamily Metastrongyloidea (tissue parasites; inconspicuous buccal capsule; with intermediate host)
Angiostrongylus, Morerastrongylus.

Superfamily Syngamidoidea (adults live *in copula* in trachea and bronchi; no intermediate host)
Syngamus.

Order Ascaridida (large worms of gut lumen; mouth with three lips; direct or indirect life cycle)
Ascaris, Toxocara, Anisakis.

Order Oxyurida (live in colon and rectum; oesophagus with posterior bulb; direct life cycle)
Enterobius.

Order Spirurida (tissue parasites; arthropod or crustacean intermediate hosts)

    Superfamily Gnathostomatoidea (body spiny, with prominent head bulb)
      Gnathostoma.

    Superfamily Filaroidea (viviparous female produces microfilariae; insect vector)
      Wuchereria, Brugia, Onchocera, Loa Dipetalonema, Mansonella, Dirofilaria, Meningonema.

    Superfamily Dracunculoidea (female very long; viviparous, larvae escape from ruptured uterus; *Cyclops* is intermediate host)
      Dracunculus.

Subclass Adenophorea ('Aphasmidia') (no phasmids; no caudal papillae in male)

    Superfamily Trichuroidea (anterior region of body narrower than posterior, male with one spicule or none; female with one ovary)
      Trichuris, Trichinella, Capillaria.

    Superfamily Dioctophymatoidea (huge parasite of kidney; indirect life cycle)
      Dioctophyma.

Phylum ANNELIDA (worms with true metameric segmentation)

Class Hirudinea (Leeches) (bear perioral and posterior suckers)
    Haemadipsa, Hirudo, Poicilobdella, Dinobdella, Limnatis.

Phylum ARTHROPODA ('arthropods'; chitinous exoskeleton; jointed appendages)

Class Crustacea

    Order Pentastomida (Tongue worms) ('degenerate' parasitic forms with worm-like body showing external annulations; head with 2 pairs of retractile claws; indirect life cycle)
      Armillifer, Linguatula.

Class Arachnida (Spiders, scorpions, ticks and mites) (adults with 4 pairs of legs)

    Order Acarina (Ticks and mites) (head, thorax and abdomen united; larvae with 3 pairs of legs)

    Superfamily Ixodoidea (Ticks) (mouth bears armed hypostome)

      Family Ixodidae ('Hard ticks') (horny shield covers dorsal surface)
        Ixodes, Dermacentor, Amblyomma, Haemophysalis.

      Family Argasidae ('Soft ticks') (no dorsal shield)
        Ornithodorus.

    Superfamily Sarcoptoidea (Itch mites) (parasites of epidermis in all stages)
      Sarcoptes.

    Superfamily Demodicoidea (Follicular mites) (live in hair follicles and sebaceous glands)
      Demodex.

    Superfamily Parasitoidea (Parasitoid mites) (require blood meals throughout life cycle)
      Dermanyssus, Ornithonyssus, Allodermanyssus.

    Superfamily Trombiculoidea (Chiggers or harvest mites) (only ectoparasitic as larvae which feed on tissue juice not blood)
      Leptotrombidium, Trombicula.

Class Insecta (Insects) (adults with three pairs of thoracic legs)

    Order Anoplura (Sucking lice) (wingless; body flattened dorso-ventrally)
      Phthirus, Pediculus.

    Order Hemiptera (Bugs) (adults usually with 2 pairs of wings; nymphs resemble adults)
      Cimex (bed bugs; no wings).
      Panstrongylus, Triatoma, Rhodnius (reduviids)

    Order Coleoptera (Beetles) (thickened forewings protect hinder pair)
      Onthophagus.

    Order Diptera (Two-winged flies) (posterior pair of wings minute — halteres, these function as balancing organs)

    Suborder Nematocera (small flies with long antennae composed of 8 or more segments)

      Family Culicidae (Mosquitoes)
        Anopheles, Culex, Aedes, Mansonia.

      Family Psychodidae
        Phlebotomus, Lutzomyia, Psychodopygus (Sandflies).

Family Ceratopogonidae (Midges)
  Culicoides.

Family Simuliidae (Black flies)
  Simulium.

Suborder Brachycera (large flies; antennae 4 segmented, the last being divided into annuli)

Family Tabnidae (Horse flies, etc)
  Chrysops (Deer and mango flies)

Suborder Cyclorrhapha (antennae short, 3 segmented, the last bearing an arista; some are larviparous*; larvae are maggots with no head capsule)

Family Oestridae (Bot flies and warble flies)
  Hypoderma, Cuterebra, Dermatobia, Gastrophilus, Oestrus, Rhinoestrus*.*

Family Calliphoridae (Blow flies)
  Cordylobia, Auchmeromyia, Calliphora, Chrysomyia, Cochliomyia, Lucilia.

Family Sarcophagidae (Flesh flies)
  Sarcophaga, Wohlfahrtia*.*

Family Muscidae (Filth flies, stable fly, tsetse fly)
  Musca, Fannia, Stomoxys, Glossina.*

Order Siphonaptera (Fleas) (wingless; laterally compressed; leap with hind legs)

Family Tungidae (Chigoe flea) (gravid female burrows deep in epidermis)
  Tunga.

Family Pulicidae (Human, cat and dog, and rodent fleas)
  Pulex, Ctenocephalides, Xenopsylla.

Family Ceratophyllidae (Bird and rodent fleas)
  Ceratophyllus, Nosopsyllus.

Index

ERRATUM
Pages bearing titles for chapters 11 and 12 should be transposed.
Page 164 becomes page 153; page 153 becomes page 164.